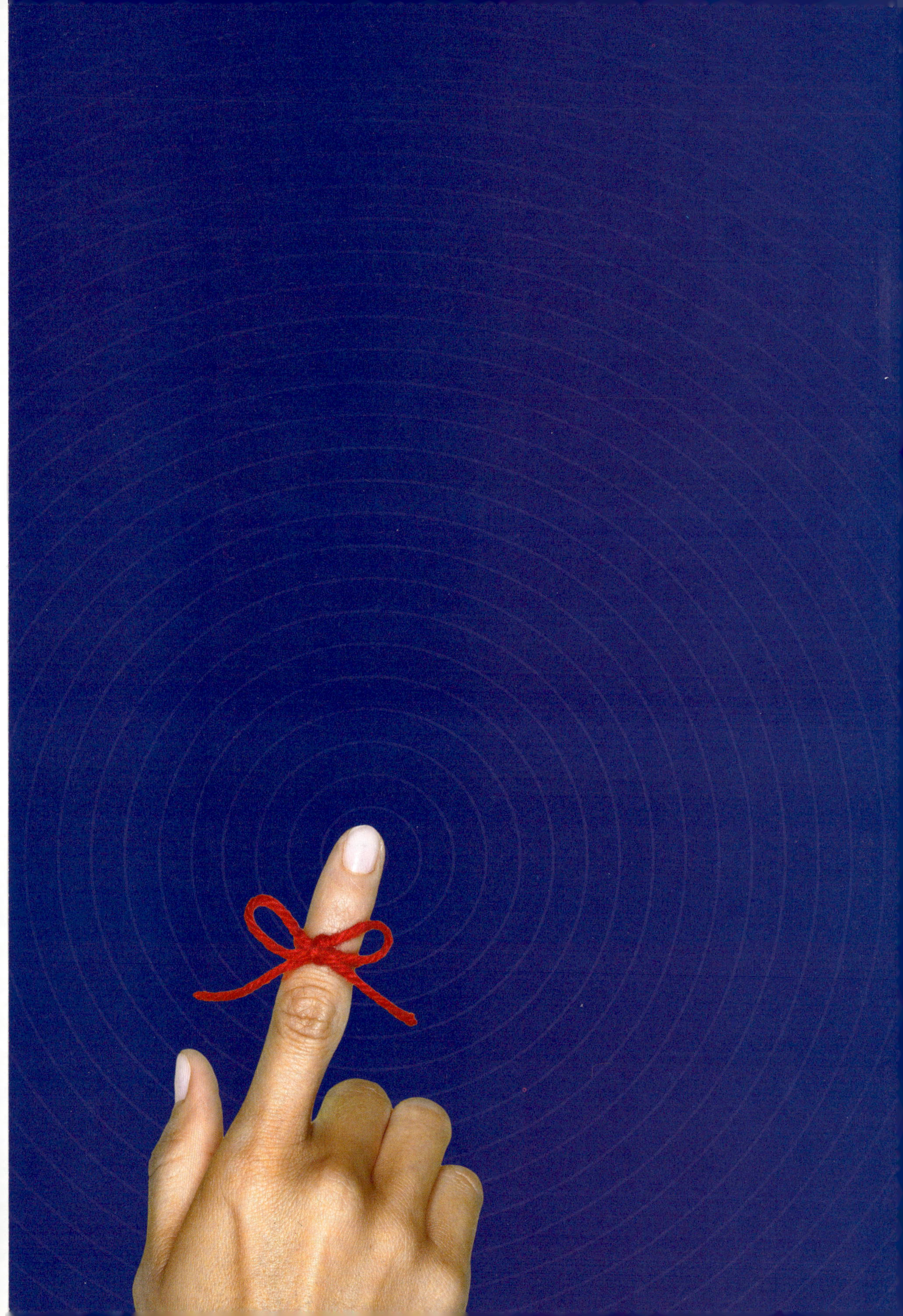

No More Brain Drain

Proven Ways to Maintain Your Mind and Memories

Reader's Digest
The Reader's Digest Association, Inc.
Pleasantville, NY | Montreal

Project Staff

Executive Editor
Marianne Wait

Senior Art Director
Rich Kershner

Writers
Sari Harrar, Carol Svec, Mariska van Aalst

Contributing Editor
Steven Slon

Illustrators
Ray Downing, Dave Phillips, Adam Raiti

Medical Advisor
David Perlmutter, MD, FACN

Copy Editor
Lisa D. Andruscavage

Indexer
Cohen Carruth Indexes

Intern
Rose DeMaria

Reader's Digest Home & Health Books

VP, Editor in Chief
Neil Wertheimer

Creative Director
Michele Laseau

Executive Managing Editor
Donna Ruvituso

Associate Director, North America Prepress
Douglas A. Croll

Manufacturing Manager
John L. Cassidy

Marketing Director
Dawn Nelson

The Reader's Digest Association, Inc.

President and Chief Executive Officer
Mary G. Berner

President, Home & Garden and Health & Wellness
Alyce C. Alston

SVP, Chief Marketing Officer
Amy J. Radin

President, Global Consumer Marketing and CEO, Direct Holdings
Dawn M. Zier

Copyright ©2009 by The Reader's Digest Association, Inc.
Copyright ©2009 by The Reader's Digest Association (Canada) ULC
Copyright ©2009 by The Reader's Digest Association Far East Ltd.
Philippine Copyright ©2009 by The Reader's Digest Association Far East Ltd.

All rights reserved. Unauthorized reproduction, in any manner, is prohibited. Reader's Digest is a registered trademark of The Reader's Digest Association, Inc.

ISBN 978-1-60652-986-7

Address any comments about ***No More Brain Drain*** to:
The Reader's Digest Association, Inc.
Editor in Chief, Books
Reader's Digest Road
Pleasantville, NY 10570-7000

To order copies of ***No More Brain Drain***, call 1-800-846-2100.

Visit our online store at **rdstore.com**

Printed in the United States of America

3 5 7 9 10 8 6 4 2

US 6069/IC

Note to Readers

The information in this book should not be substituted for, or used to alter, medical therapy without your doctor's advice. For a specific health problem, consult your physician for guidance. The mention of any products, retail businesses, or Web sites in this book does not imply or constitute an endorsement by the authors or by The Reader's Digest Association, Inc.

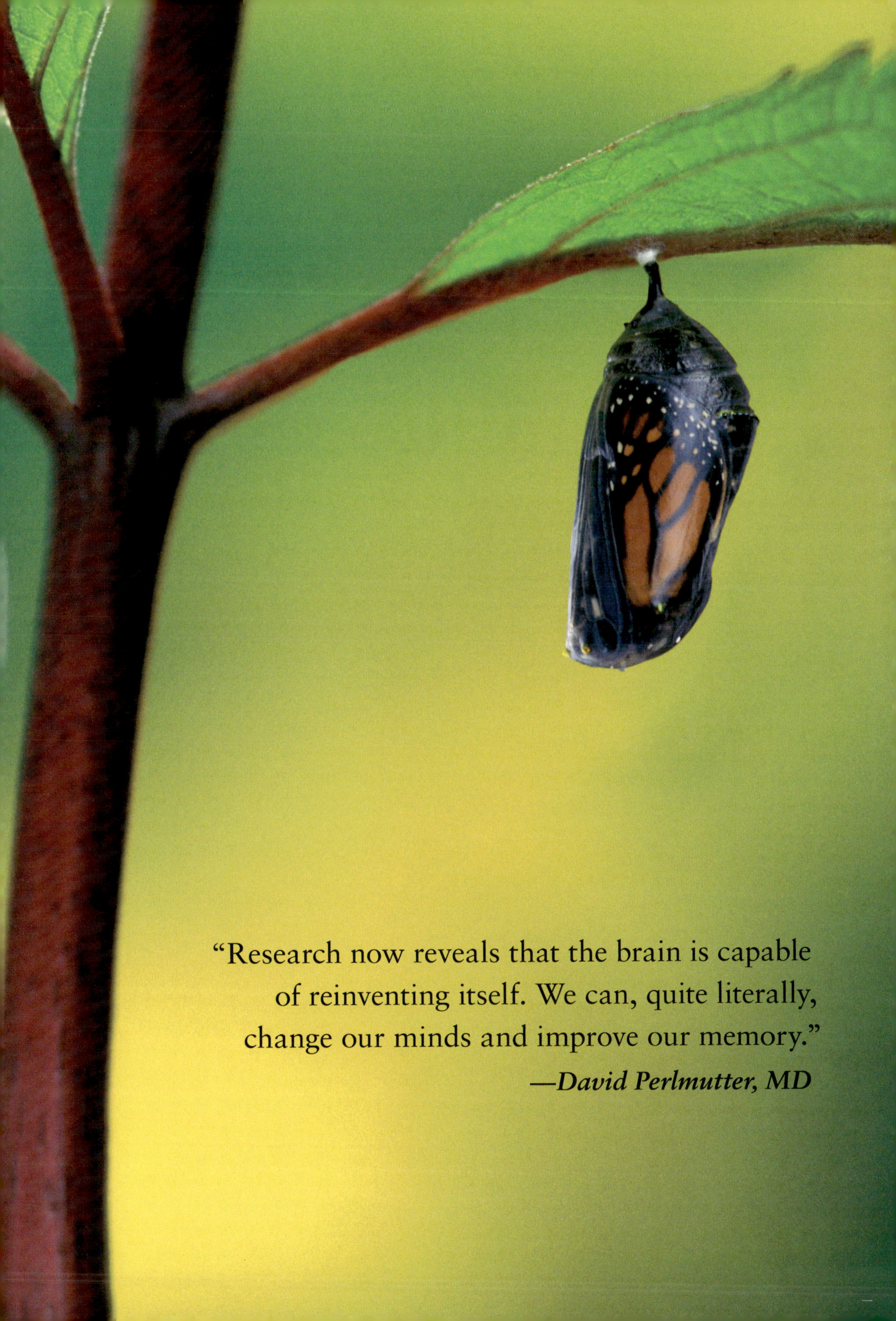

"Research now reveals that the brain is capable of reinventing itself. We can, quite literally, change our minds and improve our memory."

—David Perlmutter, MD

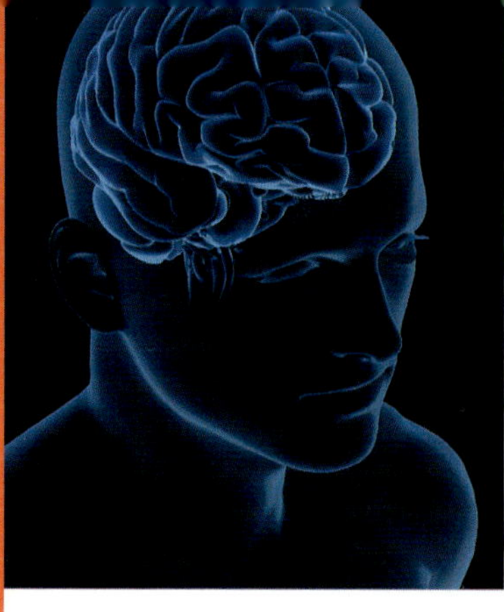

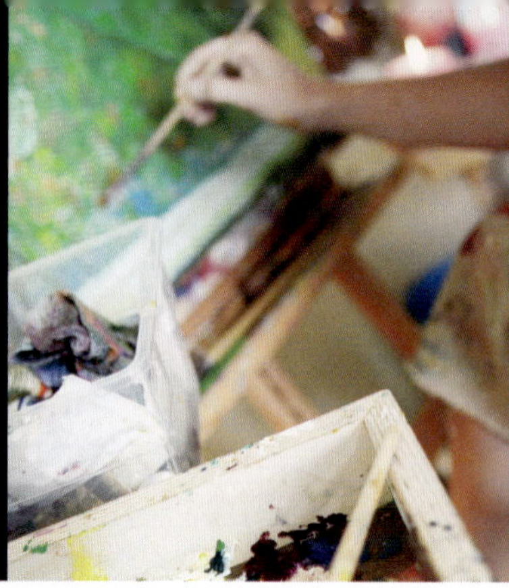

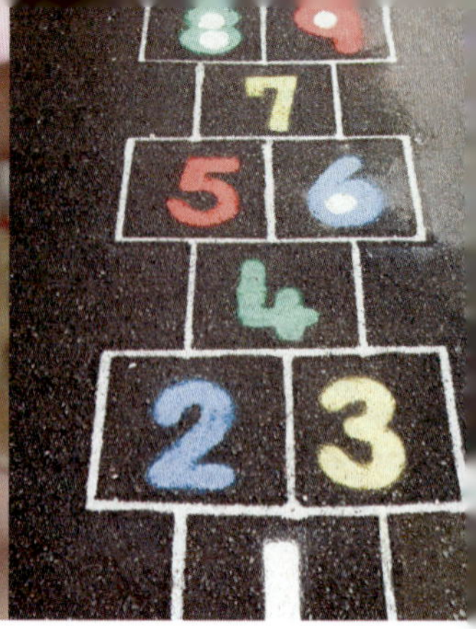

contents

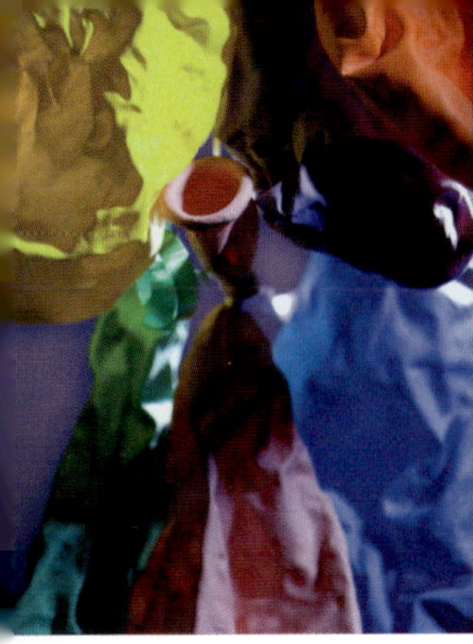
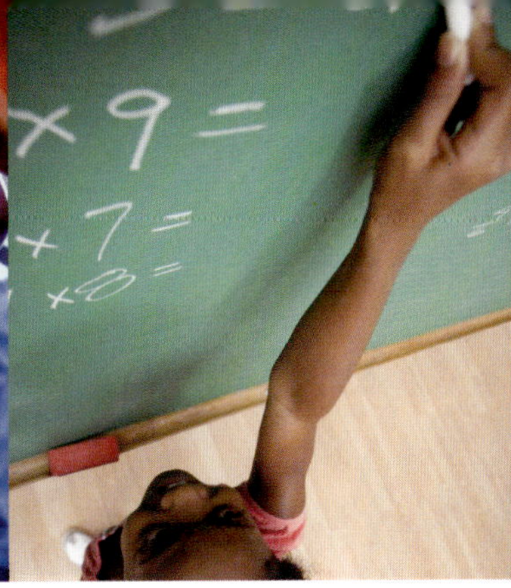
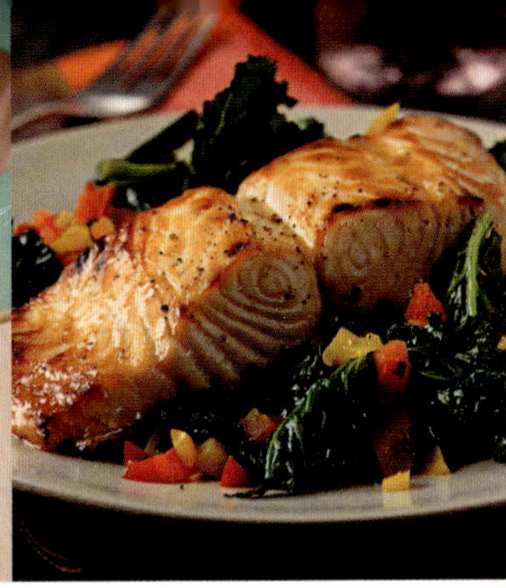

PART THREE

Six Brains Drains and How to Plug Them

PART FOUR

Your Brain Fitness Program

PART FIVE

Resources

the brain drain quiz

DO YOU HAVE

Brain Drain?

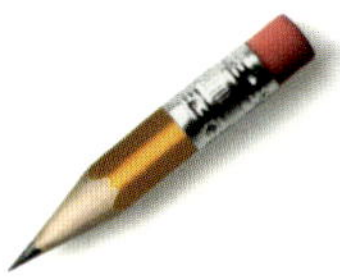

Read each statement below. If it sounds like something you would be likely to say or that generally describes your experience, check "True." If it does not describe your experience, check "False." Before you begin, try to remember this short list of words: tree, faucet, luncheon.

1. My friends and/or coworkers joke about my forgetfulness.
☐ TRUE ☐ FALSE

2. If I'm introduced to someone, chances are I won't remember his or her name an hour later.
☐ TRUE ☐ FALSE

3. When I'm having a casual conversation, I often find myself struggling to think of the right word.
☐ TRUE ☐ FALSE

4. When reading a book or long magazine article, I often have to go back and re-read passages because my attention wanders.
☐ TRUE ☐ FALSE

5. It is not unusual for me to say, "Could you repeat that, and slowly?"
☐ TRUE ☐ FALSE

6. I sometimes worry about my memory.
☐ TRUE ☐ FALSE

7. My memory isn't bad; it just might take me a little longer to think things through.
☐ TRUE ☐ FALSE

8. I frequently misplace things I use daily (keys, pens, cell phone, grocery list).
☐ TRUE ☐ FALSE

9. I don't trust myself to do even simple math without a calculator anymore.
☐ TRUE ☐ FALSE

10. I find it very difficult to add numbers in my head.
☐ TRUE ☐ FALSE

11. I couldn't function without a calendar or written schedule—I need something to remind me of important dates and appointments.
☐ TRUE ☐ FALSE

12. I have a lot of stress in my life.
☐ TRUE ☐ FALSE

13. It is not unusual for me to say, "What were we talking about again?"
☐ TRUE ☐ FALSE

14. More than once a week, I forget why I went into a particular room or closet. ☐ **TRUE** ☐ **FALSE**

15. I do better if I focus on a single thing at a time—I don't like multi-tasking. ☐ **TRUE** ☐ **FALSE**

16. I don't like adding new electronics to the house—I barely learned (or didn't learn) how to work the DVD player. ☐ **TRUE** ☐ **FALSE**

17. It feels as though the world is running at a much faster pace than I am—people seem to be constantly waiting for me. ☐ **TRUE** ☐ **FALSE**

18. It is difficult for me to hold more than three numbers in my mind. ☐ **TRUE** ☐ **FALSE**

19. My abilities in games of skill and strategy (for example, Bridge or chess) would be better if my memory were better. ☐ **TRUE** ☐ **FALSE**

20. I routinely take more than three prescription medications per day. ☐ **TRUE** ☐ **FALSE**

21. I have been diagnosed with Type 2 diabetes, depression, or heart disease. ☐ **TRUE** ☐ **FALSE**

22. I smoke. ☐ **TRUE** ☐ **FALSE**

23. I quit smoking less than 20 years ago. ☐ **TRUE** ☐ **FALSE**

24. I can't seem to find enough time to exercise—twice a week is a lot for me. ☐ **TRUE** ☐ **FALSE**

A Clue to the Colors

This quiz taps into six main facets of cognition: attention and focus, general memory, mental processing speed, verbal skills, number skills, and reasoning skills. It also looks at some lifestyle habits that affect the brain. Keep your answer to each question handy; you'll look back at this quiz when you get to Your Brain Fitness Program in Part 4. There you'll discover how to use the color coding of the questions to learn more about your particular areas of strength and weakness.

25. I have a sweet tooth and indulge in candy, pastry, or desserts almost every day. ☐ **TRUE** ☐ **FALSE**

26. I get lost often, probably because of my poor sense of direction. ☐ **TRUE** ☐ **FALSE**

27. Thank heavens for speed-dial; I can't seem to remember phone numbers anymore. ☐ **TRUE** ☐ **FALSE**

28. People often tell me that I already told them the same story or joke before. ☐ **TRUE** ☐ **FALSE**

29. When I go to the store to get groceries or materials for a project, I almost always forget something and have to go back. ☐ **TRUE** ☐ **FALSE**

Continued >>

30. It feels as though I go through life with that feeling that a name or fact is "on the tip of my tongue."
☐ TRUE ☐ FALSE

31. I know what I want to do; I just have a difficult time figuring out how to accomplish my goals.
☐ TRUE ☐ FALSE

32. Organization is not a strong point for me. ☐ TRUE ☐ FALSE

33. I often find it difficult to persuade people of my opinion, or to make a reasoned argument against someone else's opinion—my thoughts just don't come out as organized as I want them to be.
☐ TRUE ☐ FALSE

34. I often "get lost" while watching a movie or reading a book—plots seem to be much more complicated these days. ☐ TRUE ☐ FALSE

Scoring

1. Do you remember the three words you were asked to remember at the beginning of this quiz? (No peeking!)

______________ ______________ ______________

Give yourself one Memory Point for each word you missed. If you got them all, your score for this question is zero. **My Memory Points:** ________

2. Count the number of True responses for questions 1 to 34. Add this number to your Memory Points. This is your general Brain Drain Score.
My General Brain Drain Score: ________

If your Brain Drain Score is 0: Are you sure you answered all questions honestly? Perhaps you should take another pass at it.

If your Brain Drain Score is 1 to 10: Now is the perfect time to begin taking care of your brain—before forgetfulness and fuzzy thinking become a problem in your life.

If your Brain Drain Score is 11 to 20: Your minor memory problems probably pop up as little surprises in your daily life. You can definitely benefit from brain training, along with the lifestyle changes outlined in Part 3 and Part 4.

If your Brain Drain Score is 21 to 37: You probably feel as though your brain is betraying you. It is possible to reduce or eliminate many of your memory problems with the exercises in this book, along with the lifestyle changes outlined in Part 3 and Part 4.

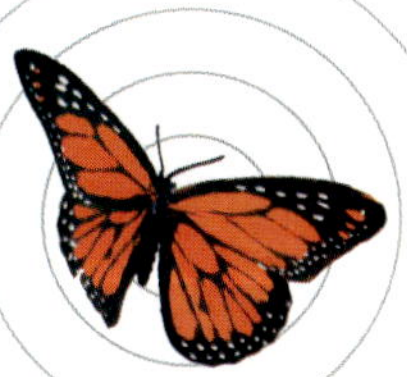

YES, YOU *CAN* change your brain

Congratulations! You picked an extraordinary time to be alive. Modern medicine has developed cures and treatments for many of the health conditions that once felled us in our prime, giving us the most valuable gift of all: more years.

Wonderful indeed—but what kind of gift is extra longevity if our minds wear out before our bodies do? After all, the brain contains everything that makes us "us": not only every talent and skill but also records of all our experiences, our hopes and dreams, the jokes and sunsets and births and achievements that give our lives purpose and meaning. It's no wonder, then, that with every little brain hiccup—the failure to remember a name, the loss of one's car keys (again), a sudden losing streak in a regular Bridge game—we see our very lives slipping away. In fact, people fear losing their memories more than they fear death itself.

Well, you can breathe a deep sigh of relief: It turns out that our deepest and darkest fears about brain drain are truly unfounded. In writing this book, we consulted some of the world's most preeminent neurologists and psychologists and studied hundreds of medical journal articles, and we found good news everywhere we looked.

Better with Age

The first piece of good news: We can tell you here and now that the old saying "You can't teach an old dog new tricks" is totally off base. In fact, aging alone does nothing to affect our capacity to learn, remember, and think clearly. (And who wants to be called an old dog, anyway?)

Another astounding finding: With age, we actually get *better* at remembering new information. That's right, better. When we're young, our memory "file cabinets" are relatively empty. There's no filing system, so the information gets thrown in willy-nilly, and it doesn't seem to make a lot of sense in there all by itself. As we age and the file cabinets are stuffed full of the fabulous record of lives well-lived, the brain makes more complex associations between ideas and puts new learnings in the context of a vast reservoir of experience, which allows new ideas to "stick" better. Additionally, as our file cabinets fill up, we learn tactics for organizing the information, and we have files already set up and ready to receive each new discovery or experience.

There's a word for this multiplicity of mental resources: "wisdom."

Another surprise: The mental file cabinets never run out of space. Its storage capacity is infinite, says James L. McGaugh, Ph.D., professor of neurobiology and behavior at the University of California, Irvine. "We are capable of learning everything and anything." One of Dr. McGaugh's research projects involves a small number of people with total recall. "I can say to them, 'What happened on May 13, 1983?' and they can tell me what the weather was like, what day of the week it was, what they ate that day, who they visited, and so forth. I simply can't stump them," says Dr. McGaugh. You may not wish to

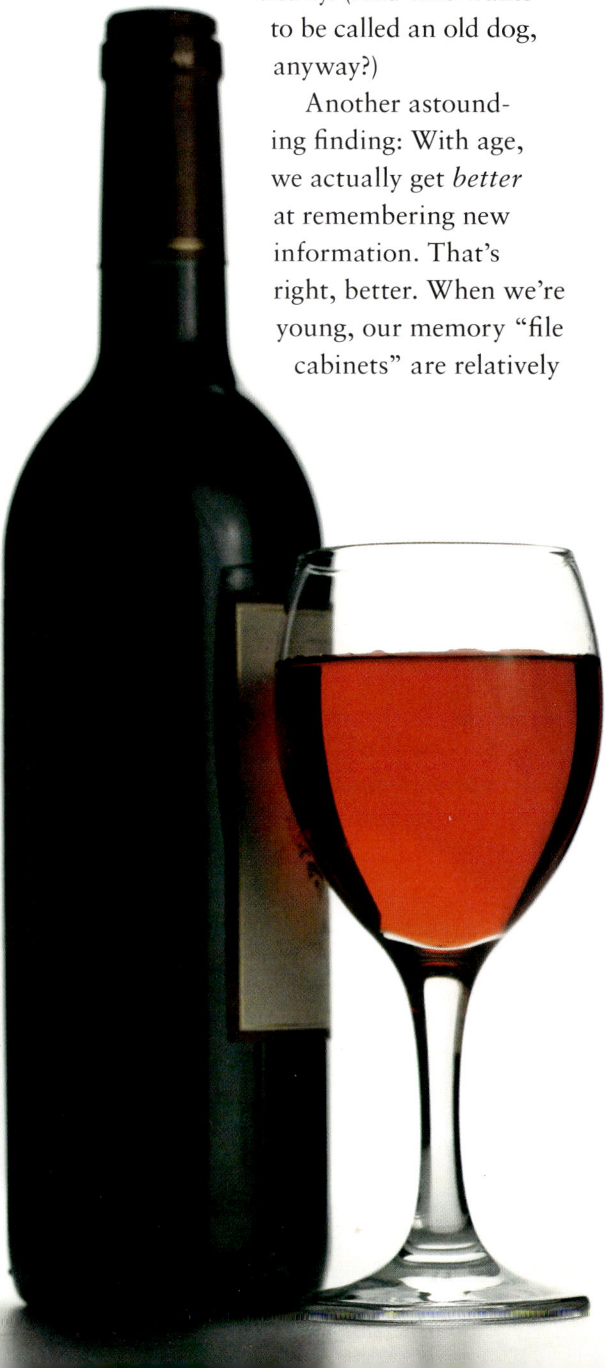

With age, we actually get *better* at remembering new information.

remember what clothes you wore on a Tuesday 30 years ago, but it's nice to know that the potential for a vast amount of memory lies within all of us.

Two Breakthroughs That Changed the Game

The brain, once a mysterious "black box" that scientists couldn't decode, is finally revealing some of its biggest secrets, and the news offers immense promise to anyone who's ever asked themselves, "Am I losing it?" High on the list of the top discoveries are these two:

WE DO GROW NEW BRAIN CELLS

Who doesn't remember tipping back a beer in their youth and joking to a friend, "Well, there goes another thousand brain cells!" It was common knowledge that infants begin life with gazillions of brain cells, then slowly lose them with time (and alcohol). There'd be fewer brain cells by our teens, we thought, fewer still by our twenties and thirties. By middle age, well, God help us! (And, back then, if we needed proof of brain decline at mid-life, all we had to do was look at our parents!) But in fact, in one of the most stunning brain discoveries ever, scientists have learned that the brain generates new brain cells every day, in a process called neurogenesis. The activities you'll do in *No More Brain Drain* can even help speed up that process.

THE MORE YOU USE YOUR BRAIN, THE GREATER ITS CAPACITY

We used to think of the brain as if it were a fixed power grid, like the kind that sends electricity to our cities. When the system gets old or overloaded, the power decreases, leading to flickering lights and dead appliances. We believed that age wore down memory and comprehension—and that there was nothing that could be done about it. Today, we know that the brain is constantly growing and adapting, expanding its capacity as needed. Not only does it generate new brain cells but it also generates new connections between those brain cells in the form of intricate nerve fibers called dendrites. The more connections, the faster and better you think. The advice and exercises in *No More Brain Drain* are designed specifically to help you expand your brain's power grid.

Cleaning Out the Mental Closet

Older people learn to be more efficient with memory, ditching useless information in order to focus on what's most important. They may not remember a stranger's name after a chance encounter, but they sure won't forget their granddaughter's birthday or their wedding day.

Use It or Lose It

Whether you're balancing your checkbook, learning how to salsa, or playing a mean hand of gin rummy, your brain's "electricity grid" is lit up like Times Square on New Year's Eve. Chemical messages zip along at speeds of up to several hundred miles per hour from one nerve cell to the next along "cables" called axons. Waiting to receive all that information are the nerve cell "branches" mentioned earlier called dendrites. And guess what? You play the most important role in keeping this complex network humming.

"When you challenge the brain with new skills and new ways of doing things, it increases connections in the brain," says Ericka P. Simpson, M.D., a neurologist at the Methodist Hospital System Neurological Institute in Houston. Forcing our brains to learn something new causes them to sprout more and more dendrites, which expands our brains' capacity to think, decide, learn, and remember.

On the other hand, being mentally lazy—getting stuck in a rut, doing everything the same way, never trying anything new—has the opposite effect. The brain, in constant cleanup mode, allows unused neurons to die and "prunes" underutilized dendrites, just as a gardener prunes dying branches on a tree.

Keeping our brains in tip-top shape even reduces our risk for serious brain problems, including Alzheimer's disease and other forms of dementia. "Use It or Lose It" declared a headline in the *New England Journal of Medicine* a few years back. The accompanying article described a 5-year study by researchers at Albert Einstein College of Medicine of Yeshiva University in the Bronx, showing that regularly partaking of leisure activities—including reading, playing board games, playing a musical instrument, and dancing—reduced the risk of developing dementia by more than half. A multitude of other studies have reached similar conclusions. To list but a few examples, you can boost brainpower simply by:

• ***Talking.*** A study found that chatting for 10 minutes a day improves memory and test scores.

• ***Walking.*** In a study published in the *Journal of the American Medical Association*, researchers looking at data from the Nurses Study, involving more than 18,000 women, found that long-term regular physical activity, including walking, is associated with significantly better

It's Bunk!

Don't believe these three common myths about the brain.

myth #1 **Our ability to remember declines with age.**

the truth The older brain loses some agility, but it gives up nothing in capacity. Remembering a complicated set of directions or a long list of words will require more time and repetition. But if we put in the effort, we'll retain the information just as well as a younger person, if not better.

myth #2 **Memories are precise photocopies of information or events.**

the truth Memories aren't so much stored as recreated every time you call one up. They live in complex networks of nerve cell pathways throughout the brain. When we commit something to memory, we are "laying tracks" along a unique memory trail. And just like a path in the woods, the more we walk down it, the more firmly established it becomes, and the easier it is to retrace our steps.

myth #3 **Our brains are less sharp starting in our forties or fifties.**

the truth Mental agility—though not capacity—actually begins to slip at about age 24. The older we are, the harder we need to work to keep our minds running at a fast clip.

cognitive function and less cognitive decline in older women.

• *Socializing.* In a Harvard study of more than 2,800 people age 65 or older, those with at least five social ties–church groups, social groups, regular visits, or phone calls with family and friends—were the most resistant to brain drain.

• *Playing video games.* A study of people in their sixties and seventies found that playing a strategy video game focused on world domination improved cognitive skills.

Your No More Brain Drain Action Plan

What's the best way to nurture your neurological garden? In Part 2, Six 'Vaccines' against Brain Drain, we'll show you exactly what small lifestyle tweaks you can make to help yourself think more clearly, retain information more effectively, and concentrate better. It can be as simple as going for a brisk walk several times a week, getting the right amount of sleep, or taking an occasional class.

Your diet is especially important. A recent study published in *Archives of Neurology* found that following the Mediterranean diet provides a powerful defense against mental decline. After 5 years, people who followed this diet—high in fish, fruits, vegetables, legumes, and monounsaturated fats like olive oil; moderate in alcohol; and low in red meat and dairy—had a 28 percent lower risk of cognitive impairment. "Nutrition is the most important tool for staying mentally and physically fit, but is the most underutilized tool," says brain expert David Perlmutter, MD, FACN. We'll point you to the very best brain foods.

You'll even discover the power of common drugs, such as medications to lower blood pressure, to help stave off brain drain and how something as simple as a getting adequate shut-eye can almost magically clear up fuzzy thinking. (Test subjects assigned to memorize lists of words in the afternoon recalled their words 30 percent better after a good night's sleep.)

In Part 3, Five Brain Drains and How to Plug Them, we'll reveal villains that can rob your brain of its power and explain how to protect yourself. Some of

> The tips and exercises in this book will challenge your brain and help nurture your "neurological garden."

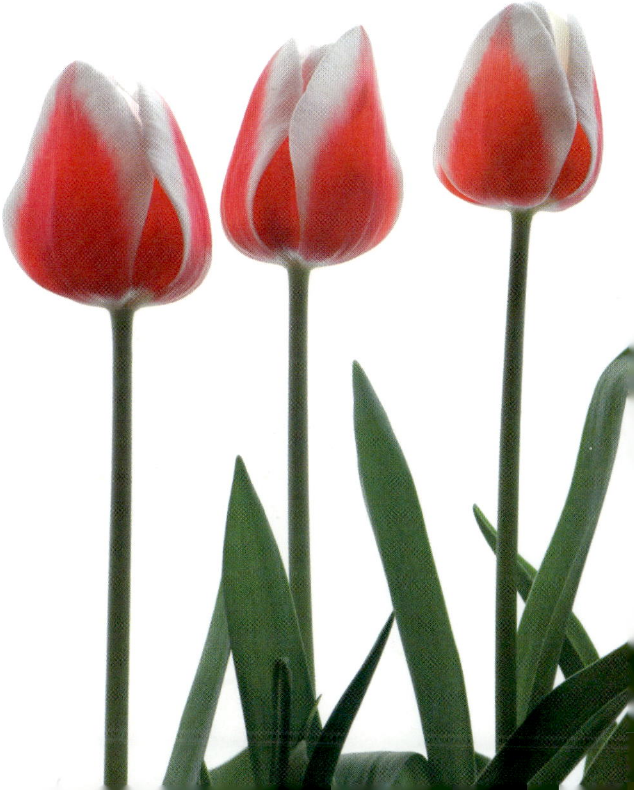

the villains are the usual suspects: Smoking and drinking to excess are just as bad for your brain as they are for the rest of your body. But others are more surprising. Scattered, fuzzy thinking? Many of us can blame it on stress. In a recent study, stressed-out medical students performed markedly worse on an important licensing exam. Depression can also rob us of brain power. When the blues turn black, the symptoms can include foggy memory, difficulty with comprehension, even slurred speech. In the elderly, these symptoms are commonly mistaken for dementia, but mental skills rebound quickly when the depression is treated. Even high cholesterol levels and belly fat can wear down your brain. We'll show you how to combat each of these drains.

Finally, we've all heard the advice to take up crossword puzzles to keep the mind fit. That's a good starting point. It'll definitely make you better at crossword puzzles—but it won't help you find your car keys, confirms Alan Castel, Ph.D., assistant professor of psychology at the University of California, Los Angeles, and an expert in memory and cognitive aging.

Leisure activities, such as playing board games, may reduce your risk of dementia.

Who'd Have Thought?

Intellectually curious people are more resistant to brain drain. They have what scientists call a cognitive reserve. This simply means that they have more nerve cells and dendrites than others to begin with, so if their brains eventually suffer damage due to a disease like Alzheimer's, they're likely to function well for a longer period of time.

Just as runners devote a portion of their training to swimming and cycling, just as boxers jump rope, you'll need to mix it up to really keep your brain in shape. Athletes call this cross-training. We've designed Part 4 of this book, Your Brain Fitness Program, to help you do just that. You'll discover a series of fun puzzles and exercises custom designed to challenge your brain in six main cognitive areas: attention and focus, general memory, processing speed, verbal skills, number skills, and reasoning. Spend a few minutes on them every day, and you

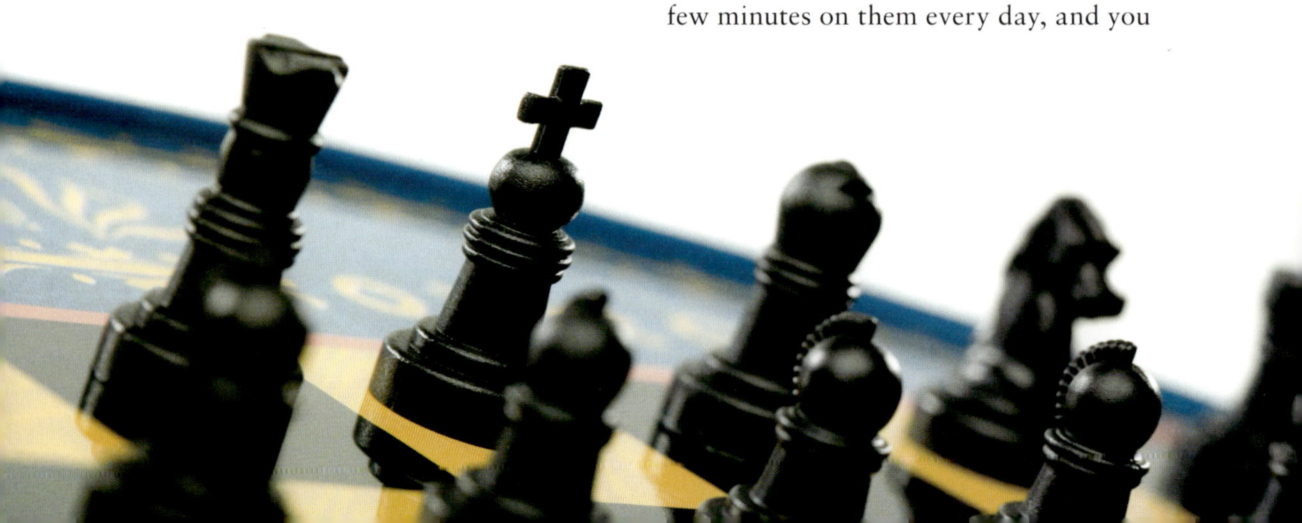

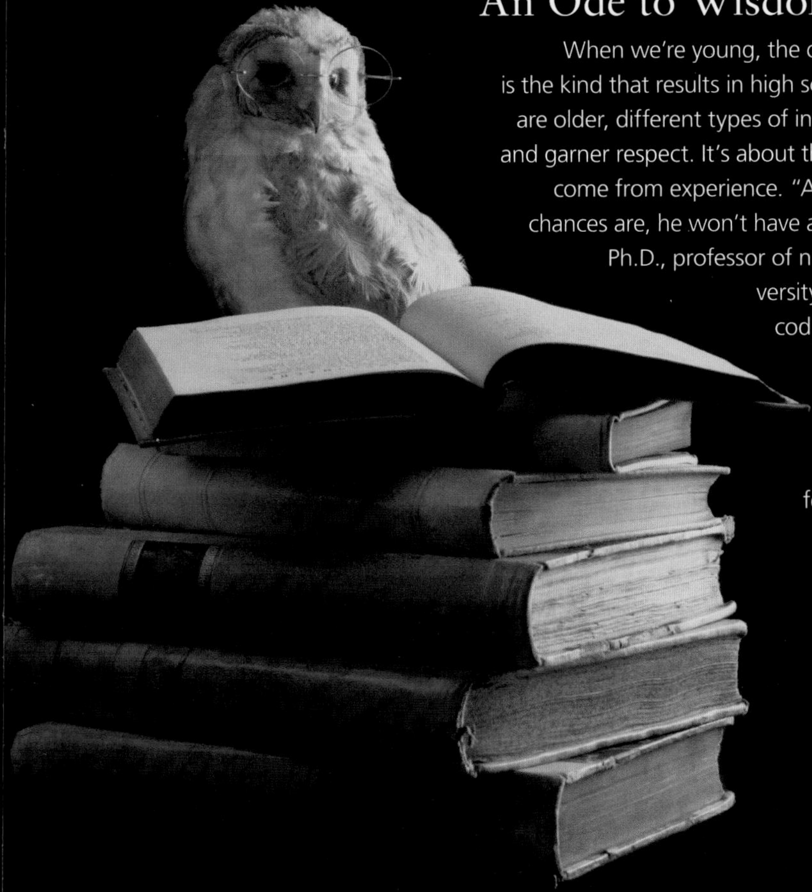

An Ode to Wisdom

When we're young, the only kind of intelligence that is valued is the kind that results in high scores on school exams. But when we are older, different types of intelligence become increasingly useful and garner respect. It's about the depth of knowledge that can only come from experience. "Ask an 18-year-old about politics and, chances are, he won't have a lot to say," says James L. McGaugh, Ph.D., professor of neurobiology and behavior at the University of California, Irvine. "But ask an old codger like me, and you'll get an earful." Wisdom isn't just about having an evolved opinion. Think of it as a kind of "street smarts" that helps an older person put different pieces of information together more effectively.

should start noticing improvements in your brain "fitness" in no time. We'll also show you useful everyday strategies for everything from remembering phone numbers to recalling those names that are always on the tip of your tongue.

Are you inspired to halt those memory slips, chase away brain fog, sharpen up your concentration and focus, reduce your dementia risk, and boost your overall confidence in yourself? You've come to the right place. Our practical, comprehensive plan is based on the latest science, but we promise to keep things fun and easy every step of the way. Do the puzzles and exercises and follow the advice to enjoy a brain that's recharged, rejuvenated, and ready to learn and remember.

As for losing your car keys, we can't guarantee that it will never happen again, but we can tell you it's something we all do, no matter what our brain health. So instead of worrying, why not use your mental energies to find a designated spot to keep them?

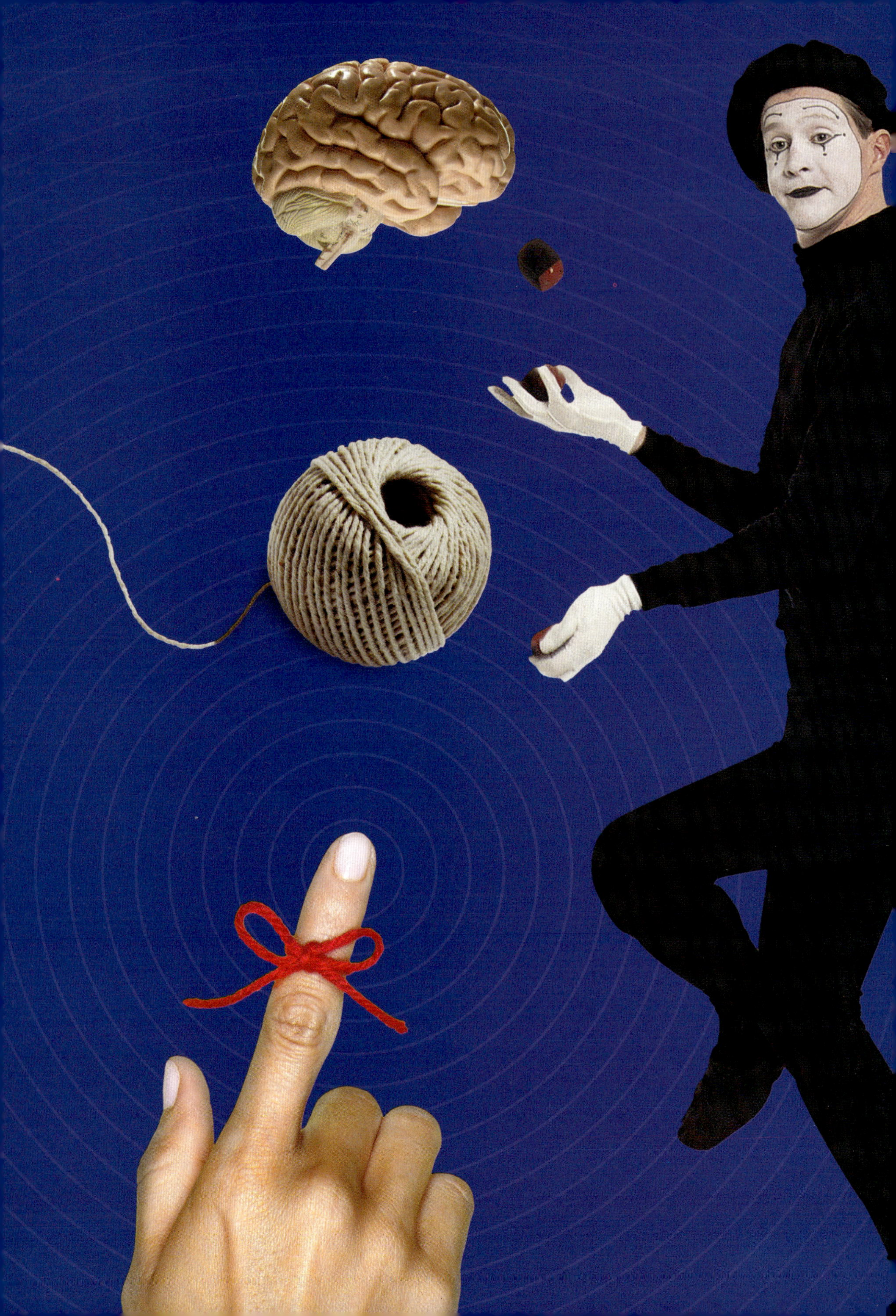

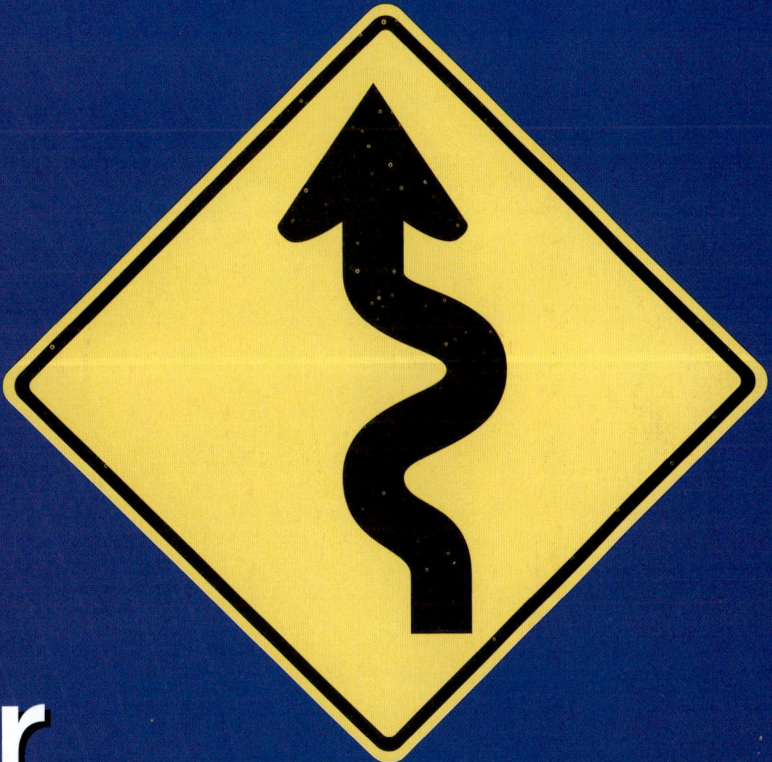

PART ONE

your amazing brain

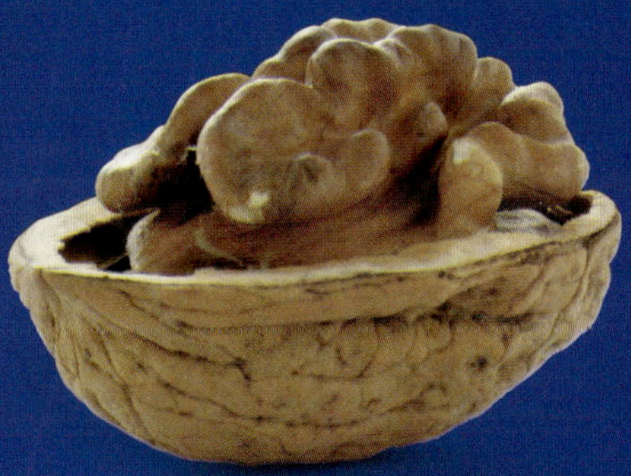

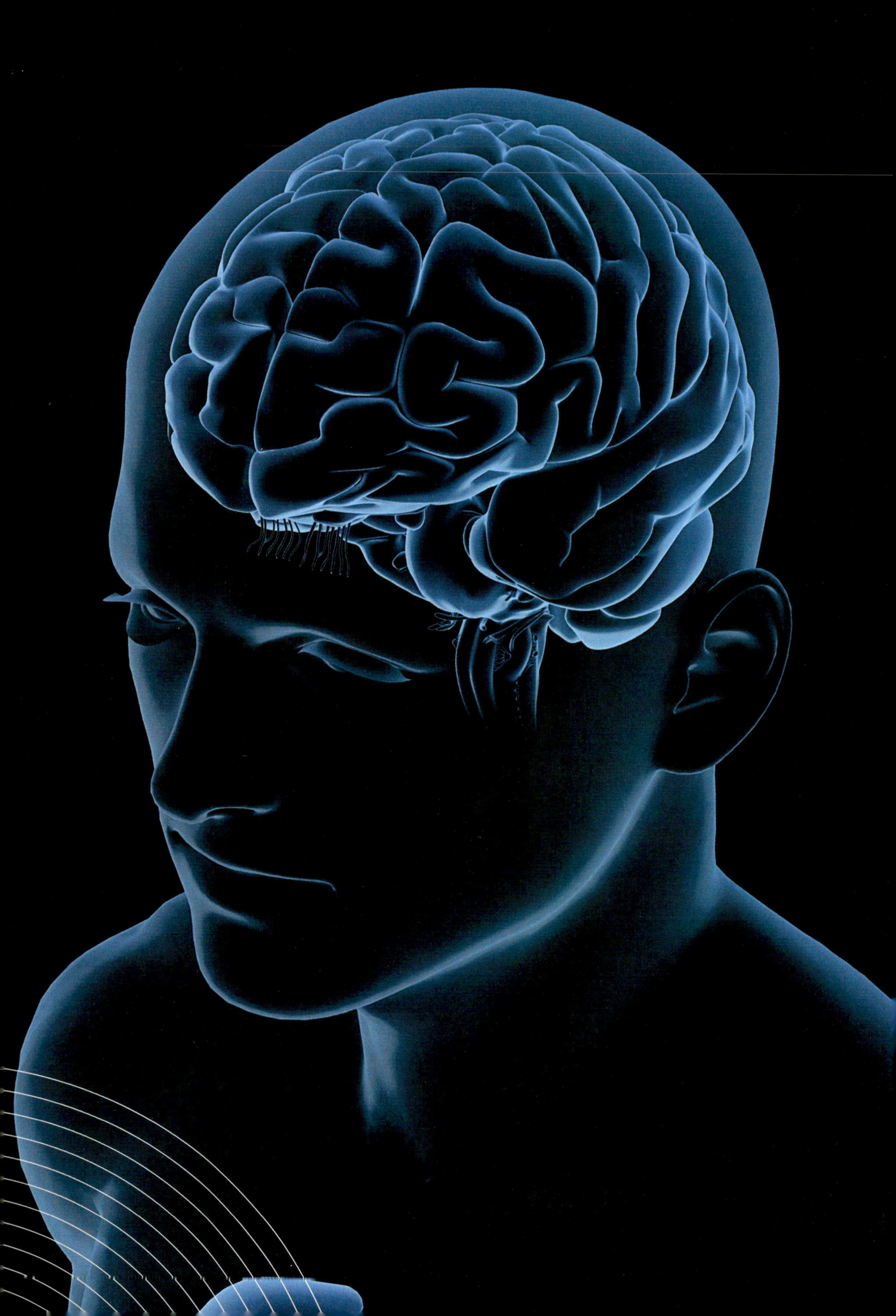

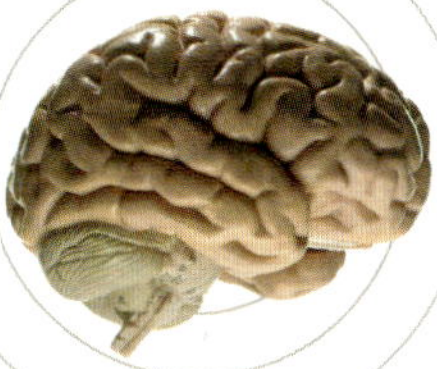

Your smart parts
A BRIEF TOUR

At first glance, the brain is less than impressive. It's a wrinkled gray mass whose surface resembles that of a walnut (that's because the brain folds itself up—just as your intestines do—to fit more matter into a small space). If you were to poke it, it would feel like a mound of soft tofu. Not very promising.

But appearances are deceiving: The brain is astoundingly complex and perpetually active. It doesn't sleep or rest, and it never loses its capacity for growth and change. In an instant, the brain can keep your heart beating, your lungs breathing, and your senses sensing, all while you drive a 2-ton vehicle 70 miles per hour down a busy highway, watch the road signs, talk on your cell phone (which, by the way, we don't recommend), eat and digest a cookie, and listen to the radio. Not too shabby for a jiggly hunk of gray Jell-O.

How does it get it all done? You'd never know it by looking at it, but the brain contains distinct regions, each with its own job to do. Much of what we know about how different parts of the brain work comes from observing how people act and react after damage to certain areas due to injury, tumors, seizures, or stroke. Without these invaluable insights, the brain would remain an utter mystery.

Gray Matter: Where It All Happens

The entire wrinkled outer layer of the brain is the cerebral cortex, also known as gray matter. Only a few millimeters thick, it contains 85 percent of all brain tissue, much of it hidden in its many folds and convolutions. The cerebral cortex (see pages 24–25 for more details) is largely responsible for all forms of conscious experience, including perception, emotion, thought, and planning.

The two sides of the brain—the left and right hemispheres—further divvy up these functions. With some exceptions, the left hemisphere controls language, while the right side controls art and spatial orientation skills. Writing a letter involves your left brain; painting a picture or finding your way back to your car in a crowded parking lot would be your right brain.

Because the body's nerves cross sides, the left hemisphere controls the right side of your body, and the right hemisphere controls the left. The two halves of your brain are connected by millions of nerve fibers bundled together in a thick cable called the corpus callosum. This "bridge" allows the brain to merge and coordinate skills so it can act as a united whole.

An interesting side note: If the corpus callosum is damaged or severed, the two sides of the brain can't communicate. If an apple is placed in the left hand of a blindfolded person with this kind of brain damage, the right side of his brain would recognize it as an apple using smell and touch. But because the brain hemispheres aren't talking, the right side can't relay the concept to the language center on the left side. It would be impossible to for this person to come up with the word "apple."

Amazing Brain Facts

- The adult brain weighs about 3 pounds, about the same as a full-grown Chihuahua.
- Size isn't everything: Albert Einstein's brain weighed in at a mere 2.71 pounds.
- The average brain is comprised of 100 billion neurons.
- The brain greedily uses 20 percent of the energy we burn and the oxygen we breathe. Brain cells will start dying after only 4 to 6 minutes without oxygen.
- More electrical impulses are generated in 1 day by a single human brain than by all the telephones in the world.
- Neurons send signals at speeds of up to 200 miles per hour.
- The brain can't feel pain because it lacks the sensory nerves that register those sensations. (That's why neurosurgeons can poke around a brain while the patient is awake and alert.)
- The human brain can perceive about 10,000 different smells.
- A newborn's brain weighs about 12 ounces, but by age 5, a child's brain is nearly the same size as an adult's brain.
- The human brain produces 70,000 distinct thoughts in an average day.

Your Brain's Communication Network

Every thought, idea, and memory you have forges a unique electro-chemical path among the billions of neurons in your brain.

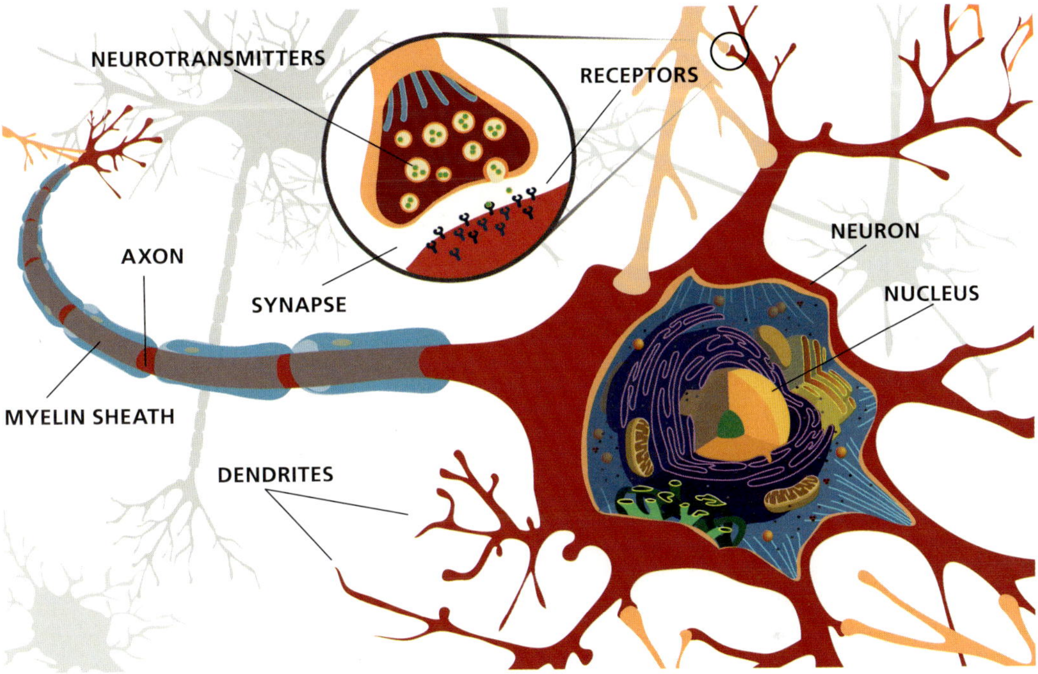

Gray matter is not a single material but a biological compote of capillaries (which carry oxygen and nutrients throughout the brain), nerve cells (also known as neurons), and glia, the cells that support, feed, and communicate with nerve cells. If you suck away the glia, you are left with a communications network wired from billions of nerve cells. This lacey structure underlies everything in your physical, mental, and emotional life.

Life depends on neurons passing messages to other neurons. The messages are transmitted along a single fiber called an axon. They're received by a multitude of short branches called dendrites. As the information passes from one neuron to the next, it must jump across countless infinitesimally small gaps called synapses. This is where brain chemicals called neurotransmitters, such a serotonin and dopamine, come into play. When the information reaches the end of a neuron's axon, neurotransmitters carry it across the gap.

As with any communications network—think about your internet service provider, or your cell phone service provider and the satellites it uses to send information from one place to another—the better the network, the clearer the messages are and the faster they get through.

To transport information from one area of the brain to another area that's far away, the brain uses special high-speed cables—bundles of axons coated by a fatty substance called myelin. Myelin stands out from the rest of the brain like

Continued on page 26

Your Gray Matter at Work

We call brainy people cerebral for good reason: The cerebral cortex, also known as gray matter, is where complex thought, attention, and memory (including muscle memory) take place. Different functions happen in different areas.

1. DECISION MAKING, PLANNING, AND PROBLEM SOLVING

The large portion of the brain called the frontal lobe is the brain's command center. It controls decision making, planning, organizing, and problem solving. It also creates our personalities, sharpens our attention, and keeps us focused on goals. It allows civilized societies to exist by putting the brakes on some of our baser instincts.

▶ Damage Report

The Caveman Effect Damage to the frontal lobe can result in wildly fluctuating emotions and difficulty performing even simple tasks. Think about it: Just brewing a cup of tea requires dozens of individual steps, including finding the tea, turning on the stove, waiting for the kettle to boil, turning off the stove, and more. Without planning abilities, this would be impossible to pull off.

2. SHORT-TERM MINI-STORAGE

The part of the frontal lobe closest to your forehead is the prefrontal cortex, the primary area for keeping short-term memories (also called working memory). Think of it as a temporary filing system that holds facts for just a few seconds—a phone number you are about to dial, for example. Thoughts or ideas reside here briefly unless you make the effort to commit them to long-term memory.

3. MOVEMENT

At the rear of the prefrontal cortex is the primary motor cortex, controlling all movement. Brain scientists can now identify the locations in the motor cortex associated with distinct patterns of movement, such as the hand motions of musicians. In fact, it's even possible to know what instrument a musician plays by looking at changes in this part of the brain.

4. PHYSICAL SENSATIONS

The parietal lobe is responsible for the body's physical sensations, such as the perception of being touched on the back of your neck. A disproportionate amount of the parietal lobe is dedicated to some of the smallest—but most sensitive—parts of the body, such as the tongue, hands, face, and the genitals. The parietal lobe also plays a role in spatial recognition, language, and our ability to focus attention.

▶ Damage Report

Half the Story Damage to the parietal lobe can cause distortions in the way a person perceives space and objects. If the damage is on the left side of the brain, the person may be totally unaware of anything on the right side of their visual field, including the right side of a computer screen, the right side of someone's face, or even their own right leg.

5. REMEMBERING NAMES

The temporal lobe connects directly to the ears and processes and interprets sounds. It also has a role in memory, particularly for words, phrases, ideas, and names of people or objects. When you forget someone's name, blame your temporal lobe for sleeping on the job.

▶ Damage Report

Subtotal Recall If the temporal lobe is damaged, a person is unable to learn new facts or remember events. Life seems eternally new (and frustrating) because no new memories can be formed—every day is an absolutely blank slate. A person with this type of damage could read the same newspaper over and over without getting bored.

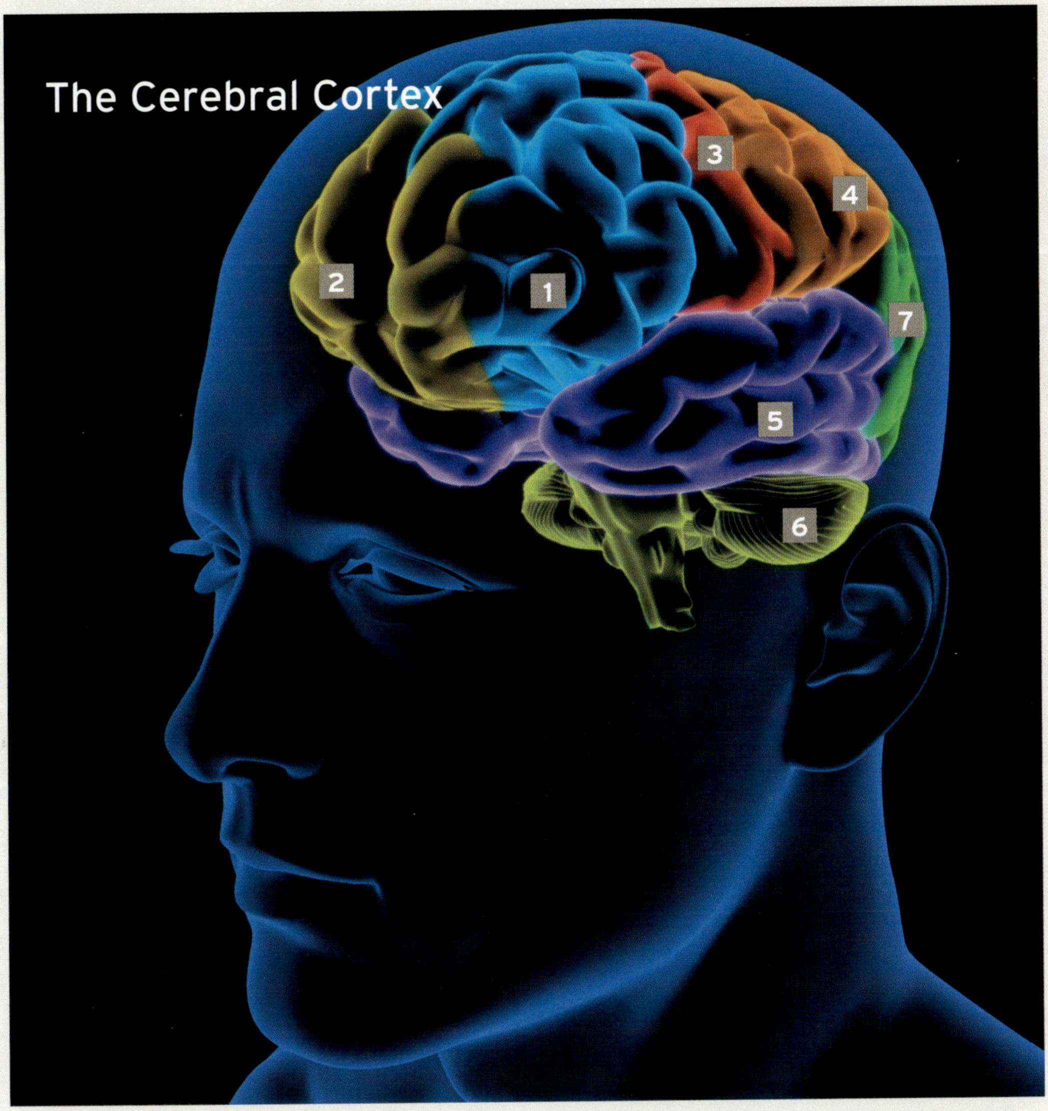

6. COORDINATION

The cerebellum (the "little brain") is a wrinkled bit that looks like it was tacked onto the brain as an afterthought. Don't let its small size fool you—it contains half the neurons in the brain. While the motor cortex in the cerebrum is the area that sends messages to muscles that cause them to move ("put your right foot forward!"), the cerebellum acts like a conductor, coordinating all the movements that let you successfully swim a lap in the pool, knit a sweater, or even walk down the street and not fall over.

▶ **Damage Report**

Drunk While Sober Damage to the cerebellum can cause dizziness, slurred speech, and nausea as well as uncoordinated movements. People with injury to the cerebellum are often mistaken for being drunk.

7. VISION

The occipital lobe manages vision. It focuses the eyes, interprets the meaning of all those shapes and colors we see, and records short-term visual memory.

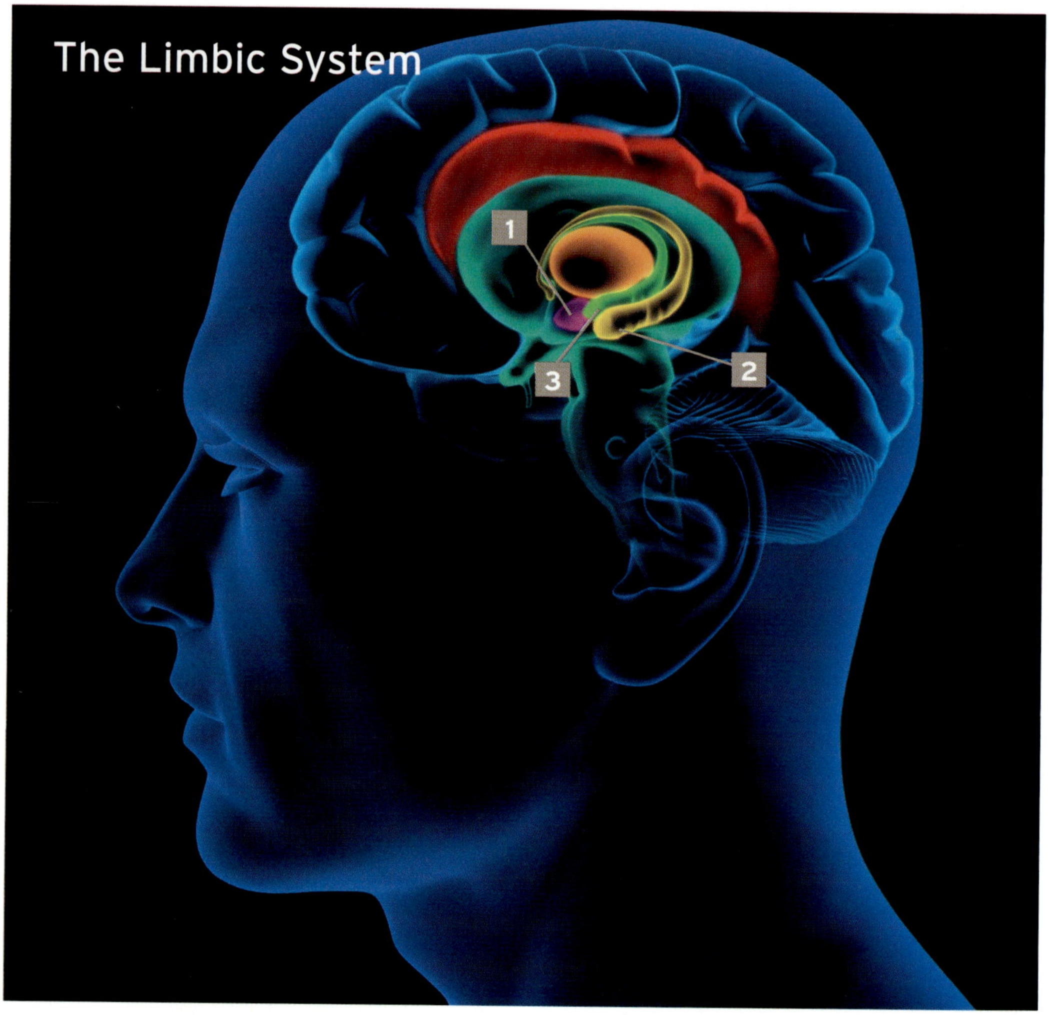

ribbons of fat in a thick rib-eye steak—and gives the brain's white matter its name. The myelin coating insulates the bundles and speeds the transmission of electrical signals along this communication expressway, allowing for faster cognitive processing.

The Limbic System: Basics Instincts

Buried deep under the cerebral cortex is the limbic system, a set of primitive structures responsible for some of our most basic human instincts and drives. Craving a piece of chocolate cake? Blame, in part, the limbic system, which regulates our response to pleasure. Bolting down the street to escape a rabid dog? Thank the limbic system, largely responsible for our survival instincts. Terrified of bees since being stung badly as a child? The limbic system is responsible, since it won't let you ever forget that event. It's also in charge of our most primal urges, including the sexual kind.

Damage to this part of the brain leaves appetite, aggression, and sex drive completely unregulated.

The limbic system consists of three main structures:

1. THE HYPOTHALAMUS.

Does your heart beat faster when you think about a scary upcoming event? That's the hypothalamus at work. About the size of an almond, this region has an amazing amount of control over what happens in our bodies, and even over our moods and actions. It not only controls sexual arousal and behavior but also regulates hunger and thirst, sleep and wakefulness, responses to pain and pleasure, levels of anger and aggression, and even body temperature, pulse, blood pressure, and other physical responses to emotional events.

2. THE HIPPOCAMPUS.

This tiny area of the brain, whose shape first reminded scientists of a seahorse (*hippocampus* is Greek for "seahorse"), converts short-term memories into long-term ones. It shares responsibility with the hypothalamus for aggressive behavior, sex drive, and appetite. And it's largely responsible for spatial memory and navigation. It's one of the first regions to become damaged in cases of Alzheimer's disease, causing memory problems and disorientation.

new thinking

A brain in your belly? What sends and receives information along a complex neural circuit, communicates with the help of chemical messengers called neurotransmitters (such as dopamine and serotonin), and is capable of functioning independently? Yes, it's the brain—but it's also the stomach!

The brain and the gut are intimately linked. For example, when you imagine something fearful, you raise your heart rate and make your stomach do backflips. Did you know that:

- An upset stomach can lead to a headache?
- Stomachs get their own form of "migraines?"
- Antidepressants can calm the guts of people with irritable bowel syndrome?

Your gut also acts on its own. Some experts hypothesize that the brain in our bellies may even hold sensory memories that we don't consciously recall, but that nonetheless guide us. Gut instinct? Maybe so!

3. THE AMYGDALA.

This part of the brain helps regulate fear, anger, and sexual response. The old thinking was that it played a special role in processing emotional memory, taking highly charged events, like a traumatic attack, a flubbed job interview, or a first kiss, and making sure they are stored permanently in your mind. The new thinking is that the amygdala may actually play a role in all long-term memory formation.

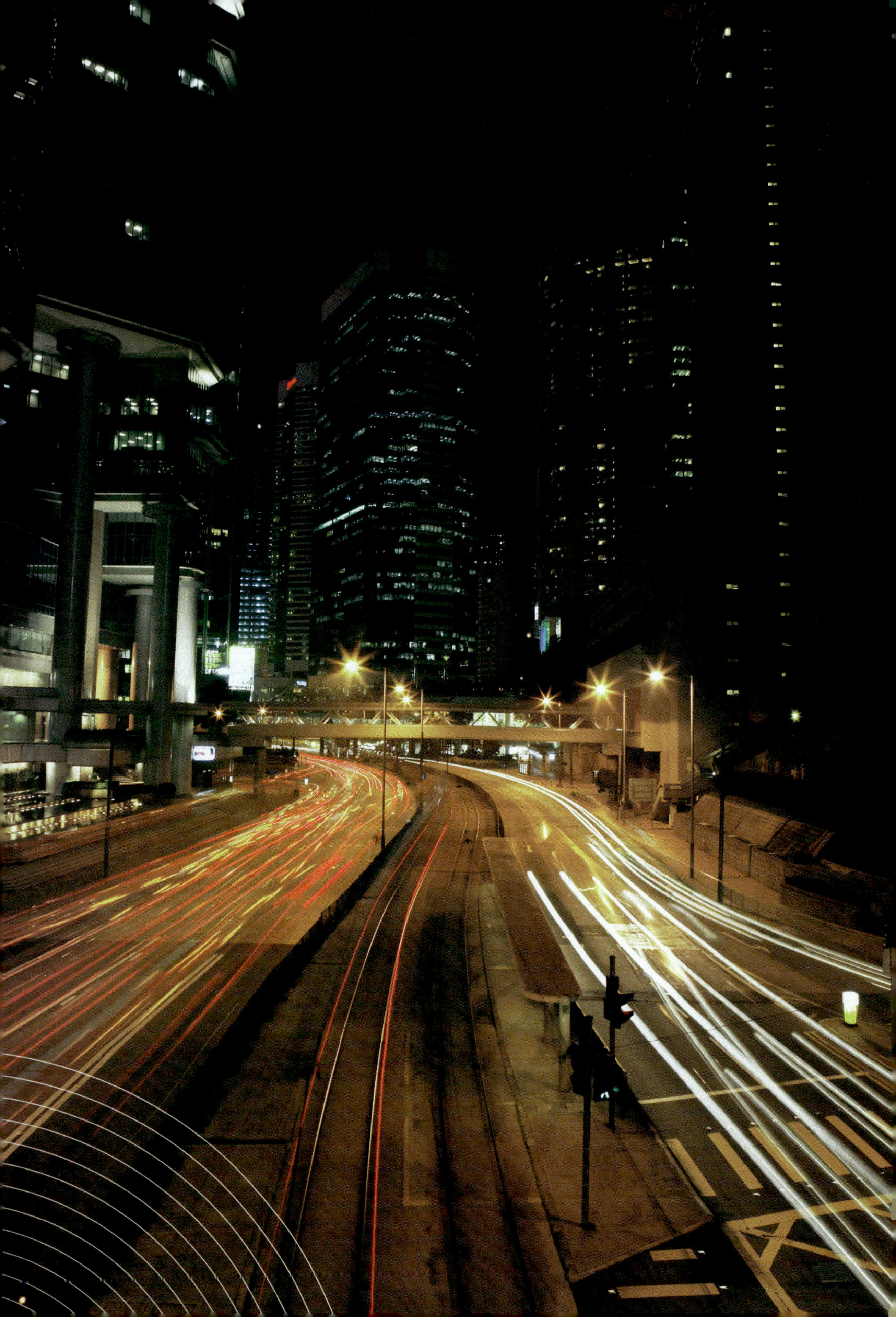

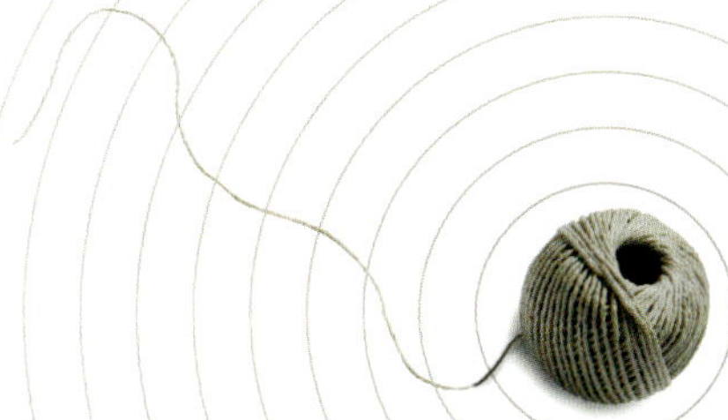

How memory and learning work

Remember the geometry equations you learned in school? Can you still recite a poem all the way through? Do you recall what you had for breakfast last Tuesday? We didn't think so! Some bits of information just seem to slip away. But others stick in the brain with startling clarity and little or no effort. It's a good bet that you remember the words to the theme song of your favorite childhood TV show, the exact time of day your children were born, the name of your favorite grade school teacher, and the price you paid for you first house. (Admit it, as you were reading that last sentence, didn't you find yourself pulled back into a detailed reverie?)

No matter how hard we try, we are never totally in control of our memories. But neurologists are gradually learning exactly what happens in the brain to allow us to process and record our experiences—and why some ideas, facts, and images stay with us as others dissolve in the mist.

Memory: The Long and Short of It

Certain kinds of information in our brains are captured and released without our even knowing it. Other types stick around very briefly, long enough for the knowledge to be used and forgotten—or, if we commit to learning it, transferred to longer-term storage.

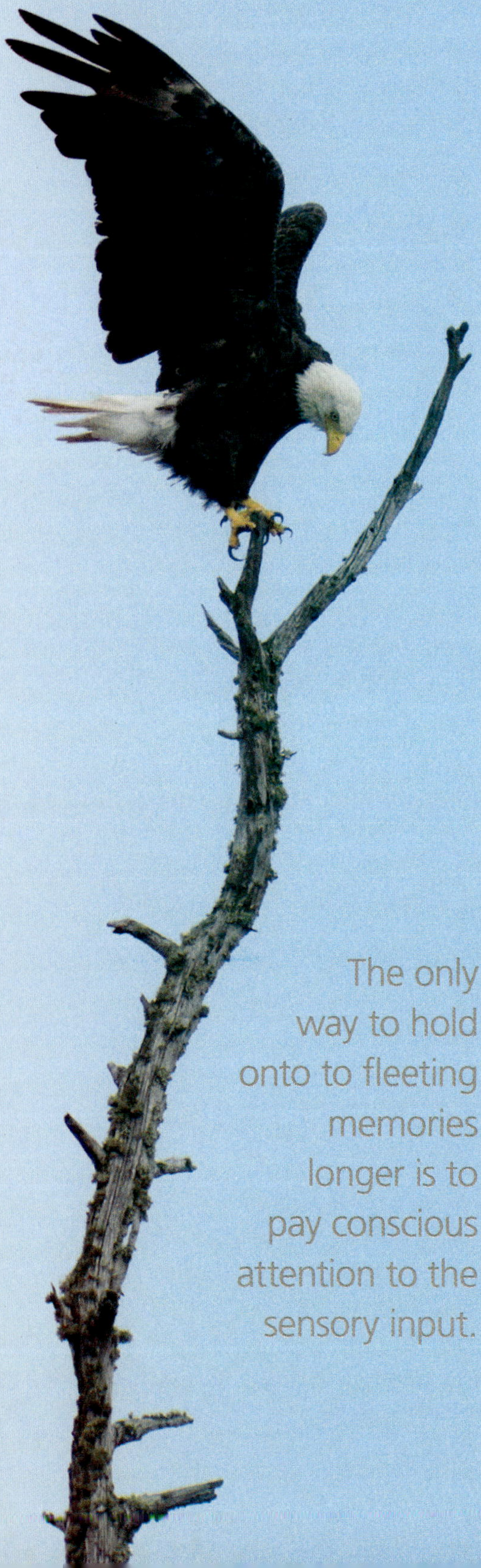

The only way to hold onto to fleeting memories longer is to pay conscious attention to the sensory input.

HERE AND GONE: BELOW THE RADAR

Memory begins with experience, and we're drenched in a sea of experience every second of every day. There's no getting away from it. If you close your eyes, you still can hear. Block your ears and you can nevertheless taste. Close your mouth and you still can smell. Hold your nose and you still can feel. Registering these sensory experiences is effortless and automatic—it doesn't even require your attention. Stop reading for a second and look around the room. Without any conscious effort on your part, your brain is registering everything within the scope of your vision. This first level of memory is called sensory memory.

So where does all that sensory information go? Pretty quickly, it vanishes. If you look out the window and see a bird alight on a branch of a tree, then fly away again, within just 60 seconds, you wouldn't be able to point out which branch the bird landed on. You saw it, your brain registered the information, but the sensory memory (the visual image of the bird on the tree) melted away.

While you may not notice sensory memory, it's essential for navigation, not to mention safety. (For example, a big crashing sound means danger!)

The only way to hold onto to these fleeting memories longer is to pay conscious attention to the sensory input. In the example of the bird, if you knew in advance that you'd be asked which branch it had landed on, you'd pay more attention, focusing on that bit of information and taking it to the next memory level, working memory.

TEMPORARY STORAGE

Working memory, or short-term memory, requires paying a bit of attention, unlike sensory memory. As you're reading this passage, you're using short-term memory to remember the gist of the sentences that came before so that what we're telling you makes overall sense.

True to its name, short-term memory lasts only a few seconds to a few minutes. Think of all the times you looked up a phone number, got briefly distracted before making the call, and had to find the phone number all over again. Not only is the storage time for working memory short, the storage space is

Truth or Excuse?

We all know lots of excuses for forgetfulness. When we say, "I'm sorry I forgot your birthday because [insert reason here]," are we just making up a phony excuse? A quick legitimacy check on the most common excuses:

EXCUSE	LEGITIMATE?	EXPLANATION
"I'm under too much stress."	Yes	Chronic stress is like poison to the brain. Stress increases production of a natural steroid called cortisol, which damages the hippocampus—the memory center of the brain. Studies show that a high-stress lifestyle even increases the risk of Alzheimer's disease.
"I'm pregnant."	Yes	Pregnancy entails many changes in the body that can affect your mental clarity, including dramatic hormone shifts, fluid shifts that can trigger headaches, an increase in coritsol, and sleep deprivation in the later months.
"I'm going through menopause."	No	With apologies to women who feel blitzed by menopause, the decline of estrogen that marks menopause does not cause much—if any—change in memory or cognitive function. (If you're not getting enough sleep, that's different story.)
"I'm on a diet."	Yes	People intent on losing weight quickly often put their bodies in a state of near starvation. Memory and thinking suffer as the brain is deprived of needed glucose (blood sugar). Very low-carb diets can also make you feel tired, lightheaded, and headachy.
"I'm having chemo."	Yes	Cloudy thinking in chemotherapy patients is so common, there's even a term for it: chemobrain. The medicines themselves can act like a brain-rattling smack on the side of the head. But chemo side effects, such as anemia, fatigue, insomnia, and worry can make concentration difficult. And one often-neglected cause is poor nutrition, since patients frequently lose their appetite.

small. For example, when scientists test working memory for numbers, they find that we can hold only about seven digits at a time—not coincidentally, the same number in phone numbers. Sure, some people can remember eight or nine, but remembering more than that requires knowing and using specific memory strategies. (More about those in Part 4).

With only a small capacity and short storage time, what's the point? Actually, short-term memory plays a vital role in our daily lives. Those slivers of temporary information allow us to write down doctor's appointments, make everyday decisions, and even have a conversation. Think about it: You have to recall what someone said to you 5 seconds ago in order to respond, though you don't need to remember it forever. This is information you use and forget...and good riddance.

Of course, it would be nice if some details didn't disappear before we could make use of them. When people say that they feel as if they are losing their memories, often they are referring to short-term memory. Do you forget where you put your keys or lose your train of thought during a conversation? Blame your working memory for those brain hiccups. And yes, working memory does tend to weaken with age. In fact, all those "senior moments" may, in fact, be related to declines in working memory. But as you'll discover shortly, the more attention you pay in the first place, the better the information will stick.

LONG-TERM STORAGE

To keep information for days, months, or even years, we need to consolidate it into long-term memory. And here's the good news: Our brains have an unlimited amount of long-term memory storage capacity. The file cabinet never gets filled up. Sure, long-term memories can and will fade with time if you don't revisit them every so often, but the potential is there to remember them forever. (Not that you'd want to remember everything. Who cares what color ink you used to write a grocery list in 1993?) The brain stores three main types of information long-term.

Words, facts, and numbers. When you're struggling to recall the name of the star in a movie, the number of feet in a mile, or the author of *Romeo and Juliet*, you're wrestling with semantic memory.

BRAIN HICCUPS

Twin Vanishing Act My worst mental slipup happened on the second day of a new school year. I was running frantic to get all the supplies, clothes, and schedules in order, while dealing with the kids' anxieties of a new school. The twins had Brownies after school, so I ironed on the patches, packed the vests, wrote a note to the teacher that the girls were not to be sent home on the bus, and told the girls three times that they had Brownies that day.

When 3:00 rolled around, I proceeded to meet the girls at the bus. The other children got off as usual, but not the twins. I screamed, "Where are my children?" My heart was pounding. The bus driver calmly called the school to ask about them. The school responded, "They are at Brownies." Of course! I walked off the bus, thoroughly embarrassed.

In Part 4, we'll show you some tricks for improving this type of memory.

Events. Episodic memory—think *episodes*—involves events or scenes from your life. Storing these memories is effortless. You don't need to work at remembering what it was like to watch your daughter get married or how you felt on the day you were accepted to college; you just do. Certain exhilarating scenes, particularly around life milestones, such as a first kiss or the first day on a job, simply captivate us—and stick around. We also remember unpleasant experiences without effort. No one forgets being robbed or cheated or fired, for example. And poker players are famous for recalling with painful clarity the biggest losing hands they've ever played, while sadly committing their wins to the dustbin of personal history.

Physical skills. They say you never forget how to ride a bike, and it's true. You can thank a form of long-term memory called procedural memory, also called muscle memory. It's responsible for acquired habits and motor skills, such as the ability to play an instrument, throw a baseball, drive a car, or even tie your shoes (something else we never forget how to do). You acquire these skills through practice.

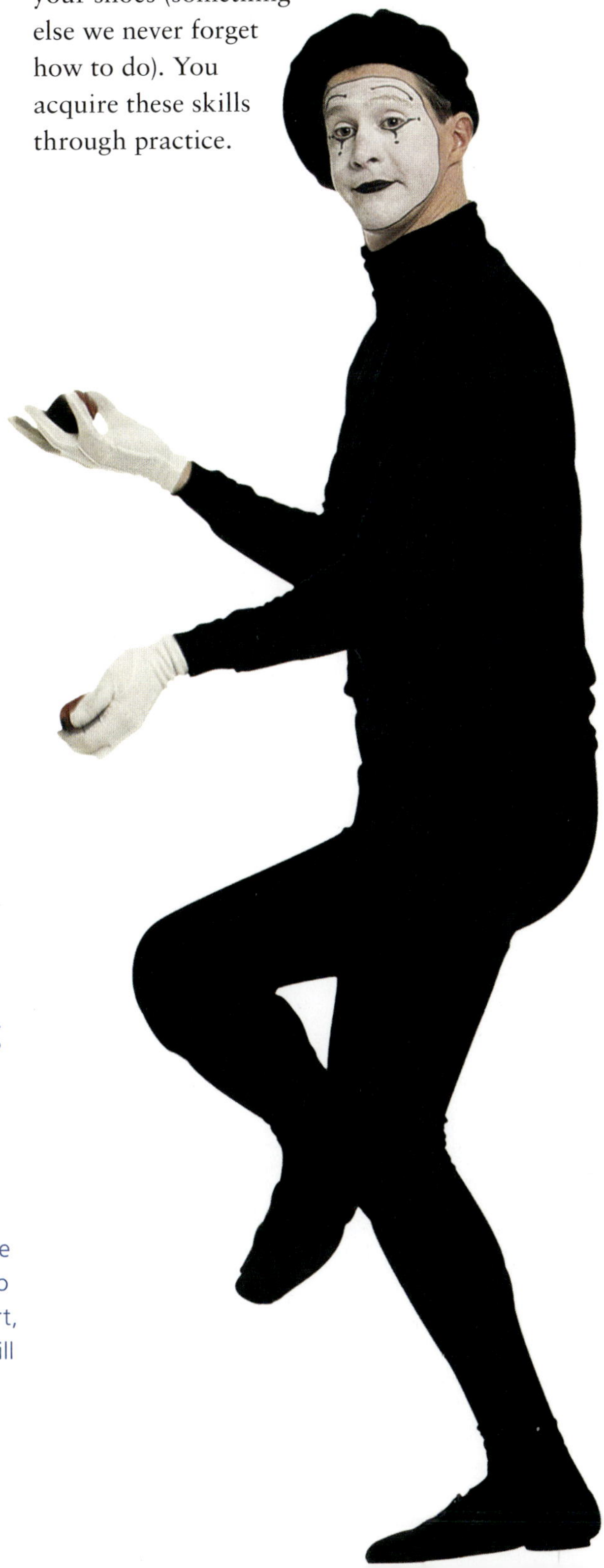

Play Ball—But Start Young

When older folks are asked to memorize lists of words or numbers, they often do as well as younger adults. But some things—especially those that involve muscle memory—are simply easier to learn when we're kids. Encoding new physical memories becomes more difficult as we get older, which means that it is much harder to learn to play an instrument, take up a new sport, or learn sign language. It can be done, but it will take longer and require more effort.

If you ever learned how to play the guitar, for example, you'll remember how difficult it was to get your fingers into position to play a chord. But finally, after hours and hours of practice, those subtle hand motions became second nature, and your fingers went right to their proper positions. Even years later, without practicing, chances are good that you could quickly find the G chord.

Muscle memory is stored throughout the brain, which makes it virtually immune to the factors that make us lose informational memories. That's why Alzheimer's patients retain their basic motor skills even when the disease robs them of the ability to recall a family member's name.

Hold That Thought–But How?

All this talk about memory storage makes it sound as though there is some kind of brain warehouse just waiting to be filled; we've even used the metaphor of a memory filing cabinet when describing the brain's capacity to keep information long-term. Yet no such cabinet or warehouse exists. Neurologists searched for decades to find it, with no luck. So where exactly do memories live—and how do they get there? Even more important, how do we make sure they stay there?

CREATING A MEMORY

Science now suggests that long-term memories aren't stored in a single place but, rather, in vast networks of nerve cell pathways. Every memory begins as a "spark" in the brain triggered when we receive input from our senses. This spark becomes an electrical signal as it travels from neuron to neuron. Each memory forges a unique pathway among the billions upon billions of neurons in the brain, as if blazing a new trail through a dense forest.

As the information passes from one neuron to the next, it jumps across gaps called synapses, with the help of neurotransmitters, such as serotonin and dopamine. Neurotransmitters are vital to memory—and, unfortunately, we produce less of them as we age. But by continuing to challenge our brains to learn new skills and information, we can create more and

ask the memory doc

My husband can drive or be driven somewhere once and remember the route months later, even if it's in another state. I, on the other hand, continue to get lost in my own city unless I follow a known route. Is there a sense-of-direction center in the brain? Or does he just have a better general memory (even though he can't remember to buy milk)?

Good observation! In fact, the right parietal lobe and other areas of the brain are specifically involved in the process of learning and remembering directions and orientation. And men seem to have a better ability at this skill than women. Women, on the other hand, are more skilled at reading human emotional cues. Different people, different talents.

—The memory doc is brain expert David Perlmutter, MD, FACN

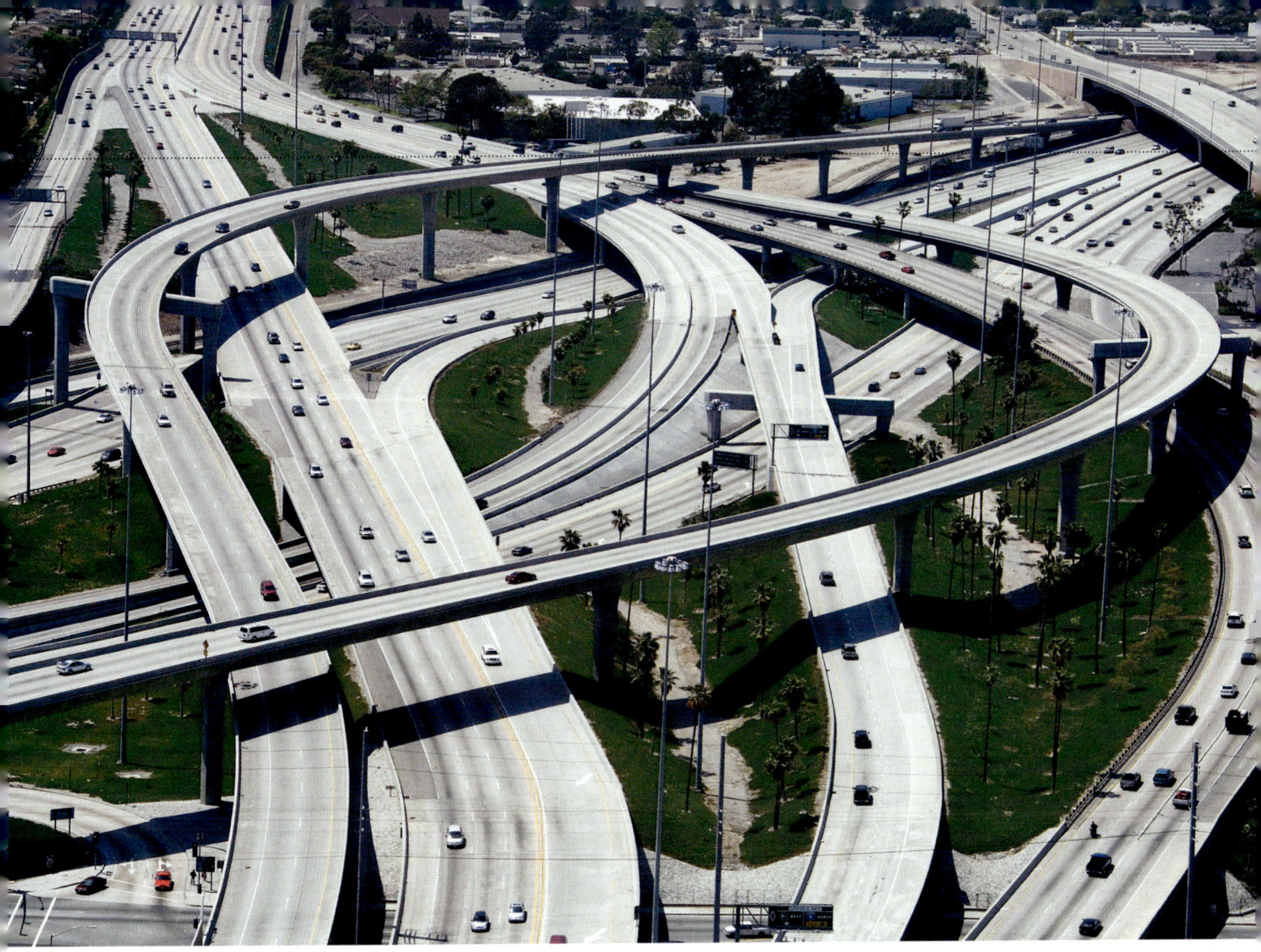

more dendrites, which help keep our brains young and spry.

Work hard enough or long enough at a given type of memory and your brain will grow and adapt in other ways, too. In a stunning 2000 study, London cab drivers, who spend their whole careers learning to navigate one of the largest, most-convoluted roadway systems in the world, underwent MRI screenings of their brains. The cabbies were found to have unusually large hippocampuses, an area of the brain that plays a major role in memory formation, particularly spatial memory.

MAKING IT STICK

Some memories naturally tend to stick better than others, but you can help any memory hang around with these two steps.

Each memory forges a unique pathway among the billions upon billions of neurons in the brain.

1. Pay attention

The first step in remembering something is paying attention to it. Unless you grab information by focusing on it, it can slip right by you.

Can't remember the name of someone you were just introduced to? You probably weren't paying enough active attention to the name (maybe you were focused on smiling and looking friendly). People who are good with names will often repeat the person's name out loud. If they meet someone named John

How One Fact Is Learned

STEP ONE	STEP TWO	STEP THREE

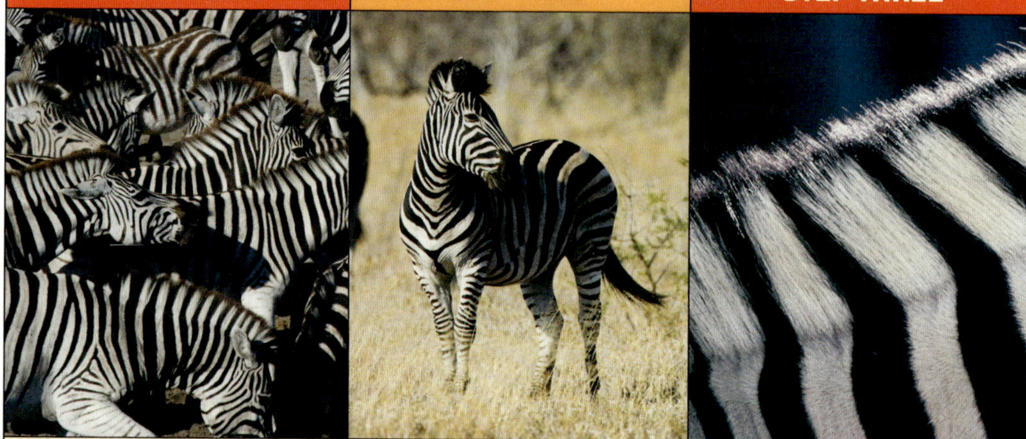

WE PERCEIVE	**WE FOCUS**	**WE REHEARSE**
Sights, sounds, sensations, tastes, smells. Our brains take in this information whether we pay attention to it or not.	If we focus on the information, it gets moved into working memory. If we don't, the information fades within seconds.	With enough repetition, studying, and review, the fact gets moved to long-term memory. Otherwise, the fact placed in working memory dissolves.

Robinson, for example, they may say: "Good to meet you, John." And silently, they may be making an association: "John is from Switzerland: Swiss Family Robinson." By repeating it, and then making the effort to come up with a rhyme, a reference, or an association, they create a nerve cell pathway—a memory trail—in the brain for the name, so it doesn't vanish without a trace. You'll learn more tricks for making names stick better in Part 4.

2. Practice and repeat.

Consolidation is the process of making a nerve cell pathway more permanent. Each time you review or revisit a fact, each time you repeat it, the pathway becomes a little stronger. This is what we typically think of as learning.

The likelihood of consolidating any particular fact or memory depends on a number of factors, including what you want to learn (whether it's a fact or a skill), your current knowledge base, your emotional state, and how well you take care of yourself. The work of consolidation is also easier if you already have a background that relates to whatever it is you are trying to learn, just as it is easier to keep track of an invoice or important tax form if you have an existing file folder for this exact type of information than if you throw the paper on the desk and vow to remember its location later.

Inexperienced chess players who look at pieces on a chess board, for example, will find it very difficult to recall where all the pieces had been placed. But chess champions can remember the placement of the pieces quite easily because they're intimately familiar with the game. Rather than just seeing individual pieces set up randomly, they see the strategic challenges illustrated by the setup of the board, and that puts the information in context, allowing for better recall.

MAKING IT STICK BETTER

In Parts 2 and 3 of this book, you'll read about how certain emotional states (such as depression), lack of sleep, and even certain medications can make it harder to consolidate memories. You'll also read about strategies, such as getting enough exercise, keeping your social connections alive, and eating brain-healthy foods, that can help you keep your brain skills at their peak.

FLASHBULB MEMORY: PERMANENT SNAPSHOTS

Every so often, the daily routine of our lives is broken by the shock of an event so surprising, so monumental, so emotional, that we remember every detail of where we were and what we were doing when we heard the news. Do you remember exactly where you were the moment you learned about the September 11 attacks on New York's World Trade Center, the assassination of U.S. President John F. Kennedy, or the death of Princess Diana? Even years later, most of us have memories so vivid that recalling those tragic days can feel as if we are looking at well-preserved photographs. The same thing can happen to an even greater extent with very personal events, such as seeing a bad car accident, being bitten by a vicious dog, or witnessing the horror of a terrorist attack. Psychologists call these intense impressions flashbulb memories.

As the name suggests, flashbulb memory is the brain's way of taking a mental "picture" of a significant emotional event. Because these memories are so vivid, accessible, and durable, they become cognitive landmarks that allow us to place other, less dramatic events into a before-or-after context. For example, you may not remember the year your favorite cousin got married, but

new thinking

We remember useful information better. Information is easier to remember, especially as we get older, if it makes sense and seems useful. In typical tests of memory, researchers ask subjects to recall lists of random numbers or words. But psychologist Alan Castel, PhD, assistant professor of psychology at the University of California, Los Angeles, and an expert in memory and cognitive aging, tried something different. He asked his human guinea pigs to memorize lists of grocery items as well as their associated prices. The pairings were either unlikely (loaf of bread, $9.71) or likely (loaf of bread, $2.19). Younger outperformed the older folks at remembering the unlikely pairings, but older folks redeemed themselves when the prices made sense. Implication: In effect, older adults have learned to compensate for the normal decline in working memory by not wasting time on useless information. "They focus on information with high value and discard the rest," says Dr. Castel.

chances are you know whether it was before or after the events of 9/11.

The closer the event hits home, the deeper the memory is embedded. Researchers from New York University interviewed 24 people who were in Manhattan at the time the Twin Towers fell, and watched brain activity light up on brain scans as the test subjects recalled their experiences that day. Some of the participants were within blocks of the Towers, some about 2 miles away, and others were more than 4 miles away. All of them had strong memories of the day. But the strongest flashes, indicating the deepest, most searing kinds of memory, only popped for those who were at or near the Towers. This group recalled the event more vividly, including specific details about sounds and smells, than people who were a few miles away.

In forming these flashbulb memories, the hippocampus (which plays a major role in long-term memory) gets help from its immediate neighbor, the amygdala, which jumps into action when triggered by stress hormones such as adrenaline to quickly process the memory. "The release of stress hormones stimulates the amygdala to send out a message: 'Hey, brain! This is really important; you better remember it,'" says James L. McGaugh, PhD, professor of neurobi-

Memory Tips from a Police Sketch Artist

How many times a week do we try to recall a fact that stubbornly eludes us, like where we put the car keys? If only we could push a button and access the information we want! It's not that simple, but you can help yourself remember better with techniques that Natalie Sweet uses with crime witnesses. Sweet is a police composite sketch artist, and every day she helps average people remember enough physical detail to create a meaningful portrait of a criminal suspect. You, too, can benefit from her techniques.

STEP 1

Try to relax.

Sweet takes the pressure off by telling the witness that the purpose of a sketch is to come as close as possible to the person in his memory. It is not intended to be perfect, and no one will be arrested based on the sketch alone.

If you lost your keys, don't panic! That will only makes things worse.

STEP 2

Cast your mind back, picturing any details you remember.

Sweet gives the witness's brain a chance to "warm up" by talking about everything about the day of the crime, except the crime itself. For example, she might ask him to go back in his mind to that day and remember everything that happened before the incident started. Does he remember what he was doing immediately before? What clothes was he wearing? What was the weather like?

Once the witness seems relaxed, Sweet asks him to close his eyes and start describing what he remembers about the environment during the crime. She asks him to look around the room and describe everything he sees, such as what might be hanging on the walls, the type of lighting, and the color of the walls.

Close your eyes and try to remember the last time you had your keys. Were you coming from an appointment? What were you wearing? Was it raining?

ology and behavior at the University of California, Irvine.

Rats in Dr. McGaugh's lab remembered how to get through a maze better when given a dose of adrenaline while learning the route. But short of injecting yourself with adrenaline, is there anything you can do to stimulate the release of stress hormones to help you remember something? Yes. In one study, test subjects improved their retention of information by immersing their hands in ice water. Another study found comparable results from squeezing a hand dynamometer, a device normally used to measure grip strength. Dr. McGaugh adds that going for a brisk walk or working out should also do the trick.

Recall on Demand

Once the new tracks of a memory are laid down and reinforced by focus and repetition, you still need a way to retrieve the goods. If memory is a path in the woods, retrieval is finding the correct path. But think about it—there are hundreds of billions of different pathways. Most people worry when they can't locate a specific memory, but given the vast multitude of pathways in our heads, the real mystery is

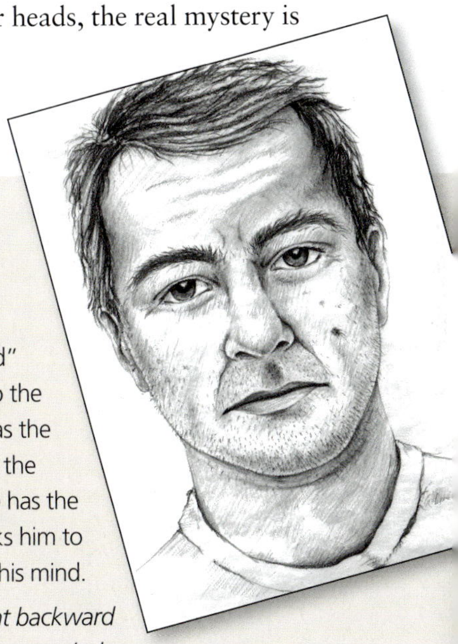

STEP 3

Pretend you were an onlooker.

Memories of any incident can be blocked by emotions, such as fear or anger. That's why Sweet gets witnesses to picture the scene as an onlooker would. "I take them out of whatever position they were in, victim or witness," says Sweet. "I tell them to think of it as though they were standing outside looking in, as though they were filming what happened, or watching it on TV. It puts them in a different mindset with a different perspective."

If you had your keys when you walked into the house, imagine watching yourself enter the house. Are the keys in your hand? Did you go straight in or did you stop at the mailbox?

STEP 4

Be flexible as you try to remember.

Our brains have remarkable abilities to revisit our memories forward, backward, from above, and in freeze-frame. The memories are there and accessible—but sometimes we have to be flexible in how we hunt for them. After the witness describes the scene and what happened, Sweet has him go back again and "rewind" the mind movie to the place where he has the clearest picture of the suspect. When he has the right view, she asks him to freeze-frame it in his mind.

Replay the incident backward and forward until your mind finds a clue that leads to the critical image: where you put your keys.

STEP 5

Don't rush yourself. Let the memory come to you.

The process of creating a sketch takes an average of 2 hours. Some take considerably longer. Most of the time, you can't rush memory and expect good results.

You will eventually remember where you put your keys; have patience!

how we ever manage to remember anything at all.

It's basically a matter of retracing our steps. "Recollection is literally *re*-collection," says Dr. McGaugh. But the route to the piece of information you want isn't a straight line. When you are having a hard time remembering the name of that actor you love, the first thing that comes to mind might be the name of his most famous film, which could lead you to the name of his co-star, which could remind you that the actor also has a famous son, which finally—Ah-ha!—triggers the memory of the actor's name. In the brain, that roundabout circuit would be completed in a split second. You probably wouldn't even be aware that it was a pathfinding process at all.

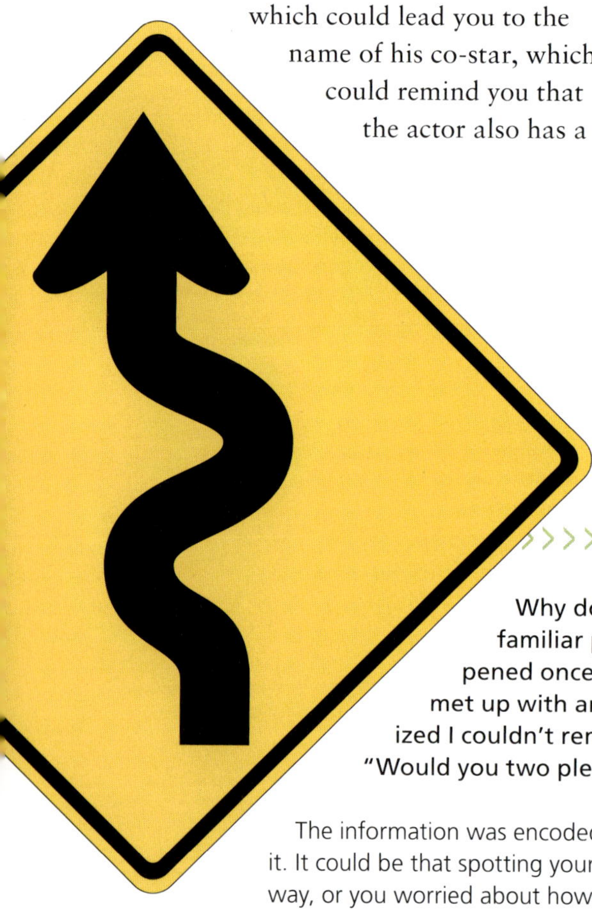

WHY MEMORY IS FALLIBLE

There is a saying that goes, "There are three sides to the story—yours, mine, and the truth." As much as we would like to think that our memories are accurate "photographs" of events, they are more like impressionist paintings. Here's why.

Perception. We all remember events differently because we perceive them differently in the first place. At your last family reunion, did you have a bad head cold? Then maybe you will remember the food tasting rather bland, while your sister might remember that it was the best

›››››››››› ask the memory doc

Why do I sometimes blank on the names of totally familiar people when I try to introduce them? This happened once when I was in the mall with my best friend, and met up with another friend. I looked at the two of them, realized I couldn't remember either of their names, and finally said, "Would you two please introduce yourselves?" Why did this happen?

The information was encoded firmly in your brain; the problem was with retrieving it. It could be that spotting your other friend in the mall shocked you in some small way, or you worried about how to handle the situation, and the emotion temporarily jammed your retrieval system. Totally normal.

Now, here's the bad news: Because this has happened to you and the experience was embarrassing, any situation that requires introductions could become a source of anxiety. Then, the brain "jam" could happen again and again. It is an everyday form of stage fright. Like any actor, try to rehearse your "lines" as you see the scenario about to unfold, and you'll be just fine.

—The memory doc is brain expert David Perlmutter, MD, FACN

dinner ever. Were you sitting at the end of the table, or in the middle? Your location affects which conversations you hear. Your sensory memory is unique to you and can never be replicated by anyone else, and it strongly colors your version of reality.

Interpretation. If your uncle gave a long, impassioned political monologue, how you remember it will depend on whether you agreed with his viewpoint. If you didn't, you probably stopped paying attention, or got busy trying to stifle your own counter-arguments. If your cousin made an observation about a new exhibit at the museum, you're more likely to remember it if you believe that your cousin is a highly intelligent person who knows what she's talking about. Your emotions, experiences, and memories will all cause you to interpret events in your own unique way, and therefore skew how you remember them.

Recall. Memories are not set in stone. The pathways we forge sometimes grow over with weeds, and even if they don't, the process of calling up the information from its disparate locations in the brain requires the brain to fill in blank spots. Consider this story: A woman was going through a family photo album with her mother. They came to a picture of a young girl on a pony, and the woman launched into her vivid memory of that day, much to the puzzlement of her mother. "But, honey," her mother said, "that's your sister. You weren't born yet." The woman had seen the photo previously and just assumed she was the one on the pony, and her brain filled in the details based on the photograph alone.

BRAIN HICCUPS

Missing the Point—And the Car My worst mental slipup happened the day I needed to drop off my car at the dealership for a minor repair in the middle of the day. My coworker Amanda volunteered to follow me to the dealership, then take me back to work. Another coworker volunteered to come along for company. At the appointed time, we met at Amanda's office. Then we all got in her car and set out for the dealership. When we were nearly there (gabbing the whole way), Amanda asked if I needed a ride back to the dealership later in the day to pick up my car. We both suddenly whipped our heads toward each other and cried, "We don't have the car!!!!" We burst into such laughter that she nearly drove off the road. ■

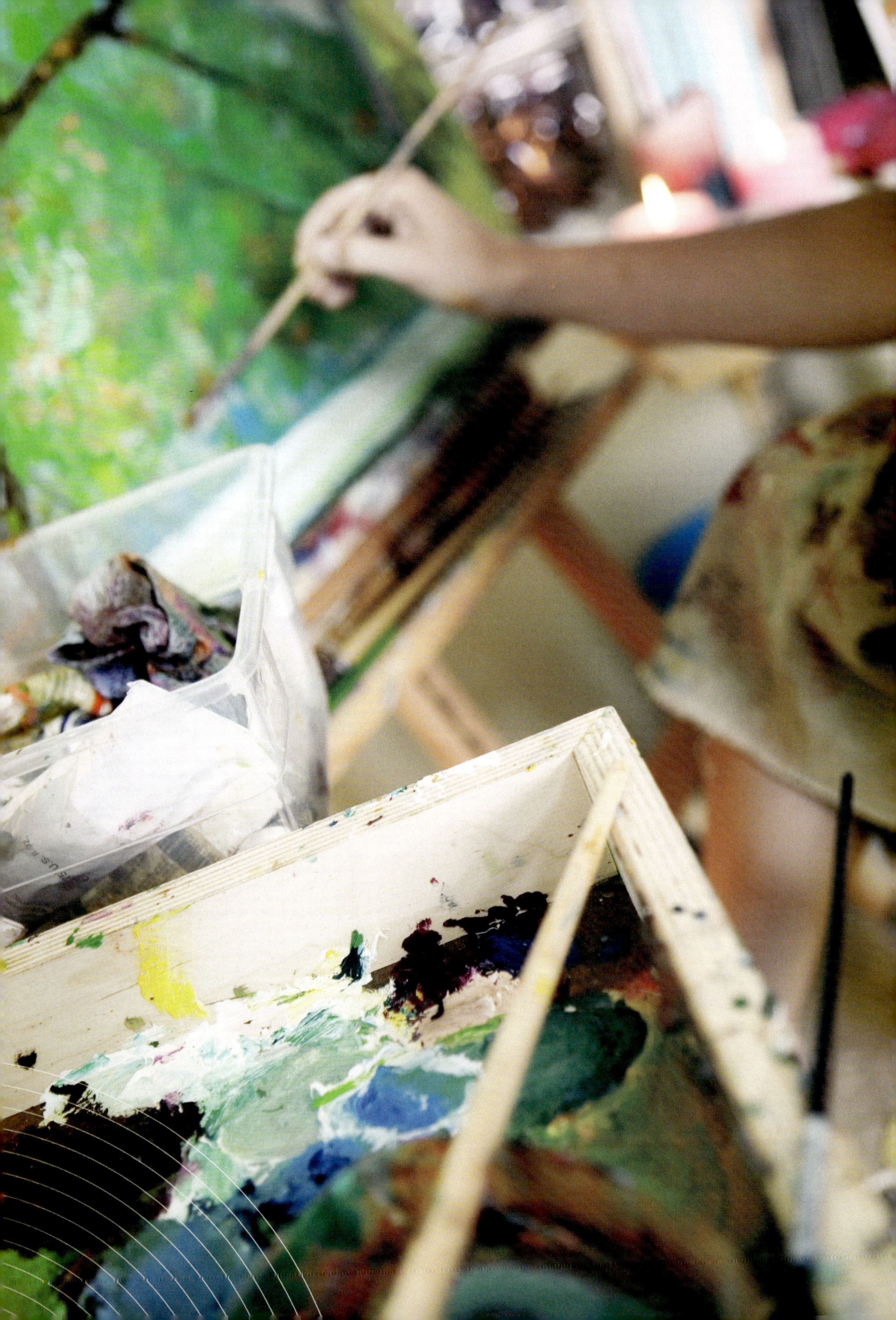

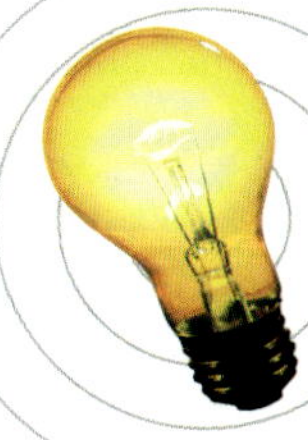

How wisdom, creativity & intelligence work

Chemical reactions, electrical impulses, gray matter, neurons—this is the language of neurologists. They can explain the brain inside and out, from cells to lobes to hemispheres and back. But what about the elusive questions humans have been asking for millennia: What is intelligence?

Where does creativity come from? What makes us truly wise? The answers don't lie in any single neuron or any single nerve pathway or any single place in the brain.

To understand these complex issues, we have to rely on psychology to make the connection between the physical brain and the intangible mind. While we may never solve all the brain's mysteries, experts are hard at work piecing together theories to explain these higher order cognitions. In other words, they are thinking hard about how we think.

Intelligence: Not Just a Number

In psychological circles, the nature and essence of intelligence has generated more theories than the origin of the universe. The debate didn't start with the invention of the infamous IQ (Intelligence Quotient) test, but that method of measurement certainly did put teeth into it. Since then, the discussion—Who's smart? Who's not? Does intelligence comes from our genes?—has turned about as heated as academic arguments get.

Researchers have theorized that intelligence is entirely inherited...entirely developed...50 percent inherited and 50 percent developed. Some say intelligence is found all over the brain or only in specific brain locations...that it includes more than 60 different abilities or is a single entity or is a subset ability within a global intelligence... that it is the single factor responsible for thought or that it is just one of many different cognitive abilities.

About 100 years ago, one psychologist devised the IQ test to evaluate students' ability to learn as a way of predicting which ones would perform well in school. This was so that precious seats could be reserved for those students who were "the best." Over the ensuing years, society latched onto IQ as a precise measure of overall intelligence. But, of course, there's much more to intelligence than one number could ever suggest. (We don't know what Albert Einstein's IQ was, for example, but we do know that he failed his college entrance exams the first time he took them.)

There are clearly different forms of intelligence, ranging from the erudition of a professor to the physical genius of the athlete. "Not all intelligence is in the head," writes Harvard professor Howard Gardner, PhD, explaining his mission to explore, identify, and define its specific realms. After years of analysis, and using a strict set of criteria, Dr. Gardner identified a total of seven intelligences. To find out what they are, see "The Seven Intelligences" on page 46.

BRAIN HICCUPS

Wrong Number My worst brain slipup happened the time my friend left his cell phone on my kitchen table. I knew he would miss it because it was the only phone he used. So I did something really dumb! I called to remind him that he had left it behind. I nearly scared myself to death when the phone on my kitchen table rang!

Who's smart? Who's not? Does intelligence comes from our genes? The academic debate remains heated.

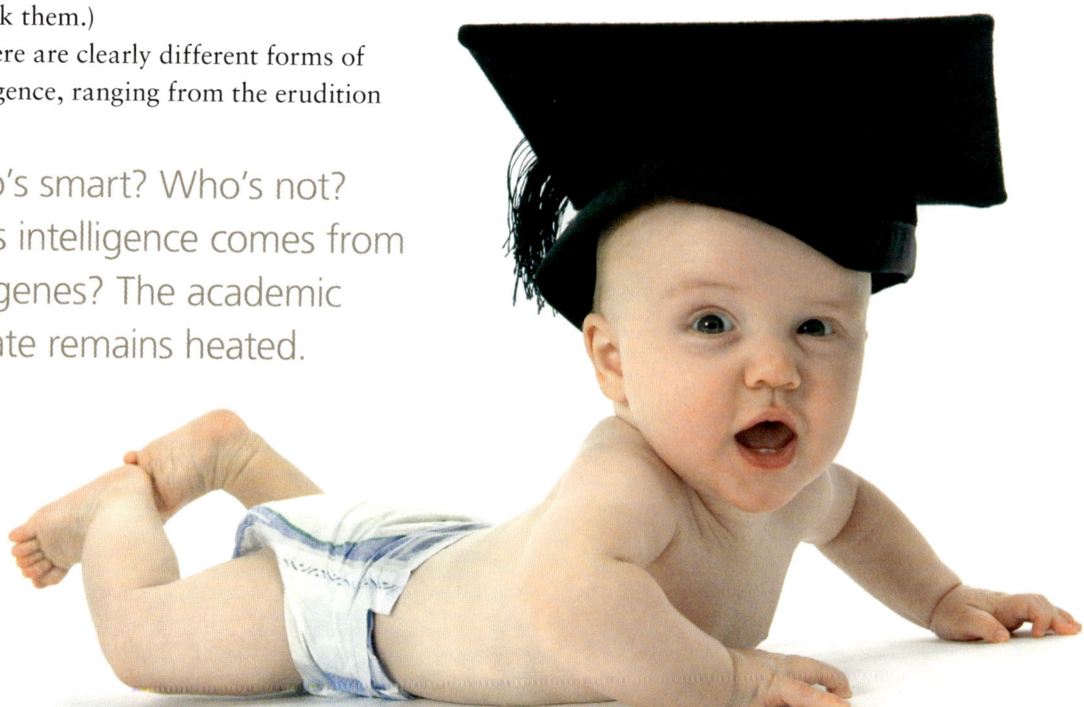

It's a good bet that another sign of intelligence—one we could actually see, if ever a sufficiently sensitive method of brain imaging were invented—would be the number of neuronal connections throughout the brain. Given that neurons can increase their connections indefinitely, theoretically, intelligence should be able to increase well into old age.

From Smarts to Wisdom

A good working definition of intelligence is the ability to learn and to use what is learned to reach your personal objectives. Although we value intelligence, the real measure of a person lies in his or her *wisdom*. Intelligence is raw and unripened. Wisdom, on the other hand, has been called the epitome of human excellence, an ancient and virtuous quality. If intelligence is knowing how to build a bomb, wisdom is knowing how to build a bomb, understanding the ramifications of using it, and being able to solve problems in such a way that the bomb is not needed.

In some ways, wisdom is like beauty—we value it, we desire it, we know it when we see it, but it is nearly impossible to pin down such an ethereal quality. Yet researchers have tried. In the late 1980s, the Berlin Wisdom Project at the Max

Continued on page 48

ask the memory doc

About a year-and-a-half back, I booked a last-minute flight to a business meeting. I slept for most of the 2-hour-and-15-minute flight and awoke abruptly when the plane touched down. I tried to recall why I was on a plane and—more important—where I was going. After several minutes, I finally reached into my briefcase and checked my calendar. Aha! A meeting in Silver Spring, Maryland.

Getting off the plane, I figured it would take about 15 minutes to grab the rental car, and about 40 minutes to drive from BWI International Airport to the Silver Spring office—enough time to make the meeting. I have flown to BWI many times, so I knew the quickest way through the terminal. I cut to the left, dipped to the right, and made a mad rush to the exit. I grabbed a seat on the passenger mover.

It was only during the 7-minute drive across the airfield that I realized I was not at BWI at all; I was at Dulles International Airport. I know I may have been a little disoriented after waking up, but why didn't I get a clue from announcements on the plane, signs in the airport, or even the layout of the airport itself?

You've already mentioned one important reason for your confusion—it's common to be confused after awakening, especially when you've slept at a time during the day that is unusual for your biological clock.

Another important factor rings clear in your query. Your descriptions of the "last-minute flight" and preoccupation with the time constraints are clear explanations of why your mind was elsewhere. With all that going on, you were obviously relieved to find the answer to your confusion in your planner, so the rest of your brain relaxed and went along with the mistaken idea that you were at the BWI airport. With less stress, you probably won't experience this again.

—The memory doc is brain expert David Perlmutter, MD, FACN

The Seven Intelligences

To deconstruct what is commonly called smarts is to recognize that every person's contribution to society is unique—and valuable. No one person has all the skills or the learning needed to accomplish society's tasks, but together we are complete. Think of the different intelligences as colors, which can stand alone or be combined, made stronger or lighter, intense or subdued. It takes only red, blue, and yellow to create the entire spectrum of color. Just think of what could be created by seven intelligences!

1 Spatial Intelligence

Brain location
Right hemisphere

Who has it
Sculptors, airline pilots, architects, theoretical physicists

What it's good for
At its most basic level, spatial ability means being able to get from your house to the grocery store and back without being confused. But people who are really gifted seem to possess an internal GPS system that tells them precisely where they are in the universe at all times. We also have a name for people who are weak in these skills: lost.

Rx for improvement
Look for puzzles that ask you to envision how a piece of paper with patterns on it will look when folded to form a box. Beyond that, we recommend buying a GPS!

2 Logical-Mathematical Intelligence

Brain location
Frontal and parietal lobes

Who has it
Scientists, engineers, statisticians

What it's good for
Even our common expressions recognize the genius of the science whiz: *"That guy's a rocket scientist!"* You might almost call this the classic form of genius; it's the kind of smarts that would show up on an IQ test. People with high levels of logical-mathematical intelligence can gather and consolidate information quickly. They tend to be methodical and organized.

Rx for improvement
Many of the puzzles in Part 4 help strengthen logic as well as number skills. Try them! And practice your everyday number skills by calculating in your head rather than on your calculator.

3 Musical Intelligence

Brain location
Right hemisphere

Who has it
Composers, musicians

What it's good for
Music is a form of communication, crossing countries, cultures, and even species—birds and whales are just two species that speak through "song." People with high levels of musical intelligence can find meaning in the rhythm, tempo, pattern, pitch, and tone of music. They often show signs of musical ability early in life and seem to intuitively grasp the mathematics behind the notes. Some can pick up an instrument and play it with barely any training; it's as if they intuitively know how to speak the language of music. At the low end are those who avoid karaoke bars like the plague; we're also the ones you'll find silently mouthing the words to *Happy Birthday* to keep from throwing everyone else off-key.

Rx for improvement
Music ability is difficult to improve; you either have it or you don't. But learning to play an instrument can't hurt.

4 Intrapersonal Intelligence

Brain location
Temporal lobes

Who has it
Philosophers, psychologists, theologians, writers

What it's good for
*Intra*personal intelligence is about self-knowledge, being fully in touch with your inner self—your emotions, beliefs, and the precise tremor and bias of your moral compass. High intrapersonal intelligence

allows us to navigate through the world without losing our sense of self, to rebound from setbacks, and to fully appreciate our fellow humans.

Rx for improvement
Keep a diary. More important, look with a fresh eye back on pages you wrote long ago and reflect on what they tell you about yourself.

5 Physical Intelligence

Brain location
Motor cortex

Who has it
Athletes, dancers

What it's good for
Although movement comes naturally to everyone, exceptional physical grace and athleticism involve their own kind of intelligence. Controlled movements are expressive and productive—consider that one of the common tests of intelligence in other species is whether they have the ability to use tools. We are fascinated by dancers and awed by superior athletes. Conversely, we good-naturedly mock those who are lacking in coordination skills. These physical dummies have a name: klutzes.

Rx for improvement
Some people are simply more physically gifted than others. But staying physically active will keep your sense of balance intact and improve your posture, which helps impart physical grace.

6 Interpersonal Intelligence

Brain location
Frontal lobes

Who has it
Salesmen, teachers, social workers, good managers

What it's good for
People with strong *inter*personal skills understand nonverbal communication and are able to read the character, emotions, and desires of others. This is a unique form of problem solving that is not as easily measured as other types of intelligence, but is critical to social success. All good leaders are interpersonal geniuses. These gifts can also be used for dark purposes by con artists.

Rx for improvement
Practice noticing other people's reactions to your words, your body language, your tone of voice. Then practice reading other people by noting *their* body language and tone.

7 Linguistic Intelligence

Brain location
Left hemisphere

Who has it
Poets, writers, orators, many lawyers

What it's good for
Everyone can speak, but some people elevate language to an art. Some of Barack Obama's speeches come to mind. This type of intelligence is also displayed by writers and every silver-tongued devil you've ever met. Shakespeare is arguably the ultimate genius in his category. The average English-speaker uses 4,000 words. Shakespeare had a working vocabulary of 29,000 words. He also coined more than 1,700 new words, including many we use today, such as "amazement", "gloomy", "zany", and "equivocal."

Rx for improvement
Doing a lot of reading can definitely build your vocabulary and lift your linguistic skills.

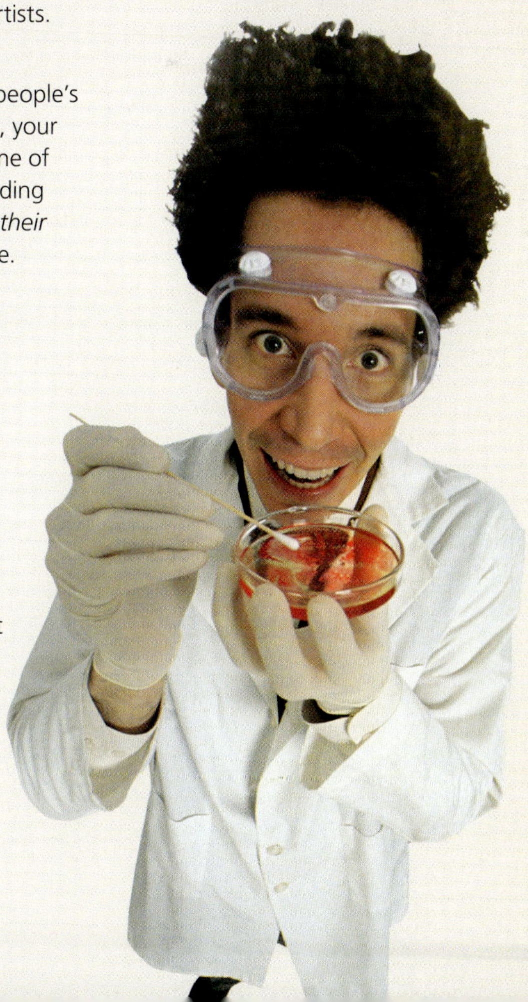

Planck Institute for Human Development set out to define wisdom. They came up with the following qualities, all of which a person must have to be considered truly wise, in their view.

- ✔ Intelligence and factual knowledge
- ✔ A deep understanding of human nature, including an empathy for people who are different or from other cultures
- ✔ Emotional resiliency, or the ability to rebound from a setback
- ✔ Humility
- ✔ The ability to learn from experience
- ✔ Openness, or the maturity to be comfortable allowing the world to see you as you really are
- ✔ Superior judgment and problem-solving skills

Put this all together and what do you have? A portrait of someone who's been around the block. Wisdom accrues from experience, so it's fair to say, you need to be older to be wise. However, it should be pointed out: Not all older people are wise. There are plenty who are painfully close-minded and set in their ways and their thinking.

In 2007, psychologist Jeffrey Dean Webster, MEd, of Langara College in Vancouver, British Columbia, updated the work of the Berlin Wisdom Project, adding the notion that true wisdom could only be measured by what you did with

How Wise Are You?

To get an idea of where you stand on the wisdom spectrum, read each statement below and check the appropriate response (T for "True" and F for "False").

1. I often reminisce about my past and am amazed at how far I've come. ☐ T ☐ F

2. Teasing is never appropriate. ☐ T ☐ F

3. Everyone is capable of dishonesty and hypocrisy. ☐ T ☐ F

4. I wear my emotions on my sleeve—if I'm upset, anxious, or sad, people know it. ☐ T ☐ F

5. Before an election, I like to hear what all parties stand for before coming to a decision about how to vote. ☐ T ☐ F

6. When I think back to my most embarrassing moments, I still feel mortified. ☐ T ☐ F

7. History is most interesting for what it can teach us about our lives today. ☐ T ☐ F

8. I think it's important to form a strong opinion—waffling is a sign of weakness. ☐ T ☐ F

9. I easily adjust my emotions to fit with the needs of the moment—it's not always necessary to let people know when I'm upset, anxious, or sad. ☐ T ☐ F

10. I make decisions easily, often on gut instinct. ☐ T ☐ F

11. I enjoy having religious discussions with people of different faiths. ☐ T ☐ F

12. If someone told me a lie, it would change my opinion of that person forever. ☐ T ☐ F

13. I have experienced a lot of change in my life, and not all of it was positive. ☐ T ☐ F

14. History is interesting as a story, but has little relevance to my life today. ☐ T ☐ F

15. I have opinions, but I am always interested in hearing other points of view. ☐ T ☐ F

it, both in terms of self-knowledge and the improvement of society at large. In other words, the proof is in the pudding. Webster's Self-Assessed Wisdom Scale (SAWS) below measures what he considered to be key traits of a wise person, including open-mindedness, the ability to control emotions, sense of humor, experience, and the ability to learn from the past. We invite you to see how you rate.

PRACTICAL WAYS TO WISE UP

Almost everyone has the capacity to become wise, given the right mindset and a little bit of effort. Wisdom requires a baseline of intelligence, but true wisdom is a mix of balance (the ability to see all sides of an issue), open-mindedness, discipline, and a concern for the greater good. There's no shortcut to wisdom, but the following strategies will lead you down the right path:

Read the newspaper. You cannot make balanced choices unless you understand world circumstances and the experiences of others. If you don't already read a paper, start by reading a single front-page article, start to finish, every day. Don't just scan or skip around; read every word. Eventually, try to read the main articles of a full newspaper every day. Most newspapers post their stories online, so you can have access to news from around the world virtually anytime you want.

16. When I try to express my emotions, I often lose control. ☐ T ☐ F

17. I laugh easily and often. ☐ T ☐ F

18. I become easily annoyed when people challenge my opinion. ☐ T ☐ F

19. I take my time before making a decision, often consulting many sources of information. ☐ T ☐ F

20. I have lived a charmed life, without much conflict or dilemmas. ☐ T ☐ F

21. I've lived through a lot, and I've had to make some difficult and uncomfortable decisions. ☐ T ☐ F

22. I'm a happy person—I never feel angry or annoyed. ☐ T ☐ F

23. It's easy for me to laugh at my most embarrassing moments. ☐ T ☐ F

24. I hate when people have a laugh at my expense. ☐ T ☐ F

25. Teasing can be a sign of affection. ☐ T ☐ F

26. My life has turned out exactly the way I thought it would. ☐ T ☐ F

SCORING

Count the number of TRUE responses for odd-numbered statements: ________

Count the number of FALSE responses for even-numbered statements: ________

To get your Wisdom Score, add those two numbers together: ________

INTERPRETING YOUR SCORE

0 to 4 Babe in the woods
Best not to wander off alone

5 to 9 Student
Keep watching and learning

10 to 14 Professor
Wiser than most

15 to 19 Leader
People depend on your guidance

20 to 26 Guru
Consider setting up shop on top of a mountain

Mind versus Mac

How does the human brain compare with a personal computer? See for yourself.

	COMPUTER	HUMAN BRAIN
Processing speed	About 5 million instructions per second	About 100 million instructions per second ✓
Work Time	Unlimited, as long as plugged in ✓	Varies by person, but the brain tires relatively easily
Memory Capacity	A powerful desktop personal computer may have 1 million megabytes	Unlimited ✓
Memory Accessibility	Every megabyte is potentially accessible at any moment ✓	Can be difficult at times
Computation	A 2GHz processor can calculate the value of pi to a million decimal places in 1 minute ✓	30 million times slower than a computer (Er, what is pi, again?)
Accuracy	Absent a bug, computers are 100 percent accurate ✓	The human brain makes many errors in all facets of calculation and memory
Adaptability	Once started on a processing problem, can't change unless redirected by human	Can change direction, task, and action in an instant ✓
Creativity	Works on a binary system for processing information—either yes/no or on/off	With at least 100 trillion neuron synapses, unlimited inventiveness is possible ✓
Energy Efficiency	Computers use about a billions times more energy than the human brain	Low energy needs—oxygen and glucose (blood sugar) ✓
Multitasking	Can work on multiple problems simultaneously and perform equally well on all ✓	Can work on several tasks at once—breathing, thinking, walking, chewing gum, etc.—but can directly focus on only one problem at a time
Learning	Computers are programmed; they can't learn on the job	Capable of learning from birth until death ✓
Free Will and Wisdom	No consciousness; no free will; can't learn, so incapable of wisdom	Has consciousness and free will; can determine its own destiny; has vast potential for wisdom ✓
And the winner is ...	5	**your brain!** 7

Read more books. While current events are important, both fiction and nonfiction books can help you expand your world view and allow you to explore new ideas and points of view without ever leaving the comfort of your sofa.

Stay social. Studies show that people who stay connected to others demonstrate higher levels of wisdom than those who are more isolated. Make an effort to join a club, sign up for Facebook, or invite an old friend or a new neighbor to meet you for coffee. And next time you're at a party or gathering, single out someone who's standing alone and start up a conversation. It's easy! Ask questions ("Where are you from?" "What kind of work do you do?") People love to talk about themselves. You, on the other hand, have the harder job: You have to really listen.

Practice being more open-minded. Wisdom is being able to understand all sides of an issue without letting emotions or personal feelings get in the way. Being open-minded means finding empathy and realizing that everyone has a life story that influences their actions. During the course of every day, take note of issues that hit your hot buttons, and take a moment to try to see the issue from the other side. It's good practice. And no one has to know!

Boost your self-knowledge. You've learned a lot just by being alive, but have you taken the time to review all that you've learned? Try this exercise: Write down your three biggest failures and your three greatest successes. For each success and failure, review the events that led up to it and what lessons you took away from the experience. Look for patterns. This is not a time for regret or pride; the goal is to learn to look at each life experience, good or bad, as more fuel for your wisdom fire.

Learn how to say these four special words: "I could be wrong." A wise person recognizes that it is impossible to

ask the memory doc

As I pulled into the office parking lot this morning, I realized that I had absolutely no recollection of the drive. I can't tell you whether I drove the speed limit, whether a particular stop light was red or green (and whether I obeyed it), whether I passed a school bus or whatever. How is the brain able to work on autopilot like this?

The monarch butterfly has a brain smaller than a pinhead, and yet it can migrate 2,000 miles to a specific location. Your big brain can certainly allow you to drive to your office without conscious involvement—although I'm not advocating brain-dead driving. Repeated activities and behaviors create packages of information stored in the brain that, over time, become instructions when those activities are repeated. Under normal conditions, we call upon these instructions for familiar tasks and then make minor modifications moment to moment as our environment changes. If you had seen a large object in the road in front of you, your brain would click back on and you would consciously be able to steer around the hazard.

—The memory doc is brain expert David Perlmutter, MD, FACN

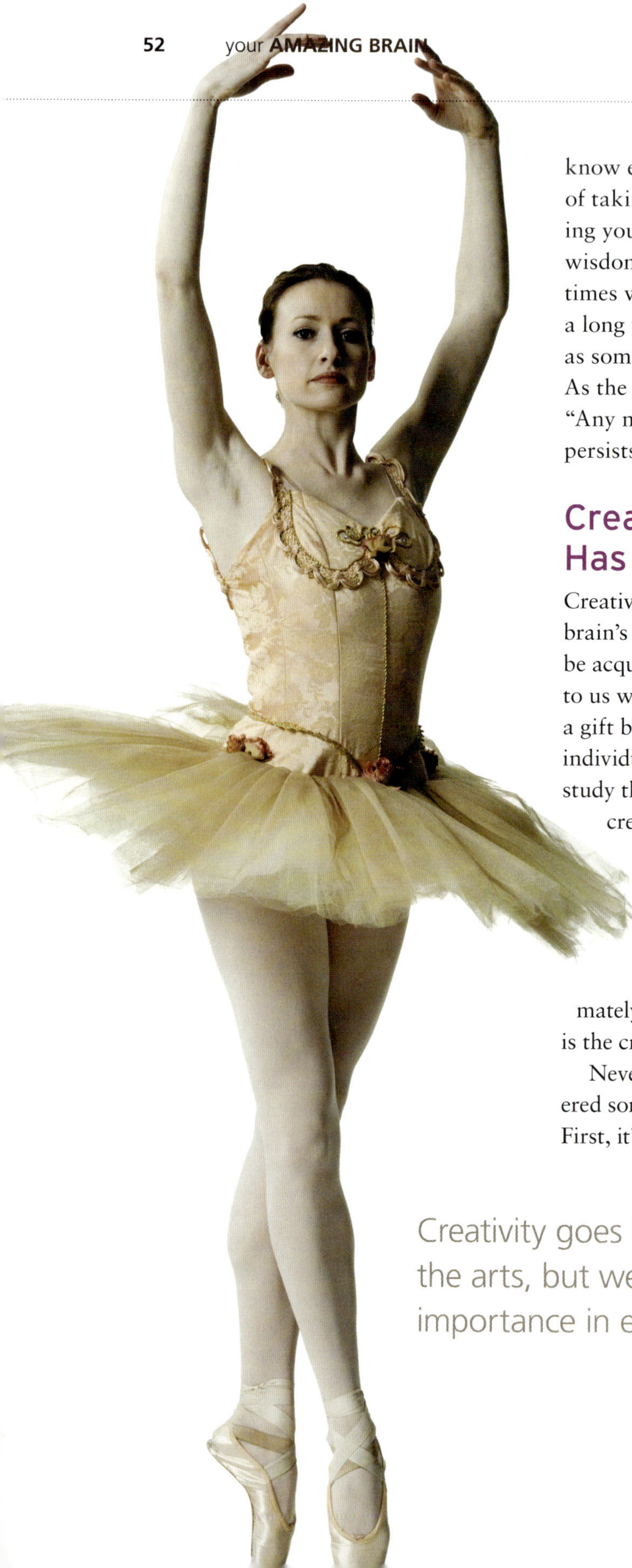

know everything and that life is capable of taking unexpected turns. Recognizing your errors can only lead to greater wisdom—and admitting that there are times when you could be mistaken will go a long way in solidifying your reputation as someone whose advice can be trusted. As the Roman philosopher Cicero said, "Any man is liable to err; only a fool persists in error."

Creativity: Everyone Has Some

Creativity is the most magical of the brain's skills. We trust that intelligence can be acquired and that wisdom will come to us with age. But creativity seems to be a gift bestowed upon only a few blessed individuals. It has proven more difficult to study than intelligence or wisdom. Because creativity comes in flashes or floods, then dries up seemingly on its own, it is difficult to harness and nearly impossible to measure. As researchers from the University of Sidney, Australia, noted: Ultimately, the only proven test for creativity is the creation itself.

Nevertheless, psychologists have uncovered some interesting facts about creativity. First, it's more evenly distributed than

Creativity goes hand-in-hand with the arts, but we often overlook its importance in everyday life.

originally thought. Yes, some people are born with more creative gifts, but just about anyone can develop and nurture creativity at any age. Verdi, for example, composed his opera *Otello* at age 73 and *Falstaff* at 79. Because creativity involves novel ways of thinking, it flourishes wherever originality is valued and individuals are encouraged to challenge traditional thoughts and styles. In other words, if you want out-of-the-box thinking, you have to, well, *step outside of the box*!

What is the "box" made of? According to legendary actor Alan Arkin, who teaches classes in creativity, the primary limitation on creative expression is expectation. We expect or wish to be successful. We wish to make others laugh. We wish to please. Creativity, he says, only shows up when you relinquish your expectations and start existing in the moment, like a child. Children play just to play, not to impress anyone. Creativity "is not about being clever or amusing," Arkin says, "it's about making a deeper connection with your creative force, surprising yourself, and letting go."

Creativity goes hand-in-hand with the arts—music, dance, theater, film, writing, painting—but we often overlook its importance in everyday life. Creativity is the ability that allows us to generate solutions to problems, to hold fresh conversations, and to plan for the future. For example, throwing a surprise party requires finding a creative way to spring the actual surprise. And plenty of non-artists show remarkable creativity when it comes to talking their way out of a traffic ticket or justifying to a spouse why they just had to buy yet another pair of shoes.

Creativity is just as strong in older people, but sometimes we have to be prompted to remember that it's okay to play the way we did when we were younger. Studies show that older folks who are involved in creative activities are more likely to remain connected to the community, suffer less debility over time, and live generally healthier lives.

FINDING YOUR CREATIVE SPARK

Creativity is about stretching your mind and coming up with solutions to unusual problems. To flex your creative muscle, try these exercises.

- Set a timer for 2 minutes and write down all the words you can think of that begin with the letter "A." Tomorrow, do the same for the letter "B," and so on throughout the alphabet.

- For each of the following sentences, imagine what happens next. (There are no right or wrong answers!)

  1. A woman wearing a red hat knocks on the front door of a large, extravagant stone house. When the door opens....
  2. A man and a woman are out on a date, holding hands as they walk down a crowded city street. The woman looks up and gasps because....
  3. A young man moves to a new country with his family, but worries that he won't fit in and will never find friends. To his surprise, on the plane over, the person seated next to him....

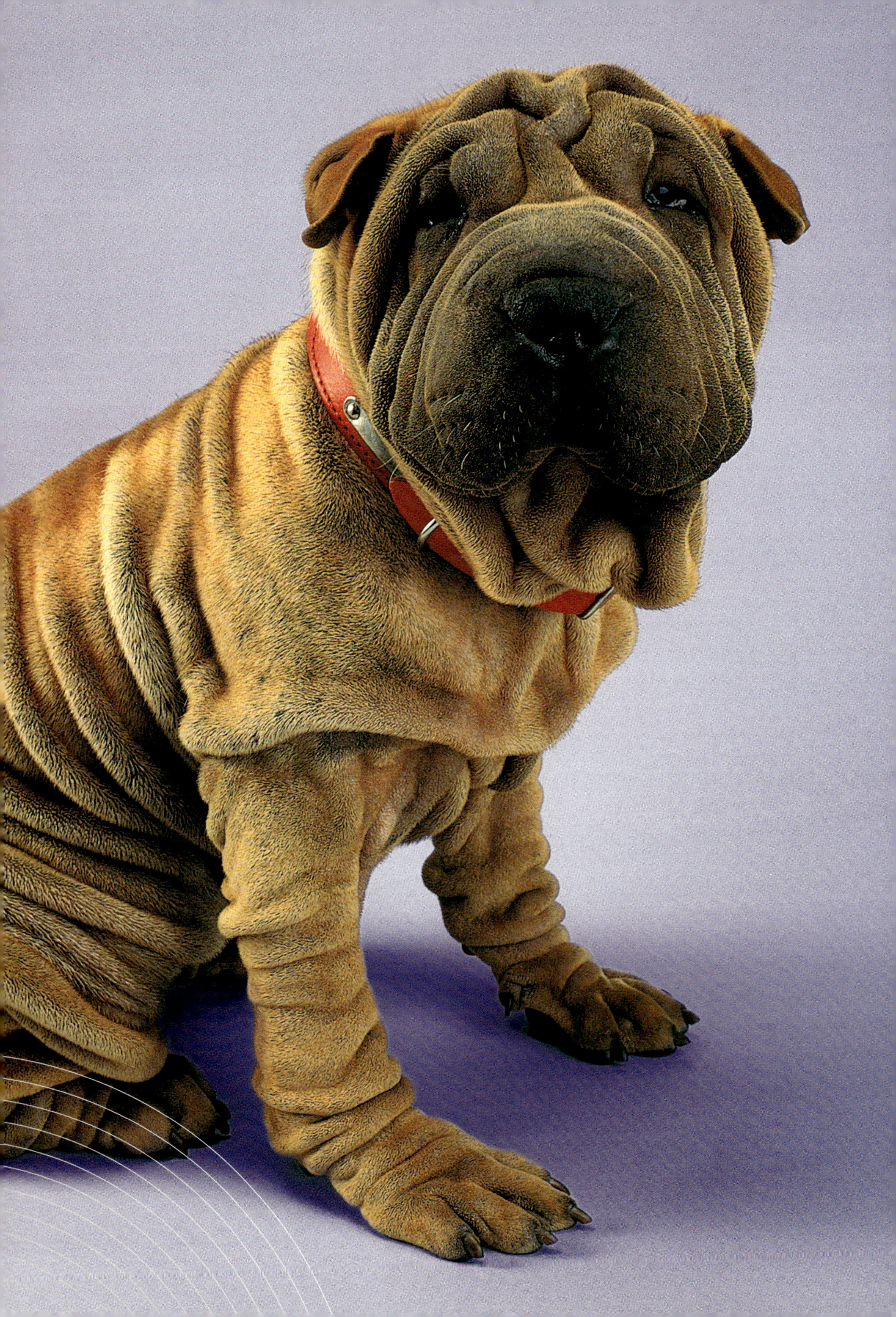

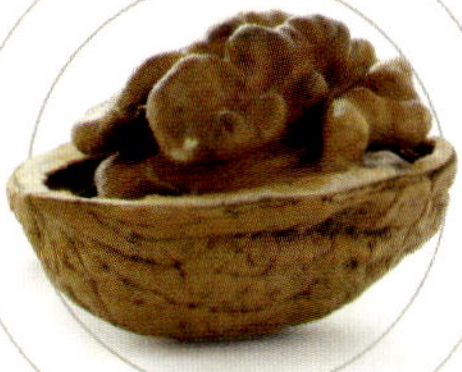

How your brain ages

As we get older, our knees start to creak, our skin starts to sag, and our brains start to...shrink? That's right: Between age 20 and 70, brain weight and blood flow to the brain decrease by 20 percent. The total number of fibers and nerves in the brain decreases by 37 percent. Sound scary?

Maybe, but the news isn't nearly as bad as you may think.

Many of these types of changes exert effects that are subtle, if they're noticeable at all. We are still capable of learning—and remembering—just about anything at just about any age, though it may take us a little longer. In addition, any small cognitive losses that do occur are easy enough to compensate for. For example, just as wearing eyeglasses can make up for a decline in vision, using the memory strategies described in Part 4 can compensate for declines in short-term (working) memory.

Want to take up the trombone at age 76? You can! Want to finally read the classics you always said you'd tackle someday? Go for it! Everything you learn to do in the rest of *No More Brain Drain*, from spending time in our "brain gym" to getting more exercise (which increases blood flow to the brain and promotes the formation of new brain cells and connections) will help you keep your brain as young as possible.

An Honest Accounting

Nearly everyone over the age of 40 worries about the state of his or her memory. We are very hard on ourselves: One missed appointment, a forgotten phone number or two, and we panic, usually for no good reason. Truth is, most of us forget where we put our keys because our lives are too busy, we're trying to multitask, we're too stressed, or we didn't get enough sleep—not because we're losing our marbles. Some of us can also chalk up memory problems and dull thinking to a medical condition, or even a prescription drug (see Brain Drain #5: Medical Issues in Part 3).

We tend to expect a lot from our memory powers—maybe more than they actually need to deliver. After all, why would day planners exist if people didn't need to write down their appointments in order to remember them? In the introduction to this book, we described a rare group of adults with total recall of every single day of their lives from adolescence on. Name a date, and these people can tell you what day of the week it was, what the weather was like, whom they met, and what they ate that day. Would you want this kind of memory? Probably not. In fact, some of those who possess this talent described it as more of an exhausting curse than a blessing.

Likewise, we may admire the sponge-like memory that children seem to possess, but it would be a mistake to feel at a loss because we can't absorb new information as quickly as children can. Consider: Most of us don't worry that we can't turn cartwheels or jump over fences in a single bound anymore. Children not only have amazing physical prowess, their little bodies, still malleable and forming, can do things most adults wouldn't want to try without a chiropractor standing by. Our bodies changed, and we barely mourned the loss. Our brains have also changed, becoming slightly less agile—but who really cares, as long as we can still perform the tasks we need to?

WHAT GETS WORSE

So, what is normal for an aging brain? Researchers tell us that we can expect slight declines in the following three areas.

Short-term memory. For reasons that science has not been able to pinpoint, our short-term memory, also called working memory, gets worse with age. Older adults have fantastic long-term memories, able to recall the names of childhood friends, details about the town they grew up in, and what movies they saw during high school, but they may not remember

It's Not All Downhill

As with most things in life, getting older means you win some and you lose some. Here's the scorecard:

Better with Age
- Long-term memory
- Emotional memory
- Untimed memory tests
- Wisdom

Worse with Age
- Short-term memory
- Timed memory tests
- Speed of processing
- Reaction time
- Focus
- Multitasking

No Change with Age
- Creativity
- Memory for important information

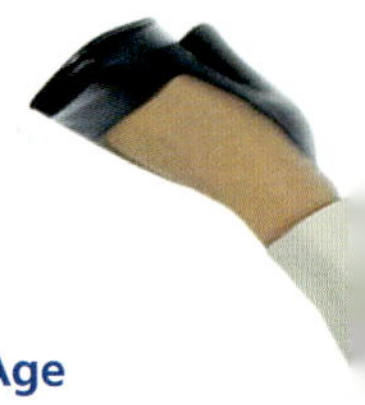

who was at a party they attended just last weekend. This shrinkage of working memory makes it more difficult for older adults to learn new things. Learning a foreign language, for example, is easier for younger people than for older people. However, older folks do as well if not better than younger folks when learning something that fits their strengths. For example, taking a history class is easier because older adults have a richer mental framework that allows them to put the facts being taught into context.

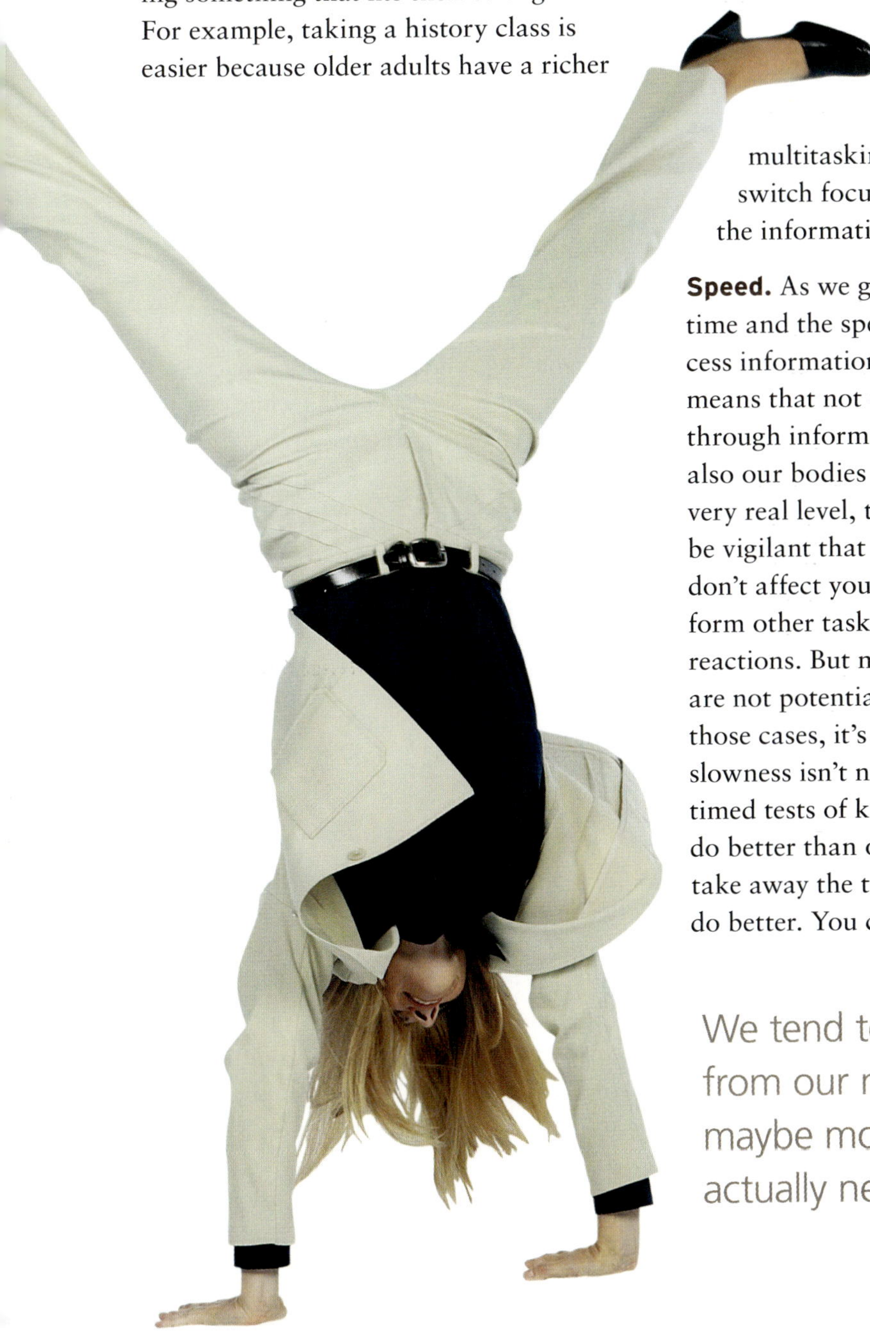

Focus. We also lose some of our ability to focus our attention, a problem that might mean it takes longer to read a book. We are more easily distracted by competing cries for attention, so reading a book with the television on can be challenging for some, impossible for others. Older adults also have a tougher time multitasking—it is difficult for us to switch focus without losing some of the information about previous tasks.

Speed. As we get older, our reaction time and the speed with which we process information both slow down. This means that not only do our brains sift through information more slowly but also our bodies react more slowly. On a very real level, this means you have to be vigilant that these normal changes don't affect your ability to drive or perform other tasks that require split-second reactions. But most of the things we do are not potentially life threatening. In those cases, it's best to understand that slowness isn't necessarily a handicap. In timed tests of knowledge, younger adults do better than older adults, but if you take away the time factor, older adults do better. You can compensate for any

We tend to expect a lot from our memory powers—maybe more than they actually need to deliver.

slowdown by simply allowing more time to learn and remember something that's important to you.

FEARING THE WORST

Most of us can deal with learning a little more slowly as we age or having to turn off the TV while we're trying to read. Our real fear is that the little brain hiccups or "senior moments" we all experience are the first symptoms of Alzheimer's disease or another form of dementia. Popular culture aggravates this fear, creating a caricature of the befuddled older person. In a self-fulfilling prophecy, we can easily come to expect that aging equals memory decline, then become alarmed whenever we forget where we put our glasses. This kind of worry may be worse than the actual forgetfulness.

Time for a reality check: Only about 5 percent of men and women ages 65 to 74 have Alzheimer's disease. The numbers do go up after 75, but we now have within our grasp the means to slow or halt the progression of dementia. We'll get to that later in the book, but first, let's take a look at what, exactly, dementia means.

To begin with, dementia doesn't necessarily have anything to do with being old. In fact, scientists no longer use the word "senile" to describe memory decline, since the root meaning of the word literally refers to old age. Instead, the experts have divided mental decline into three broad categories: age-associated memory impairment, mild cognitive dementia, and dementia.

Those darn brain hiccups. Age-associated memory impairment describes the normal state of having brief "senior moments," when your short-term memory becomes weaker and, well... shorter. By age 60, about 40 percent of us will experience this problem. What causes it? As we mentioned earlier, neurons shrink and die off, which decreases the number of synaptic contact points—those all-important brain cell connections. We also produce less of the brain chemicals called neurotransmitters, which allow communication to happen in the brain, and less of the hormones that support healthy brain function. Blood flow is reduced in all portions of the brain, but most strikingly in the frontal cortex, where our thinking, planning, and speaking abilities reside.

It's worth repeating: This is a normal part of aging, no worse than that mild ache you feel in your knee because the joint isn't as strong as it was when you were 20. These age-related brain changes explain why we forget that appointment or have trouble coming up with the right word during a cocktail party conversation. It's all part of the normal wear-and-tear of aging, and much of it can be compensated for.

When it's more serious. Unlike the everyday forgetfulness described above, mild cognitive dementia suggests a deeper problem. Typical symptoms include regularly forgetting things you really should remember, such as doctor's appointments or a weekly card game, frequently misplacing items, and having difficulty following a conversation.

Typically people with this condition are aware that they are slipping, but they possess the intelligence and social skills to cover their mistakes so well that friends and family may not even notice. Still, this could be an early warning sign of impending dementia. The probable cause: vascular problems—namely stiff and narrowed arteries—that sharply reduce circulation in the brain. (Elsewhere in the book, we'll give you plenty of advice for keeping your arteries healthy, one of the main steps you can take to help prevent dementia.)

When it's darn serious. People who are described as having dementia have memory problems that they simply can't cover up. These problems are serious enough to be noticeable to others and significantly change their ability to function in the world. They may forget how to cook, have trouble dressing themselves, and feel lost even in familiar surroundings. Some dementias can be reversed, particularly if they have been caused by dietary deficiencies, a medical disorder (such as diabetes, depression, or liver disease), or a side effect of a medication. Other dementias like Alzheimer's or Parkinson's are irreversible today—though there's evidence that with a combination of proper medication, nutrition, and fitness program, the progression of the disease may be slowed.

For Most, The Best Is Yet to Come

If the older brain is not quite as agile as it once was, it has just as much capacity as the young brain. Remember that in timed tests of knowledge, younger adults do better than most older adults, but if you take away the time factor, older adults do better. And that's not all. Those lab tests of memory skill can only ask subjects to study and spit back lists of words or numbers. That's a small part of the total cognitive picture. Scientists

Dementia: Who's at Risk?

Many of the risk factors for dementia are well-documented, and they're nearly identical to those for heart disease. The central issue is maintaining (or failing to maintain) good blood flow to the brain. Without it, brain cells don't get the oxygen and nutrients they need to function at their best. When neurons are starved or suffocated, they die.

The most common risk factors include:

- Family history of dementia
- High blood pressure
- High low-density lipoprotein (LDL) "bad" cholesterol
- Low high-density lipoprotein (HDL) "good" cholesterol
- High alcohol intake
- Smoking
- Being overweight or obese
- Uncontrolled diabetes
- Inactivity (mental and physical)
- A diet high in meat products and saturated fats
- A diet low in fruits, vegetables, and whole grains

Other risk factors:

- Hypothyroidism or hyperthyroidism
- Vitamin B_{12} deficiency
- Lyme disease
- Parkinson's disease
- Huntington's disease
- Pick's disease
- Depression
- Anxiety
- History of strokes
- Mild brain injury, including concussion

Normal or Not?

Most of us worry about the state of our brains at one time or another. But most of the time, our cognitive slips are perfectly normal. The main problem is knowing whether you should laugh it off or see a doctor. Here's how to tell a routine brain hiccup from a matter of serious concern.

PROBABLY NORMAL	SEE A DOCTOR
You frequently lose your car keys.	You look at a key and can't remember how to use it.
You walk into a room and forget why you went there.	You forget how to find the kitchen in your own home.
You forget the name of a person you were just introduced to.	You forget the name of a family member.
You momentarily forget the name of a close friend.	You don't remember the person who says she is your friend.
You put the paper towels in the refrigerator and the milk in the cabinet and have a good laugh about it.	You frequently have no idea where things are supposed to go.
Mornings can be hectic, and you sometimes find it difficult to leave the house on time because you misplaced your belt or forgot to set the alarm clock.	People comment because you leave the house without showering or because your clothes are disheveled.
You can come up with examples of times when you felt your forgetfulness was worrisome.	You know that you've been forgetful, but you can't remember details—you forget what it was you forgot.
You take a wrong turn on the way to your favorite grocery store, or get momentarily lost in familiar territory.	You sometimes leave home and can't find your way back.
You forget to go to your dentist appointment.	You forget to go to your daughter's wedding.
If asked, you could give details about yesterday's dinner or your most recent phone call. It might take awhile, but you can do it.	You have difficulty remembering recent events. You may not recall them at all.
You enjoy seeing friends at your usual level. Socializing is fun and enjoyable.	You avoid social activities because you're afraid that you'll do something embarrassing.
You find it difficult to learn how to use new appliances or electronic devices.	You find it impossible to learn to use new appliances, and you even find it difficult to use the old ones.
Sometimes you struggle to find the word you were looking for.	You often lose words and have to use substitutes or change the subject to avoid embarrassment.
You feel forgetful, but your family and friends don't notice it.	Your family and friends tell you that they are worried about your forgetfulness.

can't even come close to measuring the true intricacy—and deep reserves—of the older brain. "As people age, they are capable of more and more complex projects," says Gary J. Kennedy, MD, a professor in the Department of Psychiatry and Behavioral Sciences at Albert Einstein College of Medicine of Yeshiva University in the Bronx.

Give yourself credit. The first step in fighting brain drain is applauding the awesome potential that you already possess. Another way to put it: You're in better shape than you think. In fact, sometimes, what feels like memory decline is actually something much more benign: mental laziness. We forget a name not because our memory is on the fritz, but because our internal decision-maker judged the name of the person we've just met not worthy of our efforts.

Take action. If there's a single key lesson to be learned from the leaders in brain research, it's this: Use it or lose it. We need to flex those mental muscles in order to preserve our powers of attention, comprehension, and recall. So, the all-important second step in fighting brain drain is to consciously decide to do something about it. By reading this book, you've already begun. Congratulations!

Apply some grit and determination. The third step is to use a little elbow grease. Are you ready for a challenge? Good! Our goal in writing this book was to arm you with the most up-to-date information and advice for keeping your brain fit, capable, and ready for action. In Parts 2 and 3, we'll reveal specific brain-improving lifestyle tips and tactics to help you further armor yourself against brain drain. Later, in Part 4, you'll use our "brain gym," where you'll find specific exercises designed to increase your brain power in six areas: attention and focus, general memory, processing speed, verbal skills, number skills, and reasoning. Yes, we're asking you to do some work, but don't worry: This work is more like play. And many of these exercises are no more time-consuming than such daily grooming habits as brushing your hair and flossing your teeth. Think of it as brain hygiene!

Now, without further ado, let's get started!

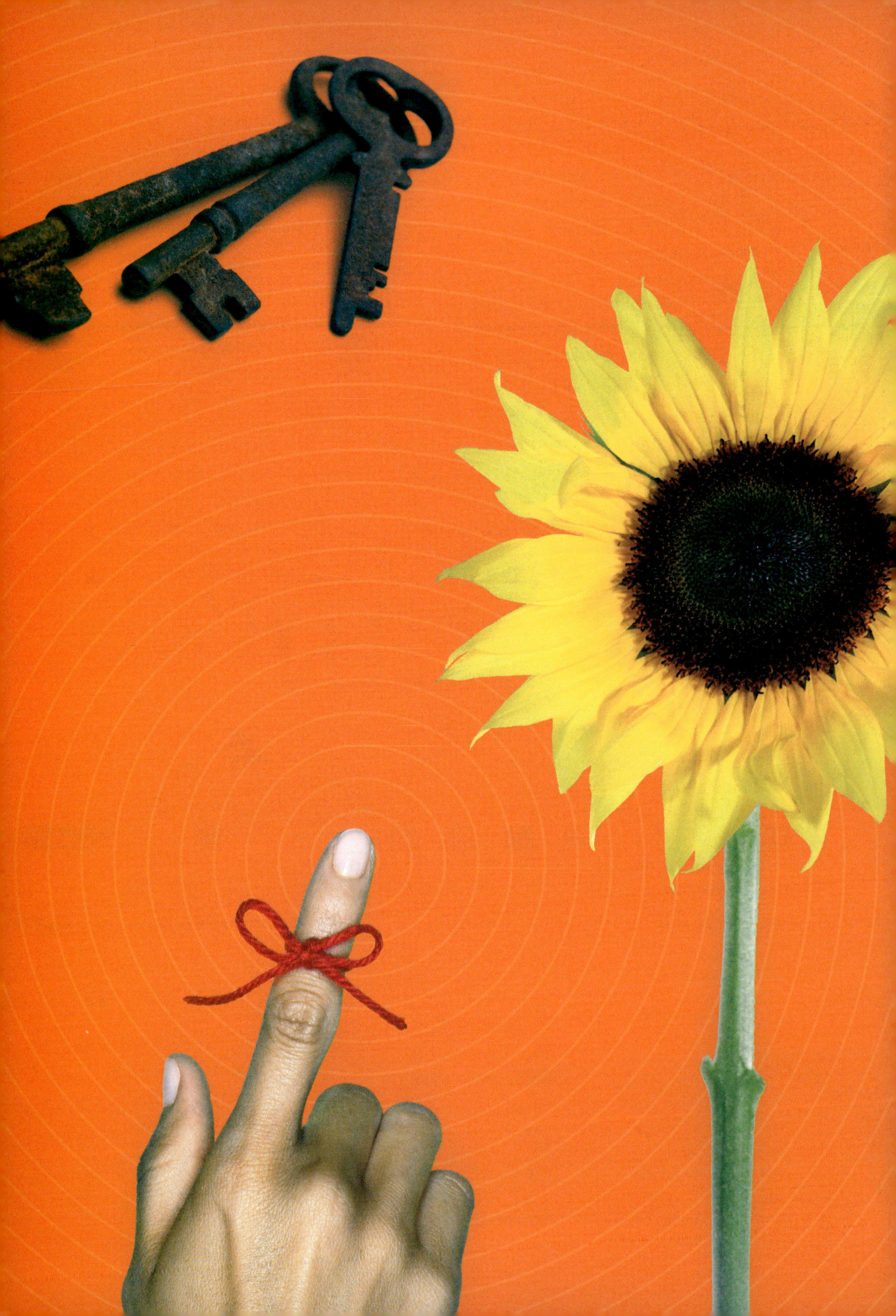

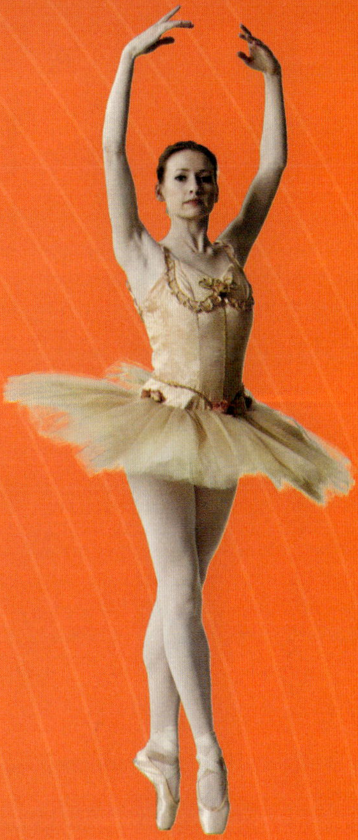

PART TWO

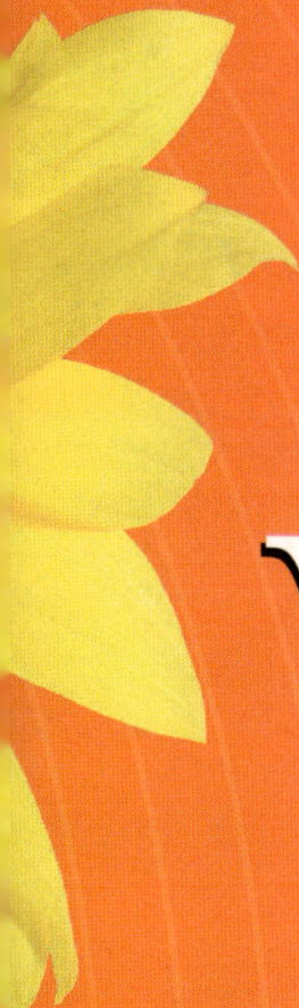

six vaccines against brain drain

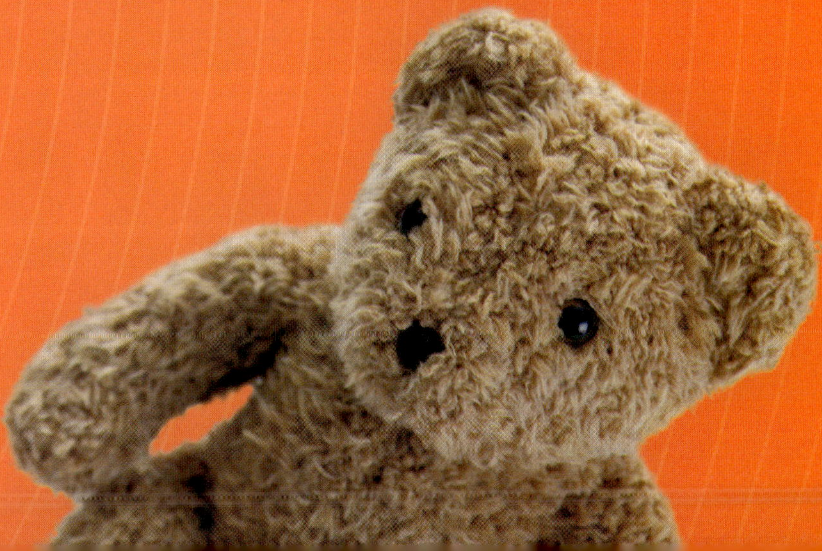

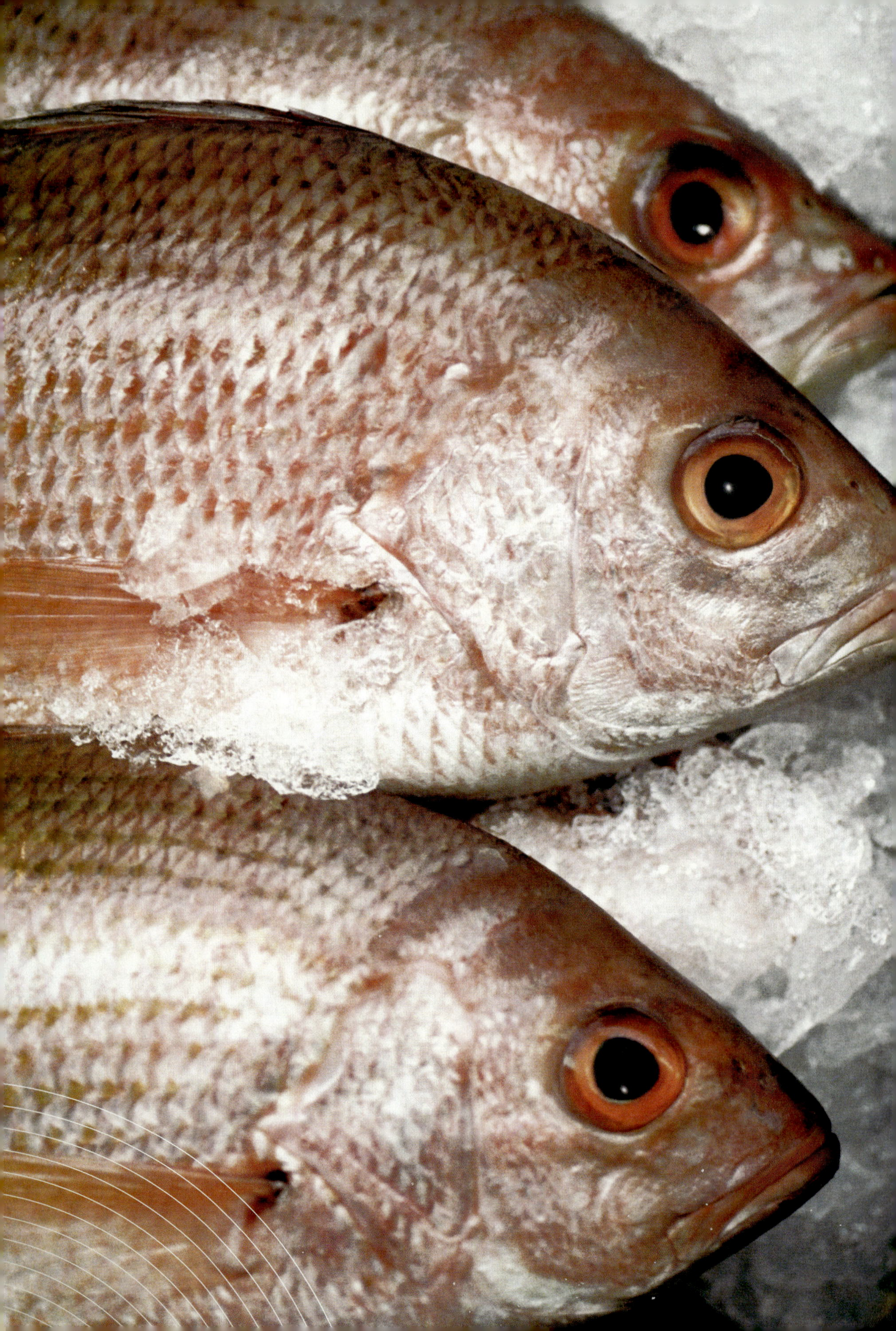

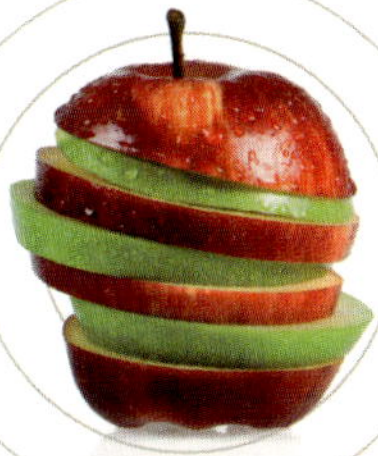

VACCINE #1

diet

We all know by now that greasy burgers are bad for the heart, while a meal of grilled salmon and sautéed greens is just what the doctor ordered. If eating heart-healthy foods, along with getting plenty of exercise, can slash your risk of heart disease in half, imagine what a brain-healthy diet can do for your brain! You probably never gave your brain a single thought as you pushed the cart down the grocery aisles but, in recent years, a stack of breakthrough research has shown that eating more of certain foods and less of others can significantly improve your memory and thinking skills and even cut your risk of Alzheimer's disease by a staggering percentage.

The ingredients for a healthy brain are as close as your kitchen. In fact, if you open your refrigerator or pantry, you'll probably see at least five brain-boosting foods. A better memory has been within your reach all along.

FOODS FOR THOUGHT

Everything your brain does—every thought and emotion it has, every calculation it performs, every memory it summons—requires energy and nutrition you can get only from food. That means your ability to feel good, think clearly, and keep a sharp memory depends in large part on what you eat for breakfast, lunch, and dinner. Who'd have thought?

To find the best brain-smart diet, look to your heart. Blood pumped from the heart delivers vital nutrients and oxygen to the brain, so it is logical that foods that are good for the heart and blood vessels are also good for the brain. In fact, the surest dietary path to better brain health may start with the same diet famous for its heart benefits: the Mediterranean diet. Research shows that people who follow this traditional way of eating have a much lower risk of heart disease, heart attack, and stroke. It helps control cholesterol, blood pressure, and inflammation, all of which contribute to heart disease. But that's not all.

Neurologist Nikolaos Scarmeas, MD, and his colleagues at Columbia University examined the effects of a Mediterranean diet on Alzheimer's disease. They found that the closer people followed the diet, the lower their risk of developing the disease. People who partially followed the diet reduced their risk by about 40 percent; those who stuck closely to the diet reduced their risk by up to 68 percent.

Rate Your Diet

Answer the questions below to help you rate your current diet. Answer honestly; no one is looking except you!

1. I eat this many different types of vegetable a day, not counting potatoes or corn:
- **0** 0 or 1
- **1** 2 or 3
- **2** 4 or more

2. I eat broccoli, cauliflower, Brussels sprouts, kale, mustard greens, watercress, collard greens, cabbage, or Swiss chard:
- **0** Rarely
- **1** Once a week
- **2** Several times a week

3. When I eat bread, it's:
- **0** White bread
- **1** Usually a smooth "white whole-wheat" bread or a stone-ground wheat bread (but not "whole wheat")
- **2** Always a coarse 100% whole-grain variety

4. When I have meat for dinner, it's usually:
- **0** A burger, a ground beef dish, or a big piece of steak
- **1** A sizable piece of tenderloin or sirloin
- **2** A small serving, more of a flavor enhancer

5. I like my chicken:
- **0** Fried
- **1** Loaded with mayo
- **2** Baked, grilled, or roasted, skin-off

6. I usually cook with:
- **0** Lard
- **1** Either butter or margarine that contains hydrogenated oils
- **2** Olive or canola oil or a heart-smart margarine

7. I eat salmon, tuna, sardines, or mackerel:
- **0** Never
- **1** At least once a month
- **2** At least once a week

8. As a side dish, I'm most likely to have:
- **0** Potatoes, corn, or white rice
- **1** Brown rice or regular pasta
- **2** Barley, quinoa, whole-wheat pasta, or couscous

People who closely followed the Mediterranean diet who already had Alzheimer's disease lived about 4 years longer than those who didn't follow the diet. Imagine keeping your mind sharp, your memory keen, your reasoning sound, and your thinking clear all because you ate the way you would on a vacation to the Greek Islands!

That means plenty of whole-grain foods, fruits and vegetables (picture a Greek salad made with tomatoes, cucumbers, and onions), fish (often grilled), olive oil, nuts, and low-fat dairy products, such as yogurt and feta cheese. Meat, poultry, and sweets are eaten only occasionally and are not a necessary part of daily meals.

The No More Brain Drain Diet

We know the Mediterranean diet works, but is it enough to protect the brain?

It's an excellent start, according to David Perlmutter, MD, FACN, neurologist and

9. I regularly eat this many of the following foods: flaxseeds or flaxseed oil, avocadoes, pumpkin seeds, walnuts, blueberries, apples, spinach, natural peanut butter (no added sugar):
   - **0** 0 or 1
   - **1** 2 or 3
   - **2** 4 or more

10. When I snack, I tend to eat:
   - **0** Cookies, candy bars, or candy
   - **1** Pretzels, crackers, or granola bars
   - **2** Whole fruit, avocado slices, or nuts

11. The cold beverages I drink most often are:
   - **0** Regular soda, "vitamin" waters, sugary iced tea or lemonade, sugary fruit drinks, or energy drinks
   - **1** Diet soda or 100% fruit juice
   - **2** Water or unsweetened tea

12. I drink alcohol:
   - **0** Liberally (more than 1 drink a day for women or 2 for men)
   - **1** Never
   - **2** In moderation

YOUR SCORE

Add up the scores associated with your answers to find out how "smart" your current diet is.

0–6 points: Elmer Fudd—You have some real work to do if you want to maintain or recapture the brain power you had when you were 40.

7–12 points: Inspector Clouseau—You've stumbled on a few healthy foods, but overall, your diet is probably doing more harm than good.

13–18 points: Marian the Librarian—Not bad! You're making some smart choices, but there's still room for improvement in other areas.

19–24 points: Albert Einstein—Congratulations! You may not have crazy hair, but your diet is going a long way toward protecting your brain.

brain expert, who helped create the No More Brain Drain Diet, which translates current research knowledge into a straightforward eating program. If you want to start eating in a way that can help save your memory—and very possibly extend your life—start here.

The No More Brain Drain Diet is easy to follow because it works on a principle of add, swap, and drop. That is, you get to *add* plenty of new foods to your menu selections, *swap* brain-healthy choices for many of the less-healthy foods you currently eat, and *drop* those foods that are downright dangerous for brain health. And you can do it all in six simple steps.

Boost Your Smarts with "Brain Fats"

In the last 200,000 years or so, the human brain underwent a critical change: It got larger and smarter. Early humans who lived near the water experienced the biggest brain advances, and scientists think they know why: seafood. Specifically, the fat contained in seafood, known as omega-3 fatty acids, and even more specifically, a type of omega-3 known as DHA, short for docosahexaenoic acid—nature's ultimate brain food.

6 Rules for a Smarter Diet

1. ADD foods rich in omega-3 fatty acids.
2. SWITCH to olive oil for cooking and in dressings.
3. DROP all foods that contain trans fats.
4. ADD more fruits and vegetables.
5. SWITCH to whole grains.
6. DROP sugary or artificially sweetened foods and beverages.

Remember that your brain is made mostly of fat, which not only forms the membranes around cells that regulate what gets in and out of them but also insulates the bundles of nerve fibers that act as high-speed communication cables in the brain. It shouldn't be too shocking, then, to learn that fat is the single most important nutrient for protecting and preserving brain function. Eating a low-fat or, worse, a no-fat diet is actually the worst thing you can do for your brain.

Of course, not just any old type of fat will do. A steady diet of cheeseburgers, for instance, won't do much to sharpen your cognitive skills, and could dull them by clogging up your arteries so that less oxygen and nutrients reach your noggin. What the brain craves most are the omega-3 fats. They turn on the genes that determine how the brain develops, repair and preserve brain cells, enable the cells to deliver signals efficiently, and may even facilitate the growth of new cells. Studies show that without enough omega-3s, the brain can't function properly. Over time, lack of omega-3s may even contribute to the development of Alzheimer's disease. Unfortunately, most people don't eat nearly enough of these good fats.

Omega-3s come in three varieties: DHA (mentioned above), EPA (eicosapentaenoic acid), and ALA (alpha-linolenic acid). Brain cells need all three kinds to maintain their structure and avoid premature aging, though the body has a much easier time using DHA and EPA than ALA. Research suggests that ALA helps to protect brain cells and is involved in neuron-to-neuron communication. EPA seems to act as an antioxidant and may help prevent brain cell damage during aging. But DHA is the brain superstar.

DHA is concentrated in the frontal lobe of the brain and is critical for clear thinking, organization, alertness, learning, and reasoning. Low levels have been linked to memory and learning problems and even Alzheimer's disease. When scientists added DHA to the diets of mice bred to develop Alzheimer's disease, the mice had less of the brain plaques associated with the disease than mice who didn't get the DHA.

Omega-3s also help prevent blood clots, which reduces the risk of heart disease and stroke, two conditions that affect brain health. When you consider that omega-3s could cut your risk of developing Alzheimer's disease by more than half, it may be worth adding some of these foods to your weekly shopping list.

DR. PERLMUTTER RECOMMENDS:

DHA Supplements

The DHA form of omega-3 is found only in fish, and most people don't get nearly enough to help with heart or brain health. About 25 percent of all brain fat is made of DHA, so you don't want to be deficient. Brain cell communication, thinking, and memory all depend on DHA. Check with your doctor before starting any new supplement.

Dose: 800 to 1,000 milligrams per day.

Type: Look for brands that are algae-based (instead of fish-based) to avoid a possible risk of mercury contamination.

Recommended brands: Nordic Naturals, Carlson.

How to take: Take with meals to avoid possible stomach upset. You can take the full dose at one meal. If you experience "fishy" burps, store the supplements in the freezer; many people report that any aftertaste disappears with frozen capsules.

EAT SMART

Eat fish twice a week. You don't need to spend a lot of time, money, or effort to get there; even canned tuna and canned salmon count. (Choose canned light tuna rather than albacore; it comes from a short-lived fish that accumulates fewer toxins than long-lived albacore.) Fish is a perfect weeknight meal because it's ready in as little as 10 minutes. When possible, buy wild fish when it's available or, if you choose farmed, opt for organic farm-raised fish if you can afford it; it may contain fewer contaminants like mercury. Incidentally, canned salmon is made from wild fish—a bonus!

Stock your freezer with frozen fish (not breaded). Let it thaw in the fridge and you'll have dinner at the ready without making a trip to the fish counter.

Make a not-tuna salad. Tuna isn't the only fish that can be used in salads. Try this basic recipe, and add your own twist: Flake or dice about 1 cup of any leftover cooked fish. Add 1/2 cup each of any three chopped vegetables, such as carrots, celery, peppers, onions, tomatoes, cucumbers, or broccoli. Add 1 tablespoon olive oil and 1 tablespoon reduced-fat mayonnaise. Season to taste with cracked pepper, red pepper flakes, turmeric, or fresh herbs. Mix well, and serve over a bed of lettuce or use as a sandwich filling.

Add walnuts to everything. They're terrific in salads, added to baked goods, and on top of cereal or even low-fat ice cream.

Invest in a bottle of walnut oil. This nut oil has a clean, delicate, slightly sweet flavor that is perfect for use in homemade salad dressings. Don't use it as a cooking oil, though, since it breaks down in heat and will turn bitter. You can also toss pasta with it. Or halve a piece of fruit, such as a peach, and brush it with a combination of walnut oil and honey, then roast or grill and serve with yogurt. Oils, especially nut oils, easily turn rancid when exposed to light, heat, and air, so store them tightly sealed in a cool, dark place and discard after 6 to 12 months.

Keep a bottle of flaxseed oil on hand. The taste is powerful and slightly bitter ... a little goes a long way! Use flaxseed oil as a nutty flavor enhancer and finishing oil on veggie sandwiches and other raw foods or instead of margarine or butter on steamed vegetables and other cooked foods (but sprinkle only after the food is moved to a serving dish; heating flaxseed oil can create harmful compounds).

Put some flaxseeds in your spice grinder. Buy whole flaxseeds in a natural foods store and grind them in a spice grinder. The whole seeds keep longer than grounds seeds. (If you eat the seeds whole, your body won't digest them and they'll come out the way they went in.) Sprinkle them on your morning cereal, your lunch salad, or a smoothie. Or add

Why We Love Fat

The human body was designed to love fatty foods in part because of the needs of the brain, but also because, ounce for ounce, fat has more than double the number of calories as carbohydrates or proteins—handy during times of famine. When food is scarce, we don't have the luxury of choice; any fat is worth eating. When food is plentiful, we still love fatty foods, but we also have the option to choose the "good" kinds of fats, skipping the dangerous ones and adding plenty of brain-healthy ones.

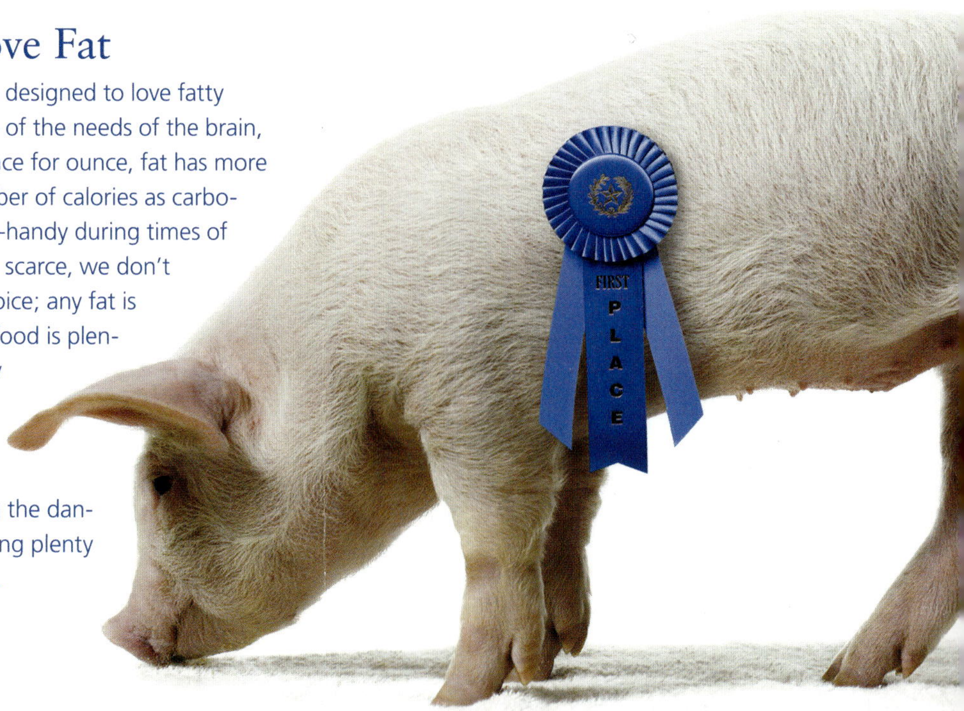

them to pancake or muffin batter. If a recipe calls for 1 cup flour, use 3/4 cup flour and 1/4 cup flaxseed meal instead. Be sure to store the seeds in the fridge or they'll go rancid fast.

Get seedy. Seeds are packed with good fat, protein, and vitamin E, and may even help you lower your cholesterol. Here's one great way to enjoy them along with another brain-healthy food, fish: Coat thin fish fillets (or chicken cutlets) with a mixture of crushed sunflower and pumpkin seeds, then panfry. Chopped seeds are also an interesting, crunchy addition to hot or cold cereal.

Use oils lightly in cooking, liberally in eating. Some of the health benefits of oils are compromised when you heat the oil (never heat flaxseed oil because it can create harmful compounds). So cook with the minimal amount of oil needed—often no more than 1 tablespoon per pan. Instead, be generous with oils as condiments, or in preparation of sauces or toppings.

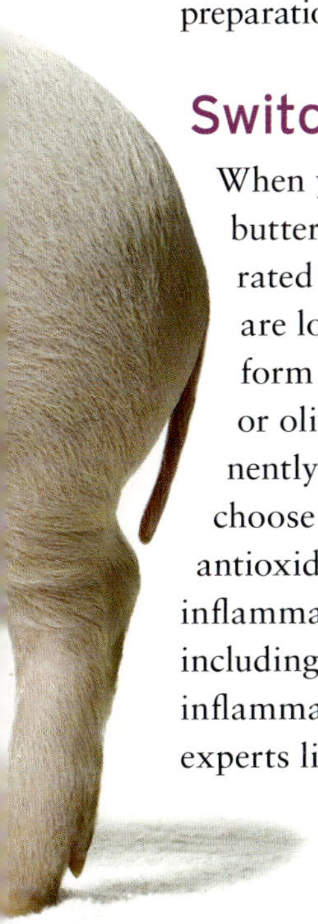

Switch to Olive Oil

When you have the choice of eating butter (full of artery-clogging saturated fat), margarine (many brands are loaded with toxic trans fat in the form of partially hydrogenated oil), or olive oil, which figures prominently in the Mediterranean diet, choose olive oil! Olive oil is a powerful antioxidant that also helps to reduce inflammation everywhere in the body, including the brain. Its powers against inflammation are so strong, in fact, that experts liken it to aspirin.

Safer Seafood

Choose fish least likely to contain mercury and other contaminants.

BEST CHOICES	WORST CHOICES
Wild Alaskan sockeye salmon	Shark
Wild Pacific salmon	Swordfish
Organic farm-raised Alaskan or Pacific salmon	King mackerel
Tilapia	Tilefish
Haddock	Halibut
Anchovies	White albacore tuna
Catfish	Chilean bass
Herring	Bluefish
Mackerel (not King)	Marlin
Freshwater trout	Orange roughy
	Any farm-raised fish (unless organic)

Olive oil also protects brain cell membranes and may help prevent age-related dementia. And it's good for your cholesterol (which in turn makes it good for your brain). One study found that when 28 men and women added 2 tablespoons of olive oil a day to their diets, they saw a 16 percent drop in LDL ("bad") cholesterol.

When you want a milder taste or an oil that survives heat better than olive oil does, go for canola oil; it's a much healthier choice than corn, safflower, or sunflower oil, all of which you should avoid because they can promote inflammation.

EAT SMART

Choose extra-virgin olive oil. Olives are crushed and then pressed to make oil. The first press yields extra-virgin olive oil, which is fruity and full-bodied and contains the most antioxidants. The second press yields refined virgin olive oil, which is of lower quality and contains fewer antioxidants.

Find your favorite flavor. Different brands and types of olive oil can have dramatically different tastes depending on where the olives where grown and when they were harvested, among other factors. Experiment until you find a brand you love. You can even become an olive oil connoisseur. Some gourmet cooking stores, such as Williams-Sonoma, have periodic olive oil tastings free of charge. Or, hold your own olive oil tasting with friends.

Store olive oil properly to avoid rancidity. Like other oils, olive oil turns rancid when exposed to heat, light, and air. Olive oil should be stored in a dark cabinet away from the stove, and always kept tightly closed. Do not store olive oil in the refrigerator; if condensation occurs in the bottle, it can ruin the taste of the oil.

Use a lower cooking temperature than usual. Olive oil burns more easily than other oils. Plus, you don't want to ruin the healthy properties of oils by heating them too much.

Buy an empty spray bottle. You can find these in department stores or kitchen specialty shops. (Do not use a bottle intended for a different use or that came pre-filled with anything except cooking oil.) This gives you the option to spritz instead of pour. For instance, toast whole-wheat baguette slices in the oven with just a spritz of oil on each slice. When golden brown and crisp, remove and top with tapenade (olive spread), pesto (basil spread), chopped tomatoes, or any topping of your choice.

Use mild yet flavorful extra-virgin olive oil in your homemade salad dressings. Using olive oil "raw" without heating preserves more of its nutrients. You can also drizzle it over pita sandwiches and use it in place of butter to flavor your cooked vegetables (including potatoes).

Substitute olive oil for butter in baking. Use light extra-virgin olive oil instead of butter or margarine in recipes for cakes, cookies, and breads. The flavor won't be exactly the same, but you'll be eliminating a lot of saturated fats. Keep this conversion information handy:

BUTTER	OLIVE OIL
1 teaspoon	3/4 teaspoon
1 tablespoon	2 1/4 teaspoons
1/4 cup	3 tablespoons
1/3 cup	1/4 cup
1/2 cup	1/4 cup + 2 tablespoons
1 cup	3/4 cup

Substitute olive oil for butter at the table. Instead of slathering saturated fats on your bread, try dipping it in oil. Pour a small amount of olive oil into a saucer or shallow bowl, and dip the bread lightly (you don't want to come away with a dripping mess). Experiment with flavors by adding a little balsamic vinegar, roasted garlic cloves, cracked pepper, or anything else you want to try.

Avoid "Bad" Fat and Lab Fat

Our bodies use the fats we eat to make cell walls. On a microscopic level, those cell walls are under continual attack from harmful oxygen molecule fragments called free radicals. Although all fats are vulnerable to attacks from free radicals, saturated fats are the easiest targets. If saturated fats are built into a cell wall, that cell is more likely to be damaged by free radicals, and that damage hastens the aging process of all cells, including brain cells.

Different fats create different types of cell walls, and the worst walls—stiff and rigid—are made from saturated and trans fats. Rigid walls can lead to insulin resistance and interfere with how well the cells function. In the brain, that means that brain cells with poor-quality walls have difficulty communicating.

To make matters worse, eating too many saturated fats can cause inflammation in the body and raise LDL ("bad") cholesterol. With all those brain-damaging consequences, you might think that eating saturated fats would cause real memory problems. You would be right. Studies show that people who eat a lot of saturated fat (think meat, butter, and cheese) have more than double the risk of age-related dementia and Alzheimer's disease as people who eat less of these fats.

It's easy to scope out saturated fats—almost all are found in animal products. Some of the worst offenders are fatty cuts of beef (especially ribs, sausage, bacon, bologna, and beef hot dogs), pork (except

Saturated Fat Content of Common Foods

FOOD	CALORIES FROM SATURATED FAT
T-bone steak, 6 ounces	106
Cheddar cheese, 1 ounce (a cube the size of a pair of dice)	82
Whole milk, 1 cup	72
Hamburger, 1 large fast food	72
Cheesecake, 1 slice	72
Croissant	63
1/2 fried chicken breast with skin	63
M&M's, 1 package	54
Pepperoni pizza, 1 slice	45
Hot dog	45
Ice cream, 1/2 cup	36
Butter, 1 pat	36
1 roasted chicken leg, no skin	18
1/2 roasted chicken breast, no skin	9
Skim milk, 1 cup	0

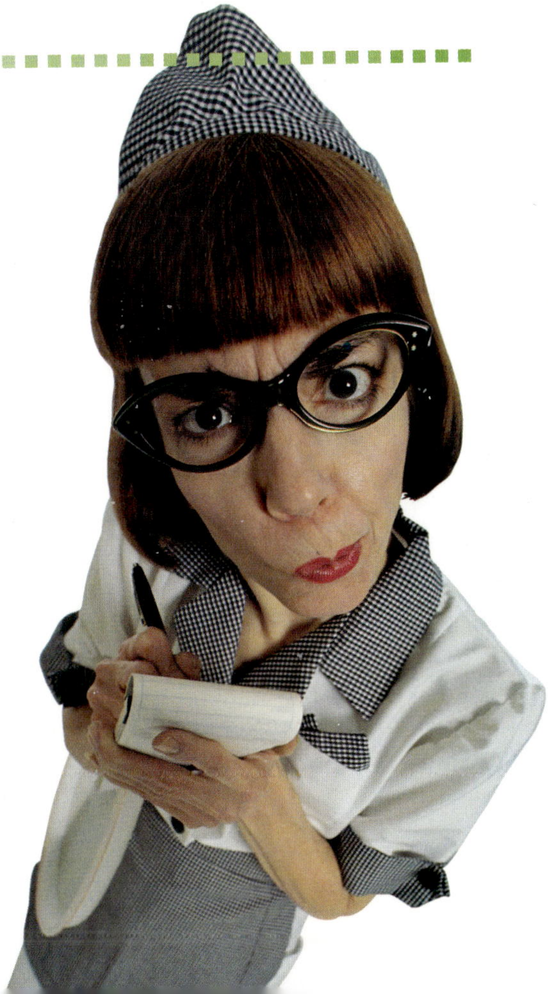

the leanest cuts), chicken skin and dark meat, whole milk, cream, cheese, butter, full-fat ice cream, and croissants. These foods should be eaten in very small quantities, and infrequently.

As dangerous as, or even more dangerous than, saturated fats are trans fats. These are found in nature only in infinitesimally small amounts. Most of the trans fats we eat are man-made. If you take a harmless liquid vegetable oil into a laboratory and twist the molecule a little, you get a form of fat that is solid at room temperature, lasts forever, and is absolute poison to the brain. Like saturated fats, trans fats make cell membranes rigid and interfere with neurons' ability to communicate with one another. Studies show that of all fats, trans fats cause the most damage and the greatest risk of developing dementia and Alzheimer's disease.

You can't cancel out the bad effects of trans fats—you have to eliminate them. If you simply add healthy fats to your diet without eliminating trans fats, the trans fats crowd out the other fats and bully their way into cell walls.

EAT SMART

Buy margarine that's free of trans fat. There are plenty of trans-fat-free brands on the market now. Read the label before you buy. Try one of the spreads made with plant stanols, such as Benecol and Take Control. These natural substances have been shown to reduce LDL ("bad") cholesterol, so they're actually good for you.

Avoid all foods with the word "hydrogenated" in the ingredients list. In the United States, food labels are required to list the amount of trans fats, so it is easier to know which products to avoid. But the system isn't perfect. Manufacturers are permitted to list trans fats as zero if the product contains less than a half-gram per serving—but even that's too much to safely consume. Bottom line: If the label says it contains hydrogenated or partially hydrogenated oil—as do most packaged baked goods, crackers, and other snack foods—don't eat it. Even if it's a seemingly healthy energy bar or granola bar. You'll find these oils in all sorts of foods masquerading as good-for-you foods.

Add avocado slices to your sandwich instead of cheese. You'll be trading brain-draining saturated fat for brain-boosting monounsaturated fat that helps control blood sugar and protect your heart and brain.

If you eat pie, make it one-crust. Unfortunately, there's no getting around the fact that pie crust is absolutely loaded with saturated fat (whether it's made from butter or lard) and trans fats (from shortening). It's nearly impossible to make a good pie crust without these ingredients, though some health-conscious bakers are turning to coconut oil for their crusts. Our advice: Make any food that involves pie crust a very special treat, and if you make pies, make the one-crust variety.

Say good-bye to fried. Many deep-fried foods are cooked in trans fats. As a rule of thumb—for the benefit of your brain and your waistline—say no to French fries, fried chicken, fried fish, potato chips, and anything else that leaves a greasy ring if it sits on a napkin.

Best Herbs for the Brain

Most herbs and spices have medicinal benefits, and a handful are thought to boost brain health. Aim to get more of these four in particular.

1 Turmeric

BRAIN BENEFIT

This mustard yellow powder is an antioxidant and a powerful anti-inflammatory. In India, where turmeric is eaten daily in curries, the risk of developing Alzheimer's is 25 percent lower than the risk in the U.S. In lab studies, mice that were fed curcumin (the active ingredient in turmeric) developed fewer amyloid plaques, associated with Alzheimer's, than rats that weren't.

EAT MORE

Add turmeric or curry powder to any curry dish and to egg salad. Include up to a teaspoonful in pea soup or your favorite lentil dish. Add turmeric to casseroles and in place of saffron in paella and Spanish rice.

2 Sage

BRAIN BENEFIT

A member of the mint family, sage is a known memory enhancer and may protect the brain against certain processes that lead to Alzheimer's. It may work by protecting acetylcholine, a chemical messenger in the brain that's critical to memory. In a British study, healthy young adults performed better on word recall tests after taking sage-oil capsules.

EAT MORE

Add to omelets, tomato sauce, butternut squash, roasted chicken or pork. Steep 2 teaspoons dried sage in just-boiled water for a strong cup of tea that provides a therapeutic dose.

3 Wasabi

BRAIN BENEFIT

Wasabi, a member of the mustard family, is the hot green condiment served with sushi. It's an excellent source (also found in horseradish and broccoli) of a compound found to help nerve cells grow extensions known as dendrites and axons, which help cells communicate with each other.

EAT MORE

Great on fish of any sort. In specialty stores, buy wasabi in a tube or as a powder. Add a little bit to ginger-, teriyaki-, or peanut-based sauces; deviled eggs; salad dressing; coleslaw; and crab cakes.

4 Garlic

BRAIN BENEFIT

Garlic thins the blood to help prevent blood clots and may slightly lower cholesterol. It contains compounds thought to protect neurons from injury and disease by stimulating the production of chemicals that help cells withstand stress.

EAT MORE

Add lots of minced garlic to just about any marinade or salad dressing. Add sautéed garlic to chicken, beef, pork, tofu, pasta, or vegetable dishes.

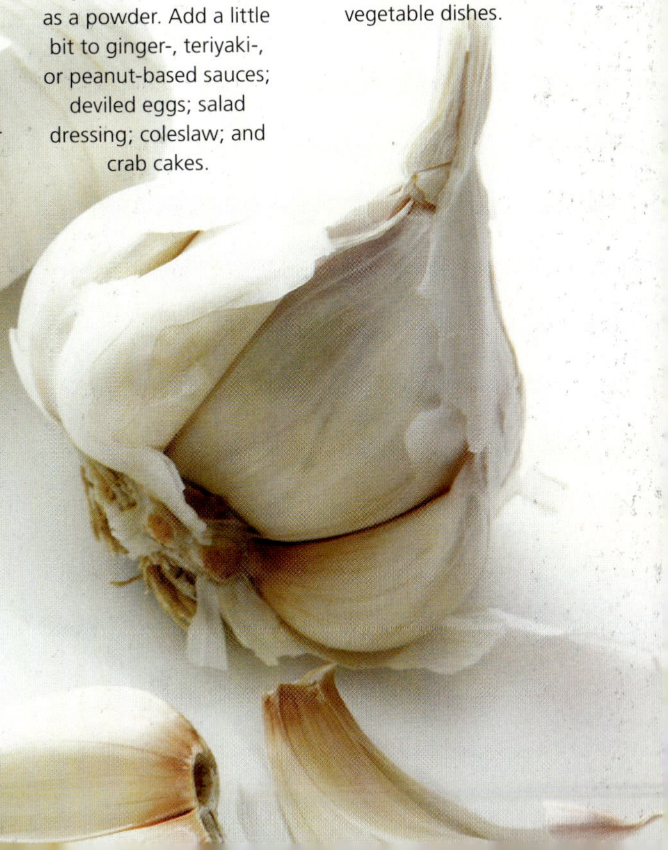

Garlic contains compounds thought to protect neurons from injury.

Limit saturated fats to less than 10 percent of your daily calories. For most people, that means no more than 150 to 250 calories per day can be devoted to saturated fats. See "Saturated Fat Content of Common Foods" on page 73 to get a sense of how much food that is. If you're counting grams of saturated fat, aim for less than 20 grams a day if you're on a 2,000-calorie-a-day diet. Bite the bullet and switch to skim milk. It contains 0 gram saturated fat per cup compared with 4.6 grams for whole milk—about as much as you'd get in a small broiled hamburger—and 1.5 grams for 1% milk.

DR. PERLMUTTER RECOMMENDS:

Vitamin E Supplements

Vitamin E is critically important for preserving brain function, yet it's difficult for people to get all the vitamin E they need from food. There have been scares about the potential for an increased risk of certain diseases linked to taking vitamin E supplements, but those studies involved synthetic vitamin E. Other studies indicate that natural vitamin E from mixed tocopherols is not dangerous and may provide significant brain benefits. Check with your doctor before starting any new supplement.

Dose: 400 IU (International Units) per day (do not take more than this).

Type: Look for labels with the words "mixed tocopherols".

Recommended brands: GNC, Carlson.

How to take: Take once a day. Store capsules in the refrigerator to keep them from becoming rancid.

Choose low-fat or no-fat dairy products. Milk, sour cream, yogurt, and cheese all come in lower-fat varieties with less saturated fat than full-fat varieties.

Eat no more than two meat servings each week. Pork, beef, lamb, and other red meats contain significant amounts of saturated fat. Chicken (skinless), turkey (skinless), bison, venison, and other game meats contain very little saturated fat, and therefore can be eaten every day.

When you eat meat, choose the leanest cuts. There are tricks to knowing the cuts with the least amount of saturated fats. Lean cuts have "loin" or "round" in the name, such as tender*loin*, sir*loin*, or beef *round*. Almost too obvious to mention: Remove excess fat before cooking.

If you eat ground beef, choose extra-lean (5% fat). You'll get 2.6 grams of saturated fat versus 6.1 for regular ground beef (25% fat).

Choose organic, free-range, hormone-free meats and poultry. They're more expensive for sure, but they're better for your brain. Artificially plumped chickens and meats may carry traces of growth drugs and hormones in their flesh—eat it and the toxins are carried into your system. Some act as direct poisons, while others simply increase inflammation in the body, including the brain.

Use nuts in place of meat. Nuts contain fats that are actively good for your brain. Try peanuts instead of meat in your next stir-fry.

Choose lower-fat cheeses. Many of us have tasted low-fat cheese in the past and proclaimed it inedible. But some perfectly good cheeses are lower in fat than others. Good choices are part-skim mozzarella, skim ricotta, low-fat feta, farmer cheese, and soft goat cheese. If you want to use low-fat cheddar, by it shredded (low-fat cheddar is difficult to shred, and doesn't taste great in blocks). Don't try to melt it in the toaster oven or broiler; it will turn rubbery. Instead, use it in sandwiches or add to casseroles. One ounce of low-fat cheddar contains 1.2 grams of saturated fat compared with 6 grams for regular cheddar.

Make Produce the Star of Your Meals

A study conducted by researchers from the Rush Institute for Healthy Aging in Chicago showed that people who ate just three servings of vegetables—any vegetables—per day slowed down the aging processes in their brains. Yes, it's that easy.

Aging anywhere in the body, including the brain, happens at the molecular level. Every day, our bodies naturally create destructive oxygen molecule fragments called free radicals. Left to their own devices, free radicals eat away at our healthy cells, damaging them through a process called oxidation. The only way to fight back is with antioxidants, plentiful in fruits and vegetables, as well as other foods, most notably, beans.

Everyone over age 5 knows that fruits and vegetables are important for good health, but we forget that "health" includes the health of our brains. Those apples and oranges and tomatoes and lettuce can help fight age-related dementia. In fact, eating plenty of fruits and vegetables can cut the risk of dementia and Alzheimer's disease in half.

Every fruit and every vegetable contains not just vitamins but also natural disease-fighting plant compounds called phytochemicals. Although scientists have known of the existence of these compounds for decades, it wasn't until the 1990s that they began to understand their enormous disease-fighting potential. There are thousands of different phytochemicals; a single apple has more than 100. That's why it's important to eat a wide variety of produce. Just about all fruits and vegetables are good for the brain, but a few seem to be especially effective against brain drain.

Broccoli and its cruciferous cousins. Sometimes called the odiferous cruciferous because of their tendency to cause gas, these vegetables include broccoli, cauliflower, Brussels sprouts, kale, mustard greens, watercress, collard greens,

Free radicals damage cells through oxidation. Fight back with antioxidants, which are plentiful in fruits and vegetables.

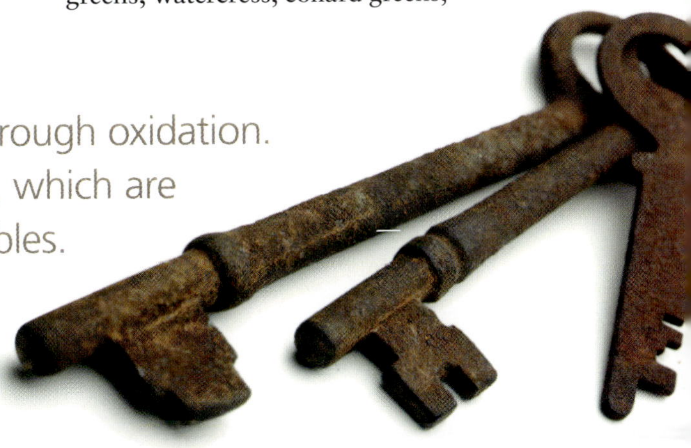

cabbage, and Swiss chard. Researchers from Harvard Medical School found that women who frequently ate cruciferous vegetables—already known to have cancer-fighting powers—had fewer memory problems than women who rarely ate them.

Blueberries, apples, and other produce rich in polyphenols. This large class of antioxidant compounds covers an alphabet soup of antioxidants including anthocyanins, quercetin, flavonoids, and hundreds of others. You don't need to know the names, just the foods, which include blueberries, strawberries, blackberries, raspberries, cherries, grapes, red onions, apples, oranges, bananas, red cabbage, red beets, onions, celery, grapefruit, avocadoes, and lettuce.

Blueberries have been celebrated as a top brain food because of studies conducted by researchers at the University of Barcelona. In the studies, old rats with memory problems were fed a diet of blueberries for 8 weeks. Even after such a short time on the blueberry diet, the rats showed improved memory, as measured by their ability to find their way through a maze. While the blueberry studies got a lot of press, that isn't the only food with brain-protective phytochemicals. Other studies have shown that neurons are protected by eating apples, bananas, oranges, strawberries, pomegranates, and spinach. So by all means, eat blueberries—but eat a variety of other fruits and vegetables, too.

Citrus fruits, nuts and seeds, and other foods rich in vitamins C or E. In a study published in 2005, researchers from the Rush Institute for Healthy Aging in Chicago reported that eating foods high in vitamin E appeared to reduce the risk of developing Alzheimer's disease by at least 25 percent. In other

Leafy greens, such as lettuce and spinach, are among the best vegetables for memory and cognition.

research, Utah State University scientists found that people who ate plenty of foods rich in vitamins C and E had better memories and cognitive function as they moved into old age than people who didn't eat such nutritious foods. Also, if they did experience cognitive decline, it happened more slowly.

Good food sources of vitamin C include citrus fruits, bell peppers, cantaloupe, strawberries, broccoli, kale, and leafy greens. Vitamin E is quite difficult to get from food but is most abundant in wheat germ, sunflower seeds, almonds, avocadoes, olive oil, and spinach.

Spinach, broccoli, and other foods rich in B vitamins. The B vitamins—especially vitamin B_6, vitamin B_{12}, and folate—are thought to help protect your memory by breaking down homocysteine, an amino acid involved in the inflammation of blood vessels. They are important for nerve health, and deficiencies can lead to sluggish thinking, memory problems, and age-related dementia. Some studies show that people who get enough of all B vitamins think faster and have better memories than those who don't. Researchers from Columbia University reported that eating a diet rich in folate (also known as folic acid or vitamin B_9) can reduce the risk of Alzheimer's disease by 50 percent, and researchers from South Korea found that folate deficiency tripled the risk of dementia.

Folate and vitamin B_6 are found in legumes, peanut butter, leafy green vegetables, broccoli and other cruciferous vegetables, strawberries, enriched cereals, and whole-grain breads. Vitamin B_{12} is found only in animal foods, which means that vegans should take supplements to avoid a deficiency. It is most plentiful in fish, shellfish, enriched soy milk, lean beef, cottage cheese, yogurt, eggs, and cheese.

The Brainiest Produce

All fruits and vegetables are good for you, but these are among the best for memory and cognition.

Cruciferous Veggies
- Broccoli
- Brussels sprouts
- Cabbage
- Cauliflower
- Kale
- Watercress

Leafy Greens
- Bok choy
- Collard greens
- Lettuce
- Mustard greens
- Spinach
- Swiss chard
- Turnip greens
- Seaweed

Legumes
- Chickpeas (garbanzo beans)
- Black beans
- Pinto beans
- Kidney beans
- White beans
- Navy beans
- Soybeans
- Peanuts

Other Vegetables
- Onions
- Tomatoes
- Peppers
- Avocadoes

Berries
- Blueberries
- Blackberries
- Raspberries
- Strawberries
- Boysenberries
- Cranberries

Citrus
- Oranges
- Grapefruit
- Lemons
- Limes
- Tangerines

Other Fruits
- Apples
- Bananas
- Cherries
- Persimmons
- Pomegranates
- Grapes
- Kiwifruit

EAT SMART

Eat at least three servings of vegetables per day. That seems to be the minimum number needed to maximize the brain-protective effects. The more you eat, the better. The exception is for starchy vegetables—including corn, potatoes, sweet potatoes, yams, and turnips—which cause a rise in blood sugar. Limit these to one serving per day.

Keep the brain doc away with apples. Apples are rich in brain-protecting polyphenols. Keep them visible—say, on the counter on a beautiful fruit plate—and you'll eat more of them.

Make leafy greens part of every day. Aim to eat a salad or steamed greens every day. And make a point to mix it up a bit—there is life beyond iceberg lettuce. Experiment a little, mixing a mild lettuce with a more flavorful variety.

- *Mild Flavors:* Boston, Bibb, Field greens, Green leaf, Red leaf, Romaine
- *Peppery:* Arugula
- *Slightly Bitter:* Belgian or French endive, Chicory, Escarole, Radicchio

Start dinner with a salad. It's a great way to squeeze in vegetables, and eating it first, before the main course, ensures that you'll get your fill.

Eat your spinach. It's an excellent source of folate, a B vitamin that helps lower levels of homocysteine. Enjoy it steamed as a side dish, in salads, and in omelets.

Serve your meals on a bed of greens. Simply steam some spinach, kale, or Swiss chard, then it put on your plate and place fish or chicken on top.

Learn to love cruciferous veggies. Put them on your menu at least once a week. If you don't eat them much now, add them slowly to your diet to avoid intestinal gas or bloating.

Dress bitter veggies in olive oil. Some people find certain vegetables—especially cruciferous veggies—too bitter. Instead of shunning these brain foods, dietitians recommend adding a little fat before serving to cut the bitter taste. And you're in luck—olive oil is a brain-healthy food. After cooking, top the veggies with a teaspoon to a tablespoon of olive oil and you'll get a double dose of memory-savers.

Shop often. If you pick an apple off the tree, it will have more nutrition than an apple you buy at the supermarket that may have spent weeks getting to the store. You may not be able to pick your own

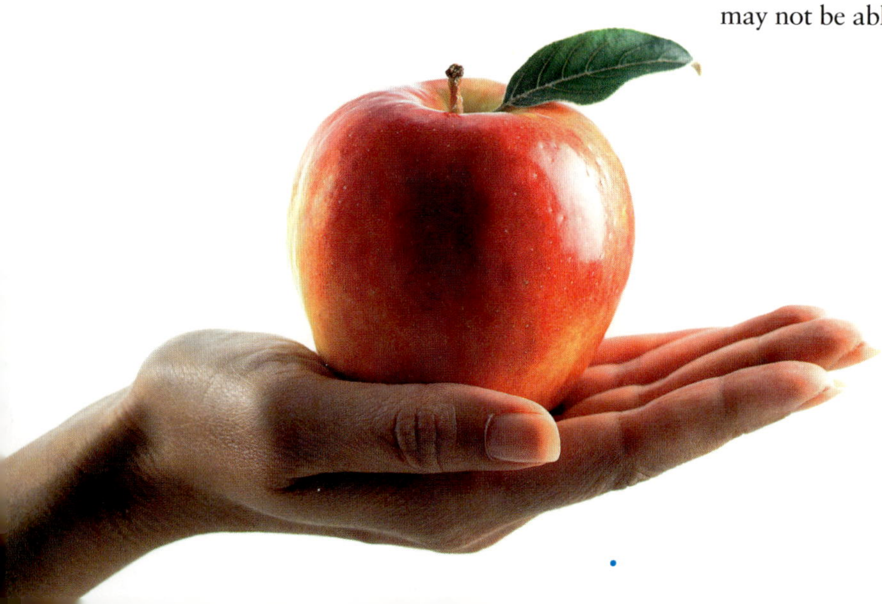

produce (though if you have access to a farmer's market, make good use of it), but you can aim to eat the produce quickly once you get it home. Shop European-style—purchase small quantities and go back to the store often rather than letting produce sit for a week in the crisper bin.

Fill the freezer. If you buy frozen fruits and vegetables with no additives—no sugar, salt, butter, cheese, sauce, or anything else—you'll have the convenience of frozen without risking rot. Because the produce is flash-frozen, nutrition experts say there is no difference in the quality of the vitamins and minerals you get.

Spend more for convenience. Vegetables come in so many pre-packaged forms now, eating them has never been quicker or simpler. Look for presliced or diced, premixed, or prewashed vegetables in the refrigerator section of the produce department. It's more expensive this way, but if it enables you to eat more produce (and perhaps keep you out of a nursing home one day), isn't it worth it?

Eat two to five servings of fruit per day. Fruit is packed with nutrition, but it is also full of natural sugar. Don't go overboard.

Experiment with different colors. Do you usually buy green bell peppers? Give red, orange, or yellow a try. Different colors indicate different phytochemicals, and it's best the get the widest variety possible.

Shred and add. Add vegetables to just about any dish by shredding them with a cheese grater or in a food processor. Shredded veggies cook quickly, and you won't have to dirty an extra pan. Add an extra handful of shredded carrots, zucchini, peppers, or spinach to egg dishes, sandwiches, casseroles, or rice.

When possible, choose organic. Organic fruits and vegetables are never sprayed with pesticides. Although there has been some question about whether the small amount of pesticide residue in and on produce grown conventionally can harm our health, recent research links food pesticides to neurological problems. For example, a 2006 study by researchers at Harvard University Medical School showed that chronic, low-dose exposure to pesticides increases the risk of Parkinson's disease by 70 percent. In addition, many studies have shown that organic produce contains higher levels of vitamins and minerals than nonorganic types. So while organic fruits and veggies are more expensive, they seem to be better for your health. If you can't afford organic all the time, spend your money on organic versions of these 10 items, found by the Environmental Working Group to contain the most pesticide residues: peaches, apples, bell peppers, celery, nectarines, strawberries, cherries, kale, lettuce, and imported grapes.

Have fruit for dessert. On those nights when you eat dessert (we suggest once or twice a week), try a roasted plum, 1/2 cup of berries with low-fat yogurt and a touch of honey on top, or a "baked" apple (core an apple, sprinkle the inside with cinnamon and a touch of sugar, and microwave for 3 minutes, or until soft).

Switch to Whole Grains

The brain is an awfully sensitive organ. One compound to which it's extremely sensitive is glucose, or blood sugar. Blood sugar is the brain's main source of fuel, but unlike muscles, the brain can't store extra sugar; it needs just the right amount at all times—a steady, even supply.

High levels are actually toxic to the brain. In 2008, researchers in the United Kingdom reported that people with uncontrolled high blood sugar had a risk of dementia that was nearly five times greater than the risk for people with normal blood sugar. And when people have uncontrolled diabetes with high blood glucose, memory loss is often one of the first symptoms.

High blood sugar levels and blood-sugar surges are bad for the brain even if you don't have diabetes. In fact, they actually shrink the hippocampus, involved in long-term memory storage. One way to avoid them and stay mentally sharp is to eat plenty of "good" fats, such as olive oil, at most meals. Another is to eat fewer refined grains (such as white rice) and more whole grains (such as oats and barley). Yes—this is again the Mediterranean diet in action.

Grains have three main parts: the bran (the protective skin, which contains most of the fiber), the germ (the unformed sprout, which contains most of the vitamins and minerals), and the endosperm (the starchy energy source). Whole-grain foods contain all three parts. When grains are refined, the most nutritious parts—the bran and the germ—are removed. All that's left is the starchy endosperm. The starch is valuable, but you need the whole grain to keep blood sugar in line.

EAT SMART

Ease into the whole-grain life. If you have had a hard time letting go of your "refined" ways, make the transition slowly. In a sandwich, start with one slice of whole-wheat bread and one slice of white bread. Mix white rice and brown rice, gradually increasing the amount of brown rice you serve. In your regular recipes for cookies, muffins, or quick breads, substitute up to one-third of the white flour with whole-wheat flour.

Start with the right breakfast. Eating breakfast in the morning is a good way to keep your blood sugar on an even keel throughout the day. But forget bagels,

What's in a Serving?

1 SERVING	EQUALS	SIZED UP AS
Chopped veggies	1/2 cup	What you can hold in a cupped hand
Legumes	1/2 cup	What you can hold in a cupped hand
Cooked leafy veggies	1/2 cup	What you can hold in a cupped hand
Raw leafy veggies	1 cup	Two handfuls, packed
Chopped fruit	1/2 cup	What you can hold in a cupped hand
Whole fruit	1	Individual piece of fruit

muffins, and white toast with jam. Instead, choose hot oatmeal or a whole-grain cereal with at least 5 grams of fiber per serving. Top it with fruit and chopped nuts or ground seeds for extra brain benefits.

Look for coarse whole-grain bread. Yes, you want to buy bread with the word "whole" in the first ingredient (as in whole wheat or whole rye). But you can go a step further. Even whole grains are digested faster (raising blood sugar faster) if they are finely ground. Coarsely ground whole-grain bread, with specks of kernels in it, is your ideal choice.

Choose whole-grain versions of everything. A lot of manufacturers have begun to make whole-wheat alternatives to your favorite foods, including breads, English muffins, buns, rolls, pitas, crackers, waffles, and pasta.

Swap barley for rice. Even brown rice, while it's still good for you, raises blood sugar levels quite a bit. Once in a while, have barley instead. Because it contains a great deal of soluble fiber, its impact on blood sugar in minimal. Add it to casseroles and soups, and use it in salads and pilafs.

Make a whole-grain side dish on Sundays. Most of us don't have as much time to cook on weeknights, so prepare a whole-grain side dish for Sunday dinner, make extra, and enjoy it through Wednesday. Try a barley and black bean salad, a barley and chickpea salad, or a quinoa salad with chickpeas and tomatoes.

Get your fill of canned beans and lentils. These contain complex carbohydrates and a significant amount of protein. And all beans, except black-eyed peas, are gentle on blood sugar.

Three Great Grains

Bulgur This quick-cooking grain is nothing more exotic than wheat kernels that have been dried and cracked. To cook, boil 2 cups water, add 1 cup bulgur, and simmer for 10 to 13 minutes, until all liquid is absorbed.

Quinoa Quinoa is a sweet, light, fluffy grain with a slightly nutty flavor. Cook the same as bulgur (above).

Whole-wheat couscous Couscous is simply spherical granules of pasta. To cook, boil 1 cup water, add 1 cup couscous and turn off heat immediately. Cover and let sit for 5 minutes, then fluff with a fork and serve.

Drop Sugar to Prevent "Brain Decay"

Could a serious soda habit or a cookie addiction be leading your brain down the path to slowdowns and decline? It's entirely possible. In fact, researchers have demonstrated exactly how bad a junk-food diet can be for the brain. They studied rats instead of people, but it's not a huge leap to see how the results apply to all of us.

Scientists from the University of California, Los Angeles, fed some of the rodents a healthy diet and others a high-fat, high-sugar diet. Some of the rats were allowed exercise, some were not. Then they all were tested in a swimming pool (rat-size, of course) to see how well they remembered the location of a platform. The junk-food-only rats who didn't exercise had virtually no memory and swam randomly around the pool. They were found to have a reduced level of the chemical known as brain-derived neurotrophic factor, or BDNF, the "Miracle-Gro" brain chemical that stimulates the growth and proliferation of brain cells and is critical to long-term memory. The junk-food rats who exercised performed somewhat better, but the rats that ate well and exercised did the best of all.

One problem with sweets and sugary drinks is their effect on glucose. Most of them trigger blood-sugar swings that are toxic to brain cells. And, of course, they can lead to weight gain and contribute to the development of diabetes, stroke, and cardiovascular disease—all bad for the brain.

EAT SMART

Eat regular meals. If you allow yourself to become too hungry by going too long between meals, you'll be more likely to reach for something sweet for a quick sugar high. You should go no longer than 4 to 5 waking hours without a healthy meal or snack.

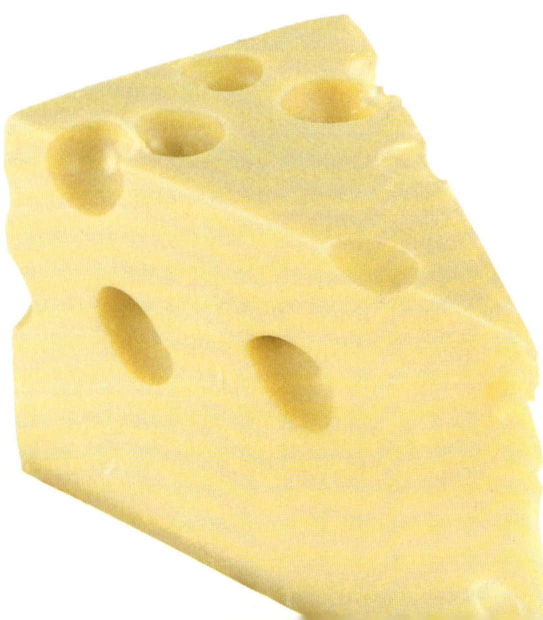

Curb Your Enthusiasm for These Foods

These send blood sugar soaring.

- Hot cooked potatoes
- White rice
- Sticky rice
- Udon noodles
- White bread
- Muffins

Keep fruit handy at all times. One reason we reach for cookies and candy is because they're available everywhere we turn. Try finding fruit in a vending machine! Surmount the problem by keeping a fruit bowl on your kitchen counter, sticking an apple in your bag when you leave the house, and stocking up on mini-boxes of raisins (they contain much more sugar than grapes, but eating them is still better than eating candy).

Keep sweets hidden. The saying "out of sight, out of mind" is true when it comes to sweets. If you keep a little "welcome" bowl of candy on your desk at work, you (and everyone else) will be certain to indulge. You'll be more likely to stay away from it if you keep it stashed away inside a drawer in another room.

Never buy in bulk. Although you may pay half as much for that giant family-

In an experiment, a high-fat, high-sugar diet poked holes in the memories of rats.

size bag of cookies, food researchers have calculated that you'll eat them twice as fast! So basically, you're saving pennies to gain more pounds. (Puts a whole new spin on "penny-wise, pound-foolish," doesn't it?)

Never do sugar solo. When you do eat sugary foods, eat them either immediately after a meal or with a food that contains fiber or protein to delay the absorption of the sugar. It will help take the top off the sugar spike.

Make dessert a special treat. Who ever said that dessert was meant to be eaten daily? Parents of young kids often serve dessert as a reward for eating dinner but, for adults especially, good food should be its own reward. When you do want a little something sweet to finish off a meal, do what the Mediterraneans do: Serve fruit. Think poached pears, berries in low-fat yogurt with a touch of honey, or cherry clafoutis (baked fruit pudding).

Booze for the Brain

While too much alcohol is poison to the brain, studies have shown that people who have one to two drinks a day have a lower risk of memory loss and half the risk of Alzheimer's disease than teetotalers. It may be because alcohol thins the blood, helping to prevent blood clots that can block blood flow to the brain. Alcohol also increases "good" (HDL) cholesterol. One drink is 5 ounces of wine, 12 ounces of beer, or 1.5 ounces of 100-proof liquor.

Avoid sodas, sports drinks, and other sugary beverages. Read the ingredient labels of beverages. If it contains sugar, dextrose, fructose, corn syrup, or other sweeteners, avoid it.

Drink water with a twist of lemon or lime. This may add just enough flavor and interest to keep you away from flavored waters that are loaded with sugar.

Avoid artificial sweeteners. Some people report side effects of artificial sweeteners that include dizziness and confusion. Even if this happens only in ultra-sensitive individuals, it is a sign that artificial sweeteners have some effect on brain cells. In rats, drinking aspartame-flavored water for 4 months caused memory problems—the rats took much longer working their way through a maze than rats who drank unflavored water.

Drink fruit juice in small doses. Fruit is full of sugar but it also has lots of fiber that helps to delay the body's absorption of the sugar. Fruit juice, on the other hand, has no fiber. It does contain vitamins and phytochemicals, making it much better for you than soda, but stick to no more than 6 ounces at a time or you may experience a blood-sugar rush.

Indulge in tea. Green and black teas are full of phytochemicals called catechins. Research has shown that green tea extracts can improve memory and learning in old rats, and may be helpful in reversing age-related deficits. Feel free to drink 2 to 3 cups of tea—green or black—every day.

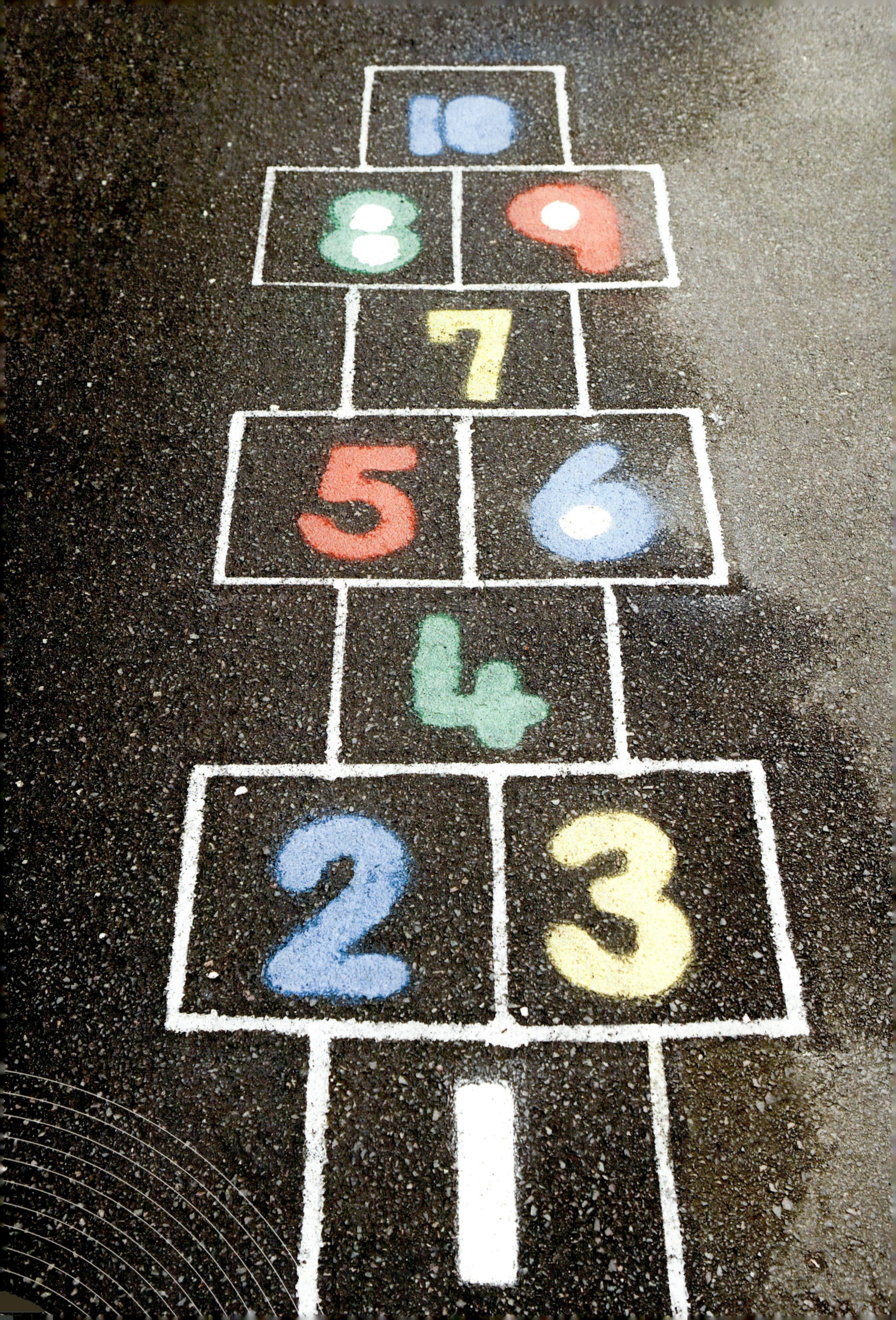
10
8
9
7
5
6
4
2
3
1

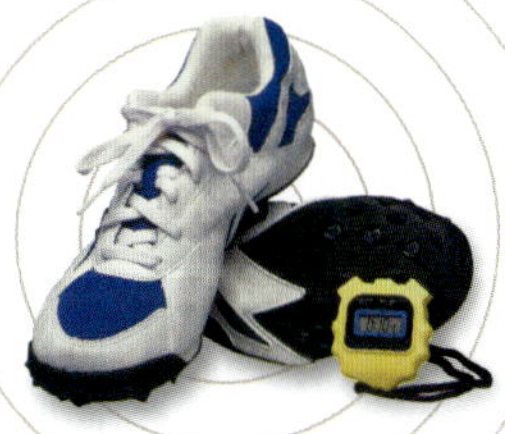

VACCINE #2
exercise

By now, you know that exercising your mind is one of the most effective ways to combat brain drain and to even help stave off dementia. Yes, a crossword a day can help keep the brain doctor away! But exercising your body may be every bit as important. In fact, just as physical exercise can make your biceps bigger and your lung power stronger, it can also increase your brain's size, strength, and endurance.

The greatest neurological benefit of exercise: increased oxygen. The brain soaks up 20 percent of all the oxygen in your body. When it doesn't get enough, brain cells can suffocate and die, causing the overall size of the brain to shrink—a warning sign of dementia and Alzheimer's disease. Exercise increases blood flow to your entire body, including your brain, and that blood carries with it the oxygen your brain so badly needs.

One way that exercise increases blood flow is by encouraging the lining of your blood vessels to produce nitric oxide, or NO. Thought to play an important role in learning and memory, NO also dilates arteries, increasing blood flow. It happens to be the biological basis of a certain sexual performance drug. Exercise is your brain on Viagra!

As critical as it is to get plenty of oxygen to your noggin, exercise does even more to help you prevent brain drain.

How Exercise Puts a Spring in Your Mental Step

Many of the same health problems that lead to heart disease—high blood pressure, high cholesterol, diabetes—also increase the risk of dementia. All of these conditions decrease blood flow to the brain, and they put you in danger of having a stroke, another major risk factor for cognitive decline. Yet all of them are either partially or completely reversible with exercise. Still, the advantages of exercise don't stop there. Here are a few more ways in which exercise can sharpen your brain power.

It grows your brain. As we get older, the birth of new brain cells slows, and our brain tissue actually shrinks. But exercise can reverse that trend. In fact, researchers at the University of Illinois found that after 3 months of getting just a few hours of aerobic exercise weekly, study subjects' brains grew to a size equivalent to that of people 3 years younger. Their number of brain cells increased dramatically, especially in the frontal lobe, where much of learning and memory making takes place. The connections between brain cells also increased, especially in the corpus callosum, a structure that connects the two hemispheres of the brain and allows them to speak to each other, enhancing creativity and efficiency of thought.

It increases your sensitivity to insulin. When you eat, your body turns most of the food into glucose, or blood sugar, the main source of fuel for your body, including your brain. In order for that glucose to enter cells, it must be escorted by the hormone insulin. Unfortunately, in some people, cells become resistant to insulin. The body has to pump out more and more of it, and still blood sugar levels rise, often resulting in (you guessed it) diabetes. Even if you don't end up with diabetes, insulin resistance is bad for your brain. When brain cells are flooded by glucose, bad things happen that can affect memory and thinking.

Regular exercise can actually reverse insulin resistance. In fact, your insulin sensitivity increases—stabilizing your blood sugar after you eat—for at least 16 hours after a single exercise session. If your brain cells are drowning in blood sugar, exercise is like pulling the stopper on the drain. The better your blood-sugar control, the less likely your brain is to develop the plaques that are the hallmark of Alzheimer's disease.

It boosts brain-building hormones. Much like Miracle-Gro plant food makes plants grow faster and lusher,

10 Brain Benefits of Exercise

1. Faster processing speed
2. Sharper thinking
3. Lower dementia risk
4. Increased rate of cell birth and growth
5. Reversal of age-related cognitive decline
6. Improved recall
7. Faster decision making
8. Enhanced focus and decreased distractibility
9. Stronger multitasking ability
10. Faster reaction time

the chemical known as brain-derived neurotrophic factor, or BDNF, stimulates the growth and proliferation of brain cells. This is especially true in the hippocampus, a brain region that is largely responsible for memory and that is particularly vulnerable to age-related cognitive decline. The more you exercise, the more BDNF you produce.

It fights depression and anxiety. Depression slows the brain's processing of information, makes it more difficult to concentrate and make decisions, and causes real memory problems. For serious depression, your doctor may prescribe antidepressants. For milder cases, however, exercise has been shown to work wonders. It cranks up the body's production of serotonin and dopamine, two neurotransmitters crucial to upbeat, motivated moods. And it boosts levels of the feel-good chemicals called endorphins.

It erases the effects of stress. If some hormones make the brain younger, others age the brain. These include the so-called stress hormone cortisol. Slow, scattered thinking and forgetfulness are caused by stress more often than we may realize. Exercise lowers cortisol levels, helping you think straight again. It is also believed to generate new nerve cells in the part of the brain called the dentate gyrus, an area linked to the creation of new memories. Brain cells in this area are seriously depleted during times of stress.

It improves your brain's "executive function." Executive function isn't reserved just for CEOs; everyone uses

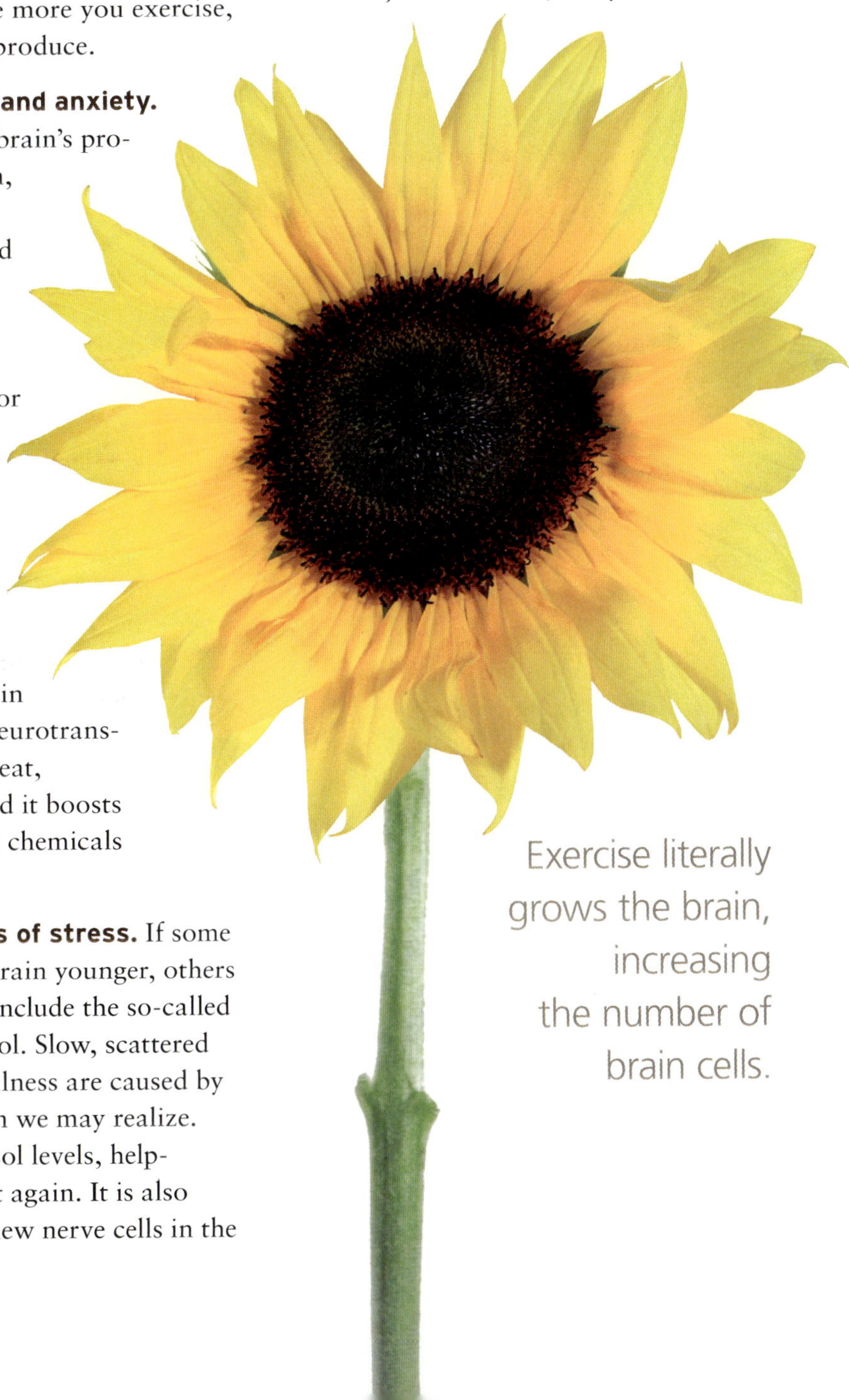

Exercise literally grows the brain, increasing the number of brain cells.

it every day. Essentially, it's the cognitive abilities that enable us to act like grown-ups, including the ability to focus on complex tasks, to organize, to choose behavior that's appropriate to a given situation, to think abstractly, to meet deadlines, and to plan for future events. It also encompasses working memory, such as the ability to keep a phone number in your head while you dial.

When researchers set out to analyze the effects of exercise on executive function, they looked at 18 well-designed studies and found that, in men and women ages 55 to 80, those who did regular exercise (particularly a combination of cardio and strength training) performed four times better on cognitive tests than the studies' control groups, who didn't exercise regularly. They improved their individual scores by a solid 50 percent regardless of the type of cognitive task. The effects were greatest among those who had exercised 30 to 45 minutes each session for longer than 6 months, but substantial benefits showed up after only 4 weeks of exercise. The caveat? Exercising less than 30 minutes per session has virtually the same brain impact—not much—as doing no exercise.

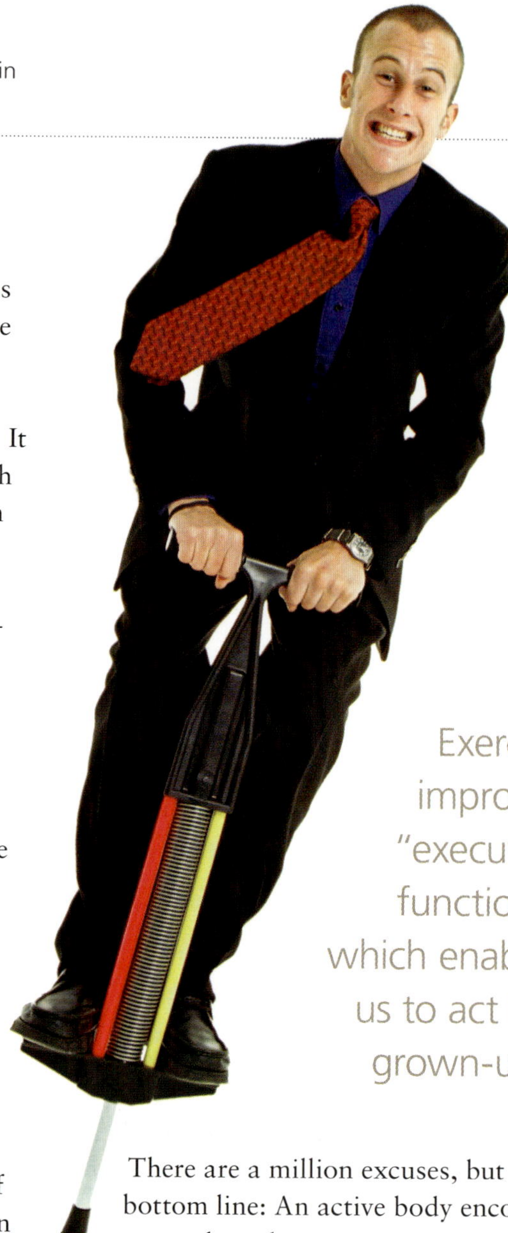

Exercise improves "executive function," which enables us to act like grown-ups.

Ready, Set, Start

We've all been there: Even when you know all the good reasons to exercise, it can still be hard to get off the couch. You can't find the time, the motivation, or the "right" sneakers to get out the door. Perhaps you haven't exercised in a while and you're afraid of looking or feeling foolish. There are a million excuses, but one bottom line: An active body encourages a sharp brain.

If you think about exercise as a chore, chances are you'll never do it. So, the trick is to find ways to make it fun, easy, and invigorating. Before you know it, exercise will become an addictive habit that makes you happier, calmer, and smarter, not to mention thinner, healthier, stronger, and more energetic.

Start with just 10 minutes. It may not be enough to boost cognitive function, but it offers plenty of other benefits. Research published in the *Journal of the American*

Medical Association found that overweight, postmenopausal women who exercised an average of 10 minutes a day had more energy, less anxiety, and were simply happier than they had been before they started their exercise programs. And their bodies' ability to use oxygen during exercise increased by more then 4 percent in 6 months.

Pull on your sneaks, walk out your door, and head down the street for 5 minutes. After 5 minutes, turn around and come home. Repeat daily, adding a minute each day. There—you're exercising!

Burn calories any way you wish. Don't like to exercise in a formal way? That's fine; anything you do to burn calories will yield benefits. One study found that for every 1,700 calories women burned in a week, they experienced a 14 percent less risk of cognitive decline. That's the number of calories you'd burn playing one round of golf, vacuuming for an hour, or dancing around your living room for a half-hour every day. As an added bonus, you'll lose 1/2 pound a week without a single change to your diet.

Do something you love. The more you enjoy your chosen form of physical activity, the more you'll do it. If you have a passion for flowers, take regular walks around the botanical garden. If used to love riding your bike as a kid, dust off the old two-wheeler (or rent a bike for a week if you don't have one) and take a spin. If you still enjoy the wind in your hair, find a way to work regular bike rides into your schedule. Like to swim? Check out the water aerobic classes at the local YMCA, or consider buying a membership to an outdoor pool in the summer. Most have "adult swim" for 15 minutes every hour, the perfect amount of time for a mini-workout. You may even make some new friends—all activities that delight and excite your brain.

Treat it like a daily prescription. If you have pre-diabetes—and many people do without knowing it—your condition can trigger changes in the blood vessels in your brain and cause problems with thinking even before you are diagnosed with full-blown diabetes. But you can stop the progression with exercise. The Diabetes Prevention Program, a major clinical trial involving more than 3,000 people, found that people with pre-diabetes reduced their risk of developing diabetes by more than 58 percent when they walked for 2 1/2 hours each week (that's 30 minutes a day for 5 days), reduced their calorie intake only slightly, and lost 5 to 7 percent of their body weight. The researchers actually had to cut the trial short by a year; the lifestyle intervention group was doing so much better than the drug intervention and placebo groups that it wouldn't have been ethical to continue.

Do 10 chair squats each time you stand up or sit down. One study in the *Journal of the American Medical Association* classified the ability to get up out of an armless chair as one of the best markers of overall health and degree of functioning as we age. Yet, as we get older, some of us tend to fall into chairs and then struggle out of them. Stay strong and in control with chair squats; they may not keep your brain sharp, but strengthening your quadriceps and stomach muscles will make other types of exercise more possible, safe, and even fun.

To do a chair squat: Position yourself directly in front of the chair, facing away from it. Keeping your back straight, bend your knees and lower your body until the back of your thighs hit the chair. Immediately straighten to a standing position and start over. Once you've done 10 squats, sit down. Repeat when you get out of the chair.

MAKE IT SOCIAL

Team up with a buddy. Exercising with a friend makes you more accountable, so you're more likely to stick to a regular routine; you may even challenge each other to walk farther or otherwise ratchet up your workouts. Your walking partner is more than just an exercise insurance policy: As you walk, you're also talking, listening, or recounting a story from last night—in short, many regions of your brain are being engaged at one time. Recruit a friend who's on a similar schedule and within walking distance of your house; you can start each walk by meeting midway between your homes. If none of your closest pals are up for walking in your neighborhood, join a walking club.

Join a club. Simply having an active social network is highly beneficial to the brain, and participating in group activities is one surefire way to cultivate yours. If you play tennis, join a tennis club or sign up at the local courts for a doubles partner. Bowling? Have a ball with the gang. There are even mall-walker clubs and stroller clubs for new moms—something for everyone.

MAKE IT CONVENIENT

Use a bike to get around town. Put a basket on the front of a cruiser bike, buy a helmet, and you have an excellent way to get around town, save gas, and keep your brain and body young at the same time. Many towns have bike safety classes in which you can learn about the basics of handling traffic, signaling, and changing a flat tire. Learning the rules and tackling fears about navigating the roads will help you gain confidence to take on other challenges, a brain-saving tactic with lifelong effects.

Do short workouts throughout the day. If you can't devote a 30- to 45-minute block of time to exercise, don't! It's that simple. Instead, walk or do some other form of physical activity, like riding a stationary bike or doing sit-ups and push-ups, for 10 minutes several times a day. Some research suggests that doing multiple workouts throughout the day yields even larger releases of growth hormone and BDNF throughout the day.

Make a list of five active things you can do in your community. Post it on the fridge and let it prompt you on weekends when you're bored. For example, you could walk or bike to a local park for a picnic, hoof it to the library and check out the used-book sale, pick your own produce, visit a local museum or flea market, or volunteer with a local charity group to paint houses or pick up trash.

MAXIMIZE THE BRAIN BENEFITS

Don't be afraid of sweat. If you've already started an exercise program, don't be afraid to push yourself a bit,

Strength Training Versus Cardio

What's better for your brain, lifting weights or cardio? For optimal overall health, you want a mix of both, but aerobic (cardio) exercise is the clear winner when it comes to stopping brain drain.

One fascinating study randomly assigned a group of 59 men and women to either an aerobics-focused program or a stretching and strength-training program. After 6 months, sophisticated brain scans using functional magnetic resonance imaging (fMRI) showed that the aerobically fit adults had significantly more activity in the frontal cortex of the brain, the region associated with executive function (planning and long-term memory storage), as well as the parietal cortex, the seat of spatial orientation—two areas often associated with age-related cognitive decline.

While cardio does increase blood flow to the brain, that's not the whole reason for aerobics' impressive effects.

Instead, the researchers believe that many of the positive changes could be attributed to an increase in BDNF, the "Miracle-Gro" brain hormone. The brain that enjoys cardiovascular training, the researchers say, is "more efficient, plastic, and adaptive, which translates into better learning and performance." Not too shabby for a daily walk around town.

with your doctor's okay. When you increase the intensity of your workouts, you boost the amount of feel-good endorphins and growth hormone your body releases. Growth hormone triggers the release of that brain-building, depression-fighting protein BDNF.

One way to increase intensity is to try a faster pace in brief 1-minute bursts during your workout. For example, you might increase the incline on your treadmill for 1 minute, then lower it again for 4 minutes, and repeat until you're done with your workout. This kind of "interval" workout burns more calories and helps your body burn even more calories for several hours afterward.

Do your exercise in the sun. Hitting the treadmill is great, but if you can get outside, it's even better. Bright sunlight exposes you to 50,000 to 100,000 lux of light, versus the 400 lux of an average living room light. This natural light helps your brain create the chemicals that stave off seasonal blues and gives you more restful sleep; it also reacts with your skin to help your body generate vitamin D. Once converted to its active form, calcitriol, vitamin D binds to receptors in the brain and spurs the release of a powerful protein, known as glial cell line-derived neurotrophic factor, or GDNF, thought to prolong the life of several kinds of brain cells. Calcitriol may also reduce the production of inflammatory chemicals, called cytokines, that contribute to age-related cognitive decline.

Mix it up. Variety is key to keeping the brain agile, whether that variety comes in the form of unique mental challenges or physical challenges. Novel exercises excite the brain in the same way that novel experiences do; any time you surprise or challenge your brain, you build new and stronger connections between nerve cells. Games like basketball or tennis, in which you have to react quickly, draw on both hemispheres of the brain and help improve your reflexes and reaction time. Your muscles love novelty, too, so switch your activities as often as possible—say, from walking to biking to swimming to gardening. Look for an aerobics instructor who changes up her routine often, or add a new class, such as yoga or Pilates, to the mix.

Learn the tango. Or ballroom dancing, line dancing—heck, the Hustle! When you learn any type of dance, you not only challenge your muscles in new ways, you also challenge your brain to concentrate and count, remember the sequence of steps and how to do them, and react to your partner, all tasks that force your brain to remain limber and make new neural connections. Many community centers offer low-cost, ongoing dance lessons. City parks sometimes offer free lessons and live music on summer nights. You'll also meet a whole new group of people with whom to socialize, an extra brain-building draw that can be an added motivation to hit the dance floor.

Try some yoga or tai chi. Chronic stress is toxic to the brain. Exercise of any sort helps reduce stress, but yoga and tai chi may be especially effective. Research has found that meditative exercises such as these help to reduce circulating levels of cortisol, a stress hormone known to hasten cognitive decline. And, of course, these exercise forms are good for you in other ways. In one small study published in the *British Journal of Sports Medicine*, participants who did tai chi and qigong (often described as moving meditation) three times a week for 12 weeks significantly lowered their body mass indexes, waist circumferences, and blood pressure levels, all risk factors for cognitive decline. Their bodies became more sensitive to insulin and they reduced their circulating blood sugar, lowering their risk of developing diabetes, another risk factor for dementia.

The Perfect No More Brain Drain Exercise: Walking

Walking is an ideal exercise for brain health. It's free, easy, and can be done virtually anywhere. The brain benefits begin virtually the moment you start and add up significantly over time. According to one American Academy of Neurology study, for every mile you walk each day, you not only burn 100 calories but you also decrease your risk of cognitive decline by 13 percent. You won't get *that* from watching the evening news!

In the famous Nurses' Health Study of more than 18,000 women, long-term regular physical activity, including walking, was associated with significantly better cognitive function and less cognitive decline in older women. The most active women were 20 percent less likely to experience cognitive impairment than the least active women. Women who walked at an easy pace for just 90 minutes a week scored much higher than those who walked less than 40 minutes a week. Even after the results were adjusted for all other

Walk This Way

You've likely been walking since you could say "Mama," but if you're like most adults, your form may not have improved much since then. When you start your walking program, follow these guidelines.

Pretend you're a marionette.
Imagine that a string is holding up your head as you walk. Keep your neck elongated and your chin parallel to the ground, your shoulders down and back.

Watch where you're going.
Many of us tend to stare at our feet as we walk, but that throws your neck and back out of alignment. Instead, point your nose forward and keep your eyes aimed about 10 feet in front of you.

Keep your core solid.
Tuck in your belly and pelvis, and feel your tailbone pull under slightly. Don't arch your back—instead, think of your entire trunk as one solid block. This stance not only helps develop your abdominal muscles but also will help prevent extra strain on your lower body.

Pretend you're on skis.
Start with your feet shoulder-width apart and aim to maintain that distance as you walk. Consider using walking poles; they help absorb shock and deflect it from your joints, improve your balance, and help you maintain proper form. Plus, you burn up to 40 percent more calories when you use them.

Think fast.
And small. Bend your arms at a 90-degree angle and pump them while you keep your stride short and quick—you'll cover more ground and burn more calories in the same amount of time.

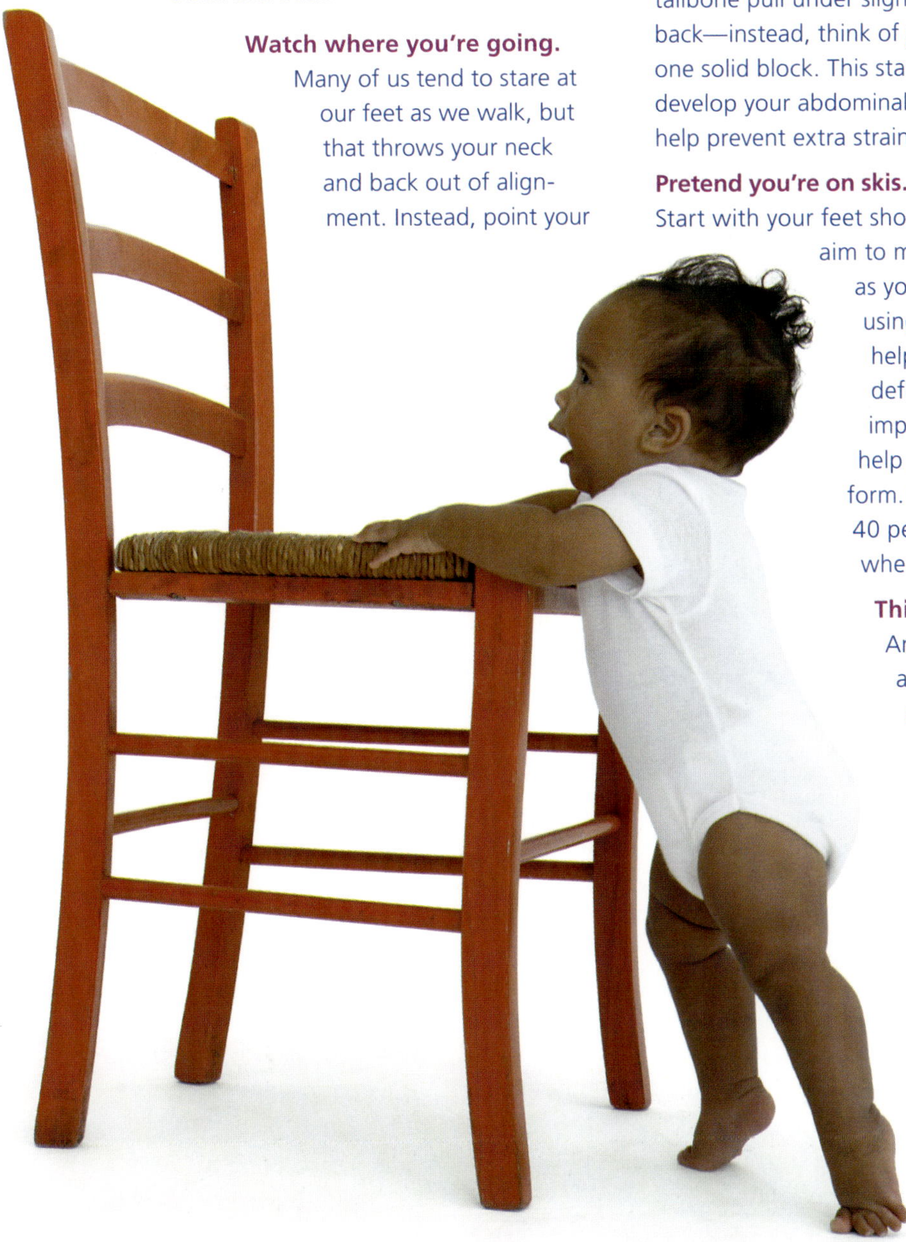

factors—age, education, smoking status, antidepressant use—those who walked the most had cognitive performance equal to that of women 3 years younger.

Sold? Good. Now, how do you get started on a regular plan? Several different paths will take you to the same destination—a stronger, healthier, younger brain.

Just open up the door. See "The No More Brain Drain Walking Program" on the opposite page to learn a simple strategy that starts with just 10 minutes of walking a day and builds up to 30 minutes a day. Or you can track miles or steps instead of minutes.

The Sole Equipment You Need

Walking requires zero equipment; you could go barefoot if you really wanted to. But having the right walking shoes can go a long way to keeping your feet happy as well as your knees and hips. To find the perfect pair, shop at a running store. Most stores that specialize in running shoes have staff members who know a tremendous amount about footwear and feet in general. They'll measure your feet, look at your old sneakers, watch you walk, ask questions, and recommend shoes that are uniquely suited to your feet. Tell them about your walking plans as well as any special issues such as diabetes or osteoporosis.

Don't skimp! Your joints depend on your shoes to absorb much of the impact when you walk, so invest in a good pair. If you can afford to, spend at least $75. Regardless of how new they might look, you need to buy a new pair of shoes every 350 to 500 miles, or every 3 to 6 months. Write a reminder on your calendar, perhaps timed to coincide with bi-yearly dentist appointments, so you don't forget.

Do a little every day. When you first start out, consistency is more important than time spent. Plan to do your 10 minutes at a time when you'll be available each day, such as after breakfast or lunch or right before the evening news—and don't skip it. Your top priority is to make it a regular part of your day. Once you've established a solid routine, then you can start adding on extra minutes.

Buy a pedometer. Who doesn't love a new toy? These gadgets are fun and provide a great gauge of how much movement you get during the day. They count every step you take, and some track miles as well. Start a mini-contest with your spouse or child to see who can pack more steps in a day. Just a 2-minute round-trip out to the mailbox can net you 200 steps; a 10-minute walk with the dog, another 1,000. Set a goal to add at least 300 extra steps each day until you reach 10,000, the equivalent of 5 miles.

Walk a 2-mile loop. A study published in the *Journal of the American Medical Association* found that older men were almost twice as likely to develop dementia if they walked less than 1/4 mile a day than if they walked 2 miles a day. Measure out a 2-mile loop in your car, and make walking that route a daily habit. If you have hills in your neighborhood, start on a downhill to make it easier to begin, or do the uphill first and "earn" that downhill stride at the end.

Shoot for 25 blocks a day. If you live in a city, walking is plenty easy—you probably have flat, well-kept, well-lit sidewalks and an easy-to-navigate city grid to work with. Start with 5 blocks a

The No More Brain Drain Walking Program

Several studies have found that a regular walking program is all you need to cut your risk of cognitive decline in half. Tracking your progress is a proven motivator, yet everyone likes to note their walks differently—some prefer to chart the minutes, others the miles. No matter how you measure them, daily walks work out to much less brain drain. The important thing is to just get out the door. Each of these three programs gets you to add roughly 2 extra miles of walking to your regular day (most people already walk 3 "base" miles) by the end of 5 weeks. Choose your metric, lace up your sneakers, and hit the bricks!

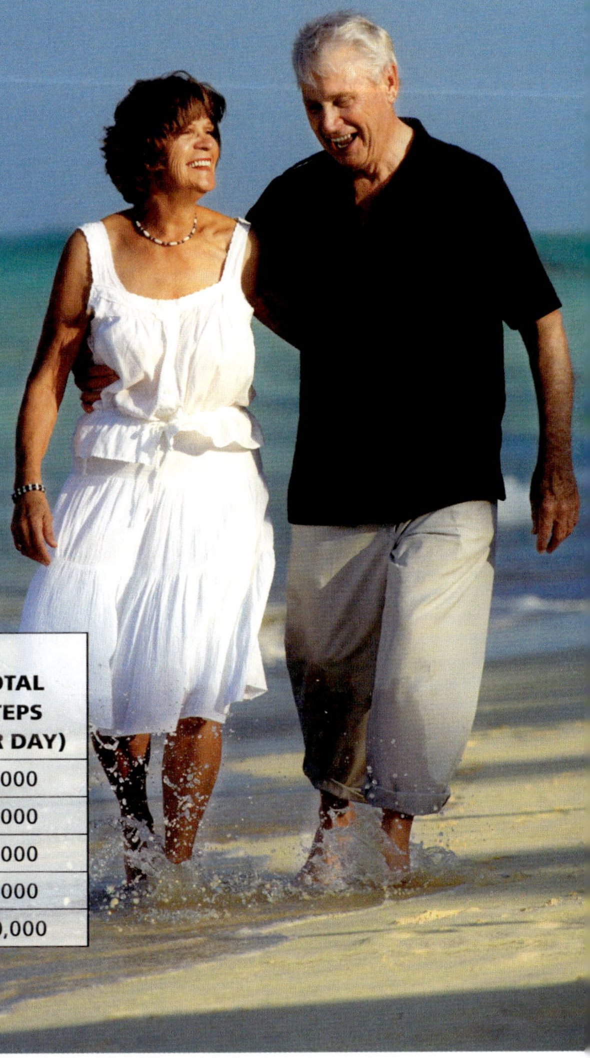

WEEK	MINUTES OF DEDICATED WALKING (PER DAY)	MILES OF DEDICATED WALKING (PER DAY)	TOTAL STEPS (PER DAY)
1	10	.25	2,000
2	15	.50	4,000
3	20	.75	6,000
4	25	1	8,000
5	30	2	10,000

day and add 5 more each week until you get to 25. Use the opportunity to scope out new restaurants or shops. Turn in a different direction each time you leave the house and challenge yourself to find a new route every day. One study of almost 6,000 women found that those who walked 175 blocks a week were 35 percent less likely to experience cognitive decline than women who walked only 7 blocks a week. If you don't live in a city, make use of your closest mall in the same way; many have walking routes marked off in 1/10-mile increments, so you can see how much distance you've covered.

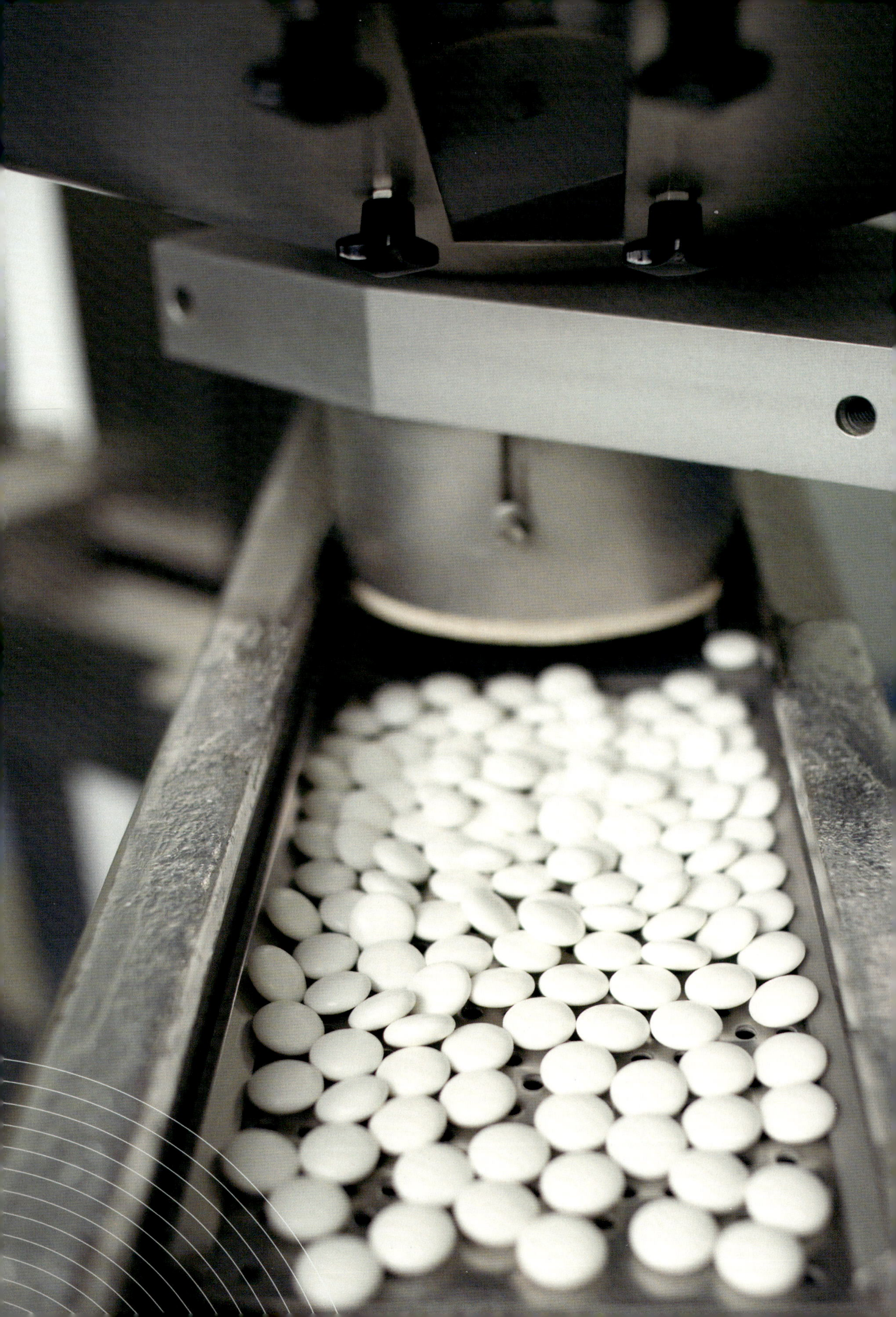

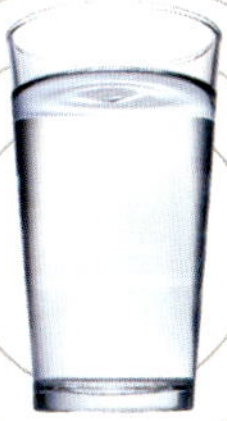

VACCINE #3

drugs

The first two brain drain vaccines taught you how to protect your cognitive powers by using the food in your fridge and the sneakers in your closet. But your medicine cabinet may be another surprising source of brain insurance.

Many researchers are hard at work developing new drug treatments to stall the progression of Alzheimer's disease (see Part 3, Brain Drain #6). Their discoveries may even result in treatments that help your grandson ace the SATs one day (speaking of school, some college students today are using stimulants such as Ritalin and Adderall to improve their focus and concentration—but unless you've been diagnosed with ADHD, these drugs aren't meant for you). But until those or other "smart drugs" come into mainstream use, medications you may already take for other health conditions, such as migraine headaches or cardiovascular disease, could have the pleasant side effect of giving you a better memory.

Any drug that helps you manage high cholesterol or high blood pressure will automatically allow more blood flow to your brain, keeping your neurons well-fed with blood sugar and energized with oxygen. Heart medication is just one class of potential allies; you could have several others lurking in your medicine chest without even knowing it.

Double-Duty Drugs

The following medications are believed to offer some cognitive benefit. If you've been taking one of them on a regular basis for a health problem, you may have been vaccinating yourself against brain drain for years. Of course, all drugs have side effects, and most of these would be inappropriate to take for their brain benefits alone.

Double-Duty Drug #1: **STATINS**

Statins, such as atorvastatin (Lipitor), simvastatin (Zocor), and ezetimibe/simvastatin (Vytorin), are prescribed to lower high cholesterol and reduce the risk of heart attack and stroke. They not only slow your body's production of cholesterol but they also remove cholesterol buildup from your artery walls, keeping your blood vessels clear and promoting good blood flow throughout your body—including your brain. In fact, some doctors use statins as their first line of defense when their patients demonstrate mild cognitive dementia.

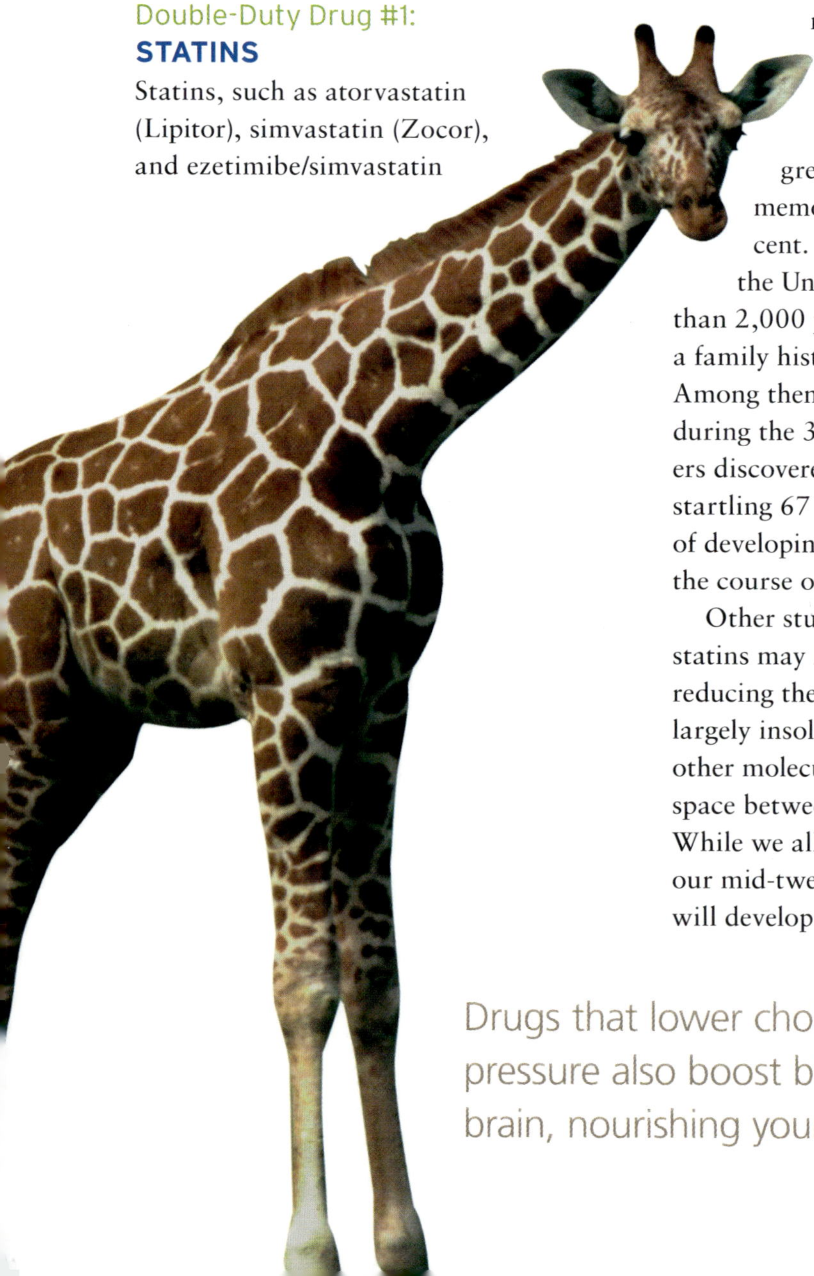

Research has shown that statin use may help reduce the risk for developing progressive dementia—irreversible memory loss—by up to 50 percent. One multi-center study in the United States recruited more than 2,000 people over age 70 who had a family history of Alzheimer's disease. Among them, 759 were taking a statin during the 3-year study period. Researchers discovered that they showed a startling 67 percent reduction in the risk of developing Alzheimer's disease over the course of the study.

Other studies have suggested that statins may help lessen dementia risk by reducing the amount of amyloid plaque, largely insoluble deposits of protein and other molecules that accumulate in the space between nerve cells in the brain. While we all accumulate this plaque from our mid-twenties onward, some people will develop Alzheimer's, while others

Drugs that lower cholesterol and blood pressure also boost blood flow to the brain, nourishing your noggin.

Brain Fog: A Side Effect of Statins?

In some patients, statins may have a dark side. For years, doctors heard stories of people, especially women, experiencing memory loss while on the drugs. One researcher investigating the side effects of statins sifted through thousands of reports of patient experiences on the drugs. He relates the story of a woman who became so forgetful that her daughter started looking into getting her Alzheimer's care and wouldn't let her babysit her granddaughter. Within 8 days of stopping the medication, the woman returned to normal.

Studies are now underway to find out if these effects are real. One theory of how the drugs might harm short-term memory goes that because statins reduce the amount of cholesterol in the body, they may also reduce myelin, a type of cholesterol that coats nerve fibers in the brain, protecting them from damage and helping to speed the transmission of thoughts from one nerve cell to the next. Myelin-coated fibers transmit information 10 times faster than uncoated fibers, increasing the brain's processing speed and decreasing reaction time. Without enough of it, the theory goes, some people might experience memory loss, or at least slower thinking.

Studies are now investigating this theory, but doctors stress that it's important to remember one thing: Any memory loss caused by statins is rare, likely short term, and reversible. Talk to your doctor; he or she will help you decide the best course of action for your situation and condition.

Research shows that statin drugs may reduce the body's production of the important brain-protective antioxidant coenzyme Q10 (CoQ10); depletion of this antioxidant may be responsible for some of the cognitive changes associated with the use of these medications. If you are taking a statin, experts recommend taking supplemental CoQ10 at a dose of 60 milligrams per day.

never will. Researchers aren't exactly sure why, but they suspect that statins may help reduce the toxic effects of the plaque, such as inflammation, in addition to increasing blood flow.

Double-Duty Drug #2: **BLOOD PRESSURE MEDICINES**

When we're young, the amount of blood that streams through our brains every minute is about 742 milliliters—a little over 3 cups. As we age, that rate declines steadily by about a teaspoon each year. When you have high blood pressure, your blood supply is even more restricted, and your poor brain is going to feel that deficit far more than other organs. Without enough blood, which brings vital oxygen and nutrients to brain cells, those cells will start to die. That's when your memory—especially your short-term memory—takes a big hit. At the same time, your risk increases for vascular dementia, the second most common form of dementia, caused by blockages in the brain's blood supply. One Dutch study of people who developed dementia after age 75 found that their brains had 20 percent less blood flow than those of healthy people their age.

In addition to following a healthy diet (rich in fruits, vegetables, and whole grains) and getting regular exercise, anything more you can do to keep your blood pressure normal is a good thing for your brain, including, if necessary, taking blood pressure–lowering medication. These medicines fall into several categories, and not all have a clear brain benefit. For example, some research suggests that beta blockers could actually aggravate cognitive decline, causing delays in memory and making dementia worse. Several medications, however, have shown real brain benefits, including the following four.

ACE inhibitors. These medications, such as captopril (Capoten), enalapril (Vasotec), and ramipril (Altace), allow blood vessels to dilate, lowering blood pressure, by blocking the effects of angiotensin-converting enzyme (ACE), which indirectly stimulates the muscles around blood vessels to squeeze. When researchers tracked 3,300 residents of Cache County, Utah, who were 65 or older, they found that those who were using any antihypertensive drug, including ACE inhibitors, at the start of the study had a 36 percent decreased risk of Alzheimer's after 3 years.

Calcium channel blockers. These drugs, such as verapamil (Calan or Covera), nitrendipine (Bayotensin), and diltiazem hydrochloride (Cardizem or Taztia), lower blood pressure by preventing calcium from entering the heart and blood vessel muscle cells. This change causes cells to relax and blood pressure to fall—and may also reduce the risk of dementia over the long haul. A European study from 106 different medical centers, involving almost 3,000 patients with an average age of 68, found that patients given the hypertension drug nitrendipine reduced their risk of developing dementia over the course of about 4 years by 55 percent when compared with a control group. The study authors projected that treating 1,000 patients with these antihypertensive drugs for 5 years could prevent 20 cases of dementia. Some doctors also use calcium channel blockers to calm the agitation of people with dementia.

Verapamil may also be effective in the prevention of migraine and cluster headaches. Doctors sometimes prescribe calcium channel blockers off-label for this purpose. Doctors don't really know the cause of migraines, but it may be related to restriction of blood flow to blood vessels in the brain—and we know that's not good for overall brain health.

Angiotensin Receptor Blockers (ARBs). These drugs block the effects of a chemical called angiotensin II, which causes the muscles surrounding the blood vessels to contract, narrowing the blood vessels. They may also have a tremendous influence on cognition. Scientists analyzed the medical histories of an incredible 5 million patients from the U.S. Department of Veterans Affairs system who were 65 years and older and being treated for high blood pressure. They found that those who took ARBs—drugs including losartan (Cozaar), valsartan (Diovan), and olmesartan (Benicar)—were 35 to 40 percent less likely to develop Alzheimer's disease or other forms of dementia than patients taking ACE inhibitors or other cardiovascular medications. Also, people who already had been diagnosed with Alzheimer's were 45 percent less likely to develop delirium, be admitted to a nursing home, or die prematurely if they were taking ARBs compared with the other blood pressure medications.

Potassium-sparing diuretics. They may not be fancy, but diuretics, sometimes called water pills, can certainly hold their own with the effectiveness rate of other antihypertensives. Diuretics flush any extra water or sodium from your blood, thereby lowering blood pressure.

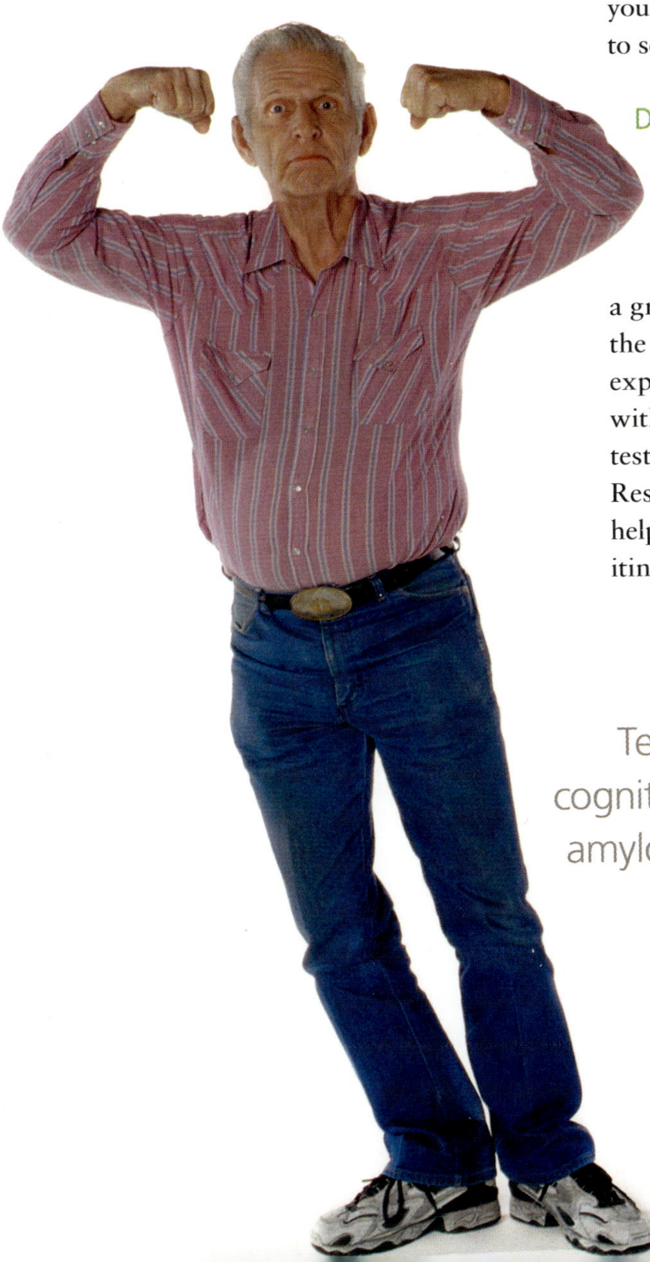

A study of older residents of Cache County, Utah, found that any use of blood pressure–lowering medicine lowered the risk of Alzheimer's disease by more than 35 percent, but that potassium-sparing diuretics such as spironolactone (Aldactone), triamterene (Dyrenium), or the generic amiloride (Midamor) lowered the risk by almost 75 percent. Considering that diuretics are some of the least expensive medicines for high blood pressure, you might discuss them with your doctor to see if they are a good option for you.

Double-Duty Drug #3: TESTOSTERONE

Male menopause, known medically as andropause, does exist. From their mid-forties on, men experience a gradual decline in testosterone (not like the steep drop in estrogen that women experience). Research has found that men with dementia tend to have lower levels of testosterone than the general population. Researchers theorize that testosterone helps prevent cognitive decline by inhibiting amyloid plaque, the deposits of

Testosterone may prevent cognitive decline by inhibiting amyloid plaque, the deposits of proteins and other gunk that are a marker of Alzheimer's.

Drugs That May Impair Memory

You're trying hard to preserve your memory, but what if one of the medications you take on a regular basis is getting in your way? All kinds of medications, both prescription and over-the-counter, can impact your ability to think clearly, although many side effects wear off once your system has acclimated to the drug, or once you stopping taking the drug. (Always discuss potential side effects, as well as the risks of stopping medication, with your doctor.) Make it a habit to ask your doctor or pharmacist about any side effects before taking a new drug. If memory loss is one of them, ask if there are any alternatives. Some of the most common memory culprits include:

1 Antacids

In an Indiana University study, older people who took H2 blockers, such as famotidine (Pepcid) and ranitidine (Zantac), long-term were 2.4 times more likely to develop dementia or some other form of mental impairment.

2 Antidepressants

Some patients taking antidepressants complain of short-term memory loss. These drugs vary in terms of their effect on cognition. Tricyclic antidepressants belong to a class of drugs called anticholinergics, which are known to negatively affect memory.

3 Antihistamines and allergy medications

Some of these, especially older drugs like diphenhydramine (Benadryl), may cause cloudy thinking. The effects wear off after the drug wears off. But all nonprescription and many prescription antihistamines have anticholinergic effects; in theory, if you take them long-term, they could speed any existing cognitive decline.

4 Bladder-control medicines

Incontinence can be seriously annoying, even life-limiting. But think twice before you take a bladder-control medication. One class of drugs used to treat overactive bladder, known as anticholinergics, may have a pronounced negative effect on cognitive function. These drugs work by blocking excess activity of acetylcholine, a neurotransmitter that helps stimulate bladder muscles to contract. Acetylcholine also helps transmit thoughts in the brain, and when you don't have enough, your brain cells can't speak to each other effectively. One study presented at an American Academy of Neurology meeting suggested that people over 75 who take anticholinergic drugs appear to have a 1.5 times faster decline in cognitive functioning than those who don't.

5 Anti-anxiety medications

These drugs, such as alprazolam (Xanax) and clonazepam (Klonopin), may cause memory impairment, confusion, and temporary speech problems.

6 Sleep aids

Some of these leave you feeling groggy in the morning, and you may not remember much of what happened after you took them. Zolpidem (Ambien) has even been associated with certain behaviors during sleep, such as "sleep-driving," that patients have no memory of in the morning.

7 Antispasmodic drugs

These drugs, which include belladonna alkaloids (Bellatal, D-Tal, Donnatal), dicyclomine (Bentyl, Byclomine, Dibent, Di-Spaz, Dilomine), hyoscyamine (Anaspaz, Cystospaz, Donnamar, Levsin), and propantheline (Pro-Banthine), may impair your thinking and slow your reactions.

8 Muscle relaxants

These drugs include carisoprodol, chlorzoxazone, cyclobenzaprine, metaxalone, and methocarbamol. Most muscle relaxants have anticholinergic effects, and therefore could negatively affect memory.

proteins and other gunk in the brain that are a marker of Alzheimer's.

A large long-term study, the Baltimore Longitudinal Study of Aging, found that the more free testosterone in a man's body, the lower his risk of Alzheimer's disease. The research team found that for every 50 percent increase in the free testosterone index in the bloodstream, the risk of developing Alzheimer's dropped by 26 percent. By the end of the study, men who'd been diagnosed with Alzheimer's had only half the free testosterone as healthy men, and the hormone declines were sometimes detectable a decade before the Alzheimer's diagnosis.

But depending on your age, taking testosterone won't necessarily improve your thinking. In one study, when men averaging age 67 were given testosterone injections, they performed better than their peers on cognitive tests. In another study, when younger men were given testosterone injections for 4 weeks, they performed better on spatial ability tests but worse on a verbal fluency test.

If you've had trauma to the testes, trouble with your pituitary gland, or one of several genetic conditions that necessitate supplementing with testosterone, chances are you're already benefiting from any brain-protective effects. Despite some drug company's ads promising increased sexual appetite and muscle tone, giving testosterone to healthy men remains controversial because of potential increased risks of baldness, sleep apnea, prostate cancer, shrunken testicles, or other unknown long-term side effects. Contact a board-certified endocrinologist for a full hormonal workup before you make any moves.

Double-Duty Drug #4: **ESTROGEN**

Estrogen makes brain cells communicate more effectively with one another, perhaps by helping information (thoughts, ideas, phone numbers) jump across gaps, or synapses, between neurons. One way the hormone accomplishes this is by boosting the amount of brain chemicals called neurotransmitters, which transmit the information across the gaps.

In women, in the decade or so before menopause, levels of estrogen start to wane, and some of the beneficial effects of estrogen wane, too. Some research suggests that hormone replacement therapy (HRT), when taken prior to menopause, might protect against Alzheimer's disease and dementia. The "critical period" theory argues that estrogen given to women during perimenopause, typically when women are in their late forties or early fifties, may stem any negative brain effects of estrogen depletion, which some research suggests leads to a 50 percent decreased risk of dementia. If you wait too long after that, scientists believe the damage may already be done. In fact, once a woman passes through menopause, supplemental estrogen may increase her risk of Alzheimer's and dementia by 50 percent. For that reason, postmenopausal women, in particular, should exercise caution when taking HRT.

HRT has not had the best of reputations in recent years. Prescriptions plummeted after the Women's Health Initiative found that taking supplemental estrogen plus progestin increased the risk of heart attack, stroke, blood clots, and breast cancer in women over 65. Yet for women who took estrogen alone, the risks were far less serious. In fact, a Danish study of more than 1,800 female OB/GYNs found that, while they'd all but stopped prescribing estrogen to their patients, the doctors still took it themselves. The study authors suggested that perhaps their reluctance to prescribe estrogen may have had more to do with a fear of lawsuits than a fear of drug-related dangers.

While estrogen replacement therapy may be helpful to premenopausal women at risk for osteoporosis or dementia, your age or health history may take the option off the table for you. Before starting any hormone treatment, speak with a board-certified endocrinologist about your particular situation.

Double-Duty Drug #5: **ASPIRIN**

Consider the humble aspirin. The little white headache pills help prevent heart attack and stroke by discouraging blood clots. They may even help stave off cognitive decline. One well-designed study of more than 6,000 women age 65 or older tested the effect of long-term use of low-dose aspirin (100 milligrams on alternate days) on cognitive decline over a period of almost 10 years. The women were evaluated at 5.6 years after the start of the study and then reevaluated 2 and 4 years later. Researchers found that women on aspirin therapy were 20 percent less likely to develop substantial decline in something they call category fluency, tests used to assess semantic knowledge, retrieval ability, and executive functioning in which subjects are asked to quickly produce words in a specified category. People who seemed to benefit the most from aspirin where those who had high cholesterol or who were smokers.

If you're already on aspirin therapy for heart concerns, you're in luck. If not, discuss the pros and cons with your doctor. People with asthma, stomach ulcers, heart failure, or a bleeding or clotting disorder may not be able to take aspirin. Before starting on aspirin therapy, be sure to tell your doctor about all the other pills you take, including prescription and

What About NSAIDs?

Many researchers believe that inflammation in the brain contributes to the development of Alzheimer's disease, which would imply there is a brain benefit from drugs known as nonsteroidal anti-inflammatories (NSAIDs). In fact, several early studies suggested that using NSAIDS such as naproxen (Aleve) and celecoxib (Celebrex) could indeed help prevent cognitive decline in people with a family history of Alzheimer's disease. However, more recent research points to just the opposite conclusion.

A double-blind, placebo-controlled study conducted at Johns Hopkins University and funded by the National Institute on Aging was suspended when evidence arose that celecoxib was linked with increased risk of cardiovascular problems. Researchers further analyzed their data and found that the NSAIDs naproxen and celecoxib not only did not prevent cognitive decline but were associated with decreased cognitive performance. Another major, multi-center study has since come to a similar conclusion.

No one is certain whether other NSAIDs, such as ibruprofen (Advil or Motrin), might have similar effects.

over-the-counter medicines and even vitamins and herbs. Some may increase the risk of dangerous bleeding when combined with aspirin.

Double-Duty Drug #6:
CAFFEINE

For many people, coffee is the favorite addictive drug of choice. Now there may be a great reason to forgo the decaf and stick with the caffeinated kind. A study involving more than 4,000 French women age 65 or older found that those who drank 3 or more cups of caffeinated coffee a day scored higher on word retrieval and spatial memory tests than those who consumed 1 cup or less. The protective effect of coffee was found to increase with women's age, especially for those over age 80.

While caffeine did not appear to decrease overall dementia risk in this particular study, drinking coffee just might reduce age-related cognitive decline and may help stall the development of mild cognitive impairment into full-blown dementia. Considering that emerging research suggests coffee might also help decrease the risks of diabetes and some types of cancer, perhaps an extra cup a day could be just what the doctor ordered.

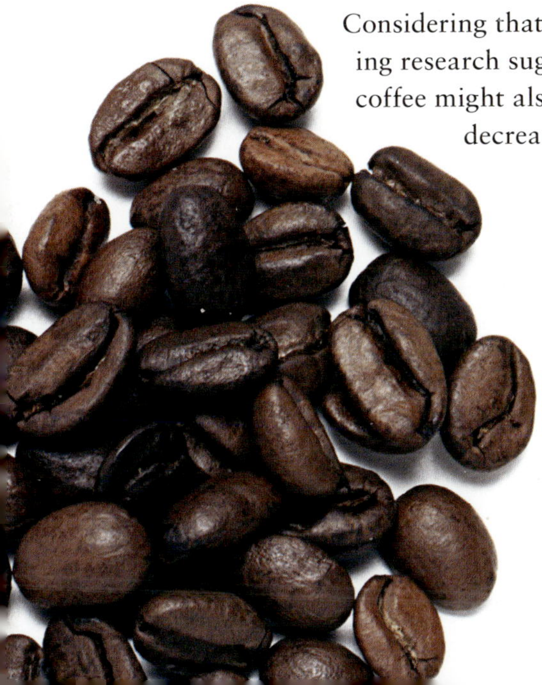

Double-Duty Drug #7:
NICOTINE PATCHES

So, you've taken the big step to rid yourself of the smoking habit—good for you! If you're using nicotine patches to help you quit, you may even be helping your brain.

A small study from Duke University Medical Center gave 11 patients with memory impairment a nicotine patch to wear for 16 hours a day. After 4 weeks, the researchers determined that the nicotine improved the patient's performance on reaction time and attention tests. In another study, Korean researchers placed a nicotine patch on 63 older men for 5 hours. They compared their performance on cognitive tests before and after the nicotine patch and found that memory functions improved significantly after receiving the nicotine.

More studies are currently underway about how to exploit the potential memory-boosting effects of nicotine. If you are not a smoker trying to quit, no one would ever recommend using the nicotine patch—and certainly no one would suggest you start smoking (after all, smoking leads to strokes, a major cause of brain drain). But if you are trying to quit and you use the patch, you may be helping your attention and memory at the same time.

Your daily coffee habit could be a boon to your brain, sharpening memory and guarding against decline.

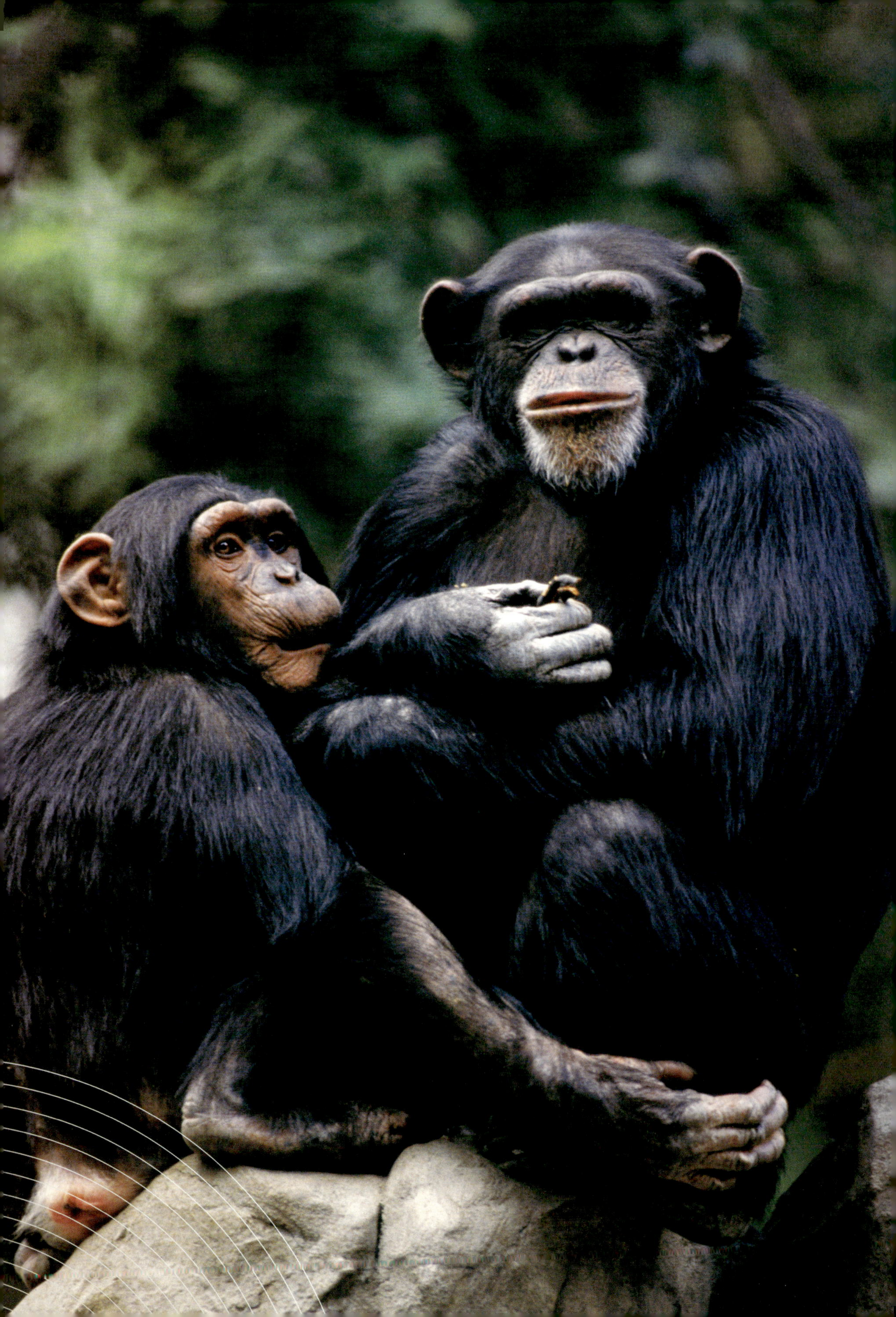

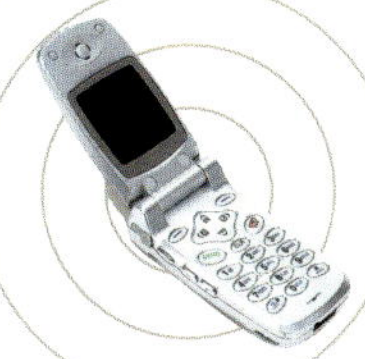

VACCINE #4

social connections

Next time you go to the zoo with your grandkids, stand outside the chimps' cage for a few minutes. Watch the animals long enough and you'll see a complex social structure emerge, every bit as subtle as the one that governs the social lives of another primate: the human being. We primates didn't get our big brains because we were itching to develop the theory of relativity. Instead, the size of our gray matter increased because of how mentally challenging it is to negotiate social relationships. And you know by now that the brain loves a challenge!

Way before we ever carved wheels out of stone, we needed to figure out our place in the pecking order of the clan, a big reason why the brain is designed to process social information first, before any other information gets through. We process this information faster than other information and are more likely to remember details about people and relationships than abstract ideas or inanimate objects. Even while we dream, our brains are more likely to toss around images of people, not things. In other words, we are wired to be social.

Our brain gets a good workout whenever we encounter another human being—even if it's just for a casual 10-minute chat. To carry on a conversation, we have to pay close attention, respond to questions, interpret vocal tone and body language, and even use short- and long-term memory to access facts that pertain to the conversation. At the same time, we have to block out the other stimuli that compete for our attention. All of these are complex executive functions, demanding extra work from the prefrontal cortex, an area of the brain particularly vulnerable to age-related cognitive decline.

Countless studies have shown that people with more active social lives live longer, enjoy better health, and are less depressed than those who go it alone—and they tend to suffer less cognitive decline later in life. No matter your age, the mere act of hanging out with friends or relatives can improve working memory and processing speed, both immediately and over the long haul. Animal studies have shown that social contact encourages brain cell growth and an increase in brain volume. In humans, a strong social network may even delay symptoms of Alzheimer's in people with the brain plaques and tangles (twisted fibers found inside nerve cells) associated with the disease.

Now, there's one caveat: The relationships have to be positive ones. Fights with your spouse and squabbles with your siblings can physically damage your brain by increasing levels of cortisol, a stress hormone believed to shrink the hippocampus, the seat of memory. Positive relationships serve the brain well, and the more diverse those relationships are, the better. Nurturing your social connections widens your support network not only by increasing the number of people who can help you when you need help but also by boosting your confidence and your ability to help yourself.

How big are the brain benefits? One study followed almost 800 Swedish seniors for 6 years and found that social activities such as attending concerts, traveling, belonging to groups, attending the theater and art exhibitions, and playing cards and other games reduced the risk of dementia by more than 30 percent. People who were social *and* challenged themselves mentally and physically with activities such as swimming or walking and drawing, painting, or reading—essentially, those who followed some of the main components of the No More Brain Drain Plan—lowered their risk almost an additional 20 percent.

Creating a No More Brain Drain Social Network

Spending quality time with friends and family just might be the most fun way you'll protect your brain! Don't worry; you don't have to become a social butterfly. If you're more of a mole, though, it's time to coax yourself out of your hole and into the world at large. Every little step counts. Not exactly the life of the party? Start with a simple phone call to a friend, or a "hello" to a neighbor, and take it from there. Researchers have concluded that even brief social interactions can have positive effects on memory and cognitive performance.

Deliberately widen your circle. Many of us tend to have fewer relationships as we get older—the kids move out of town, we retire, elderly friends and relatives start to slip away. We might not care so much about running with a hip crowd, but research shows that we should at least stick with the "crowd" part. One 12-year study followed more than 2,800 adults age 65 and older who lived in their own homes. Those who had five or six social ties had less than half the risk of cognitive decline of those who had none. The same results were shown 3, 6, and 12 years after the start of the study.

Aim for daily contact with others. Another study found that among women who were 78 or older, those who had larger social networks were 26 percent less likely to develop dementia or age-related cognitive decline. Of those women, the social butterflies—the ones with daily contact with friends and family—cut their risk in half. Researchers noted that those women were the most likely to confide in their friends and ask them for help, not just go out for lunch, which may have been key to their retaining independence. Do your best to emulate these chatty Cathies.

See your best friends at least twice a month. And talk on the phone at least once a week. The healthiest people maintain a core group of close friends over their life span. Studies that followed people from age 18 to 100 have found that, as we get older, we tend to "prune" our social circle—we keep the people we feel closest to but shed relationships that don't mean as much to us. These close relationships provide the most emotional satisfaction, so make the most of them (but don't neglect adding new friends, too).

Turn off the tube. As the song from *Cabaret* goes, "What good is sitting alone in your room?" In fact, it may do harm, especially to older folks. When we're alone for long stretches, especially in front of the television, we tend to zone out. One researcher theorizes that older people may have a hard time switching from that zoned-out state to the more focused state required to carry on a conversation or perform tasks. Therefore, the less time spent zoned out, the better. If you find yourself alone for a long stretch, walk outside and say hello to whoever's out and about, or pick up the phone and call a relative or friend.

BREAK OUT OF YOUR RUT

Interview your friends about their hobbies. Tag along with friends or family to participate in their interests: music, theater, art, even bingo. Ask them to help explain the nuances of each new discipline: What's great about this piece of music? What's your favorite painting? How do you manage five bingo cards at once? Have them introduce you to their hobby-related acquaintances, too. Hanging out with smart, interesting people usually provides terrific stimulation for your brain.

Draw courage from friends to try new things. Join a water aerobics or yoga class with a friend, or join a hiking group together. Experimenting with new activities in the safety of a close relationship helps you manage your anxiety (and prevent a negative stress reaction) while you get the brain benefits of new environments.

Make a date for something different. Mixing novelty with love is a win-win situation for your brain and your relationship. Novel experiences and adrenaline-pumping experiences switch on your brain's reward circuits and increase your levels of norepinephrine and dopamine, neurotransmitters associated with increased attention span as well as pleasure—the same brain chemicals released when you first fall in love. Act like kids and go to an arcade to play air hockey. Break out the Ping-Pong table or play badminton in the backyard. Take a day trip to a city you've been interested in, and seek out a restaurant with a cuisine you rarely try. You'll enhance both your brain power and your relationship. It's no surprise that when committed couples spent an hour-and-a-half each week for 10 weeks doing something together they both find exciting (as opposed to merely pleasant), they experienced greater marital satisfaction.

Plan an exciting getaway together. Plan a vacation with your spouse or best friend in a place neither of you have ever visited. Make each person responsible for planning one full day of the trip, and surprise the other person with every activity and meal that day.

COMBAT SOCIAL SHRINKAGE

Create a call list. Write down all the people in your social life, along with their phone numbers. In addition to your closest circle, include the people on your holiday card list, neighbors, and friends from the pool. Organize them into two lists, like the phone company does: one local, one long-distance. Then, make a point to reach out to at least one person on each list every week, if you're not very social, or once a day if you are. But don't just phone. One

How Social Are You?

Data from the MacArthur Study of Successful Aging found that the more social time a 70- to 79-year-old man had, the lower his levels of fibrinogen, a protein that speeds up clot formation, increasing the risk for heart attack and stroke—and therefore cognitive decline. Men with the two lowest levels of social activity were more than twice as likely to have elevated fibrinogen as those with the highest level. To ballpark your risk of high fibrinogen, take this test, drawn from the study.

1. Do you live with your spouse?
yes = 1; no = 0

2. How many close relatives do you have?
0 or 1 = 0; 2+ = 1

3. How many close friends do you have?
0 or 1 = 0; 2+ = 1

4. How often do you attend religious services? never or 1 time a month = 0; 2+ times a month = 1

5. How often do you do religious activities outside of attending services?
never = 0; sometimes or frequently = 1

6. How often do you participate in clubs or other voluntary associations?
never = 0; sometimes or frequently = 1

YOUR SCORE

Add up the scores associated with your answers to determine your Social Network Score. A score of 4 ("Medium-High") or above should mean a dramatically lower risk:

Low 0–2; Low-Medium 3;
Medium-High 4; High 5–6

Tap Your Marriage for Extra Brain Benefits

With your spouse in the house, you have a built-in brain-booster sitting right across the breakfast table. Get the biggest cranial lift from your relationship with these five tactics.

Marry someone similar to you, if a bit smarter. The Seattle Longitudinal Study looked at 169 couples in 7-year intervals between 1956 and 1984 and found that the most stable relationships were those in which people were similar in intelligence, flexibility of attitudes, social responsibility, and education levels. Researchers also found that after 14 years together, spouses with the better grasp of verbal meanings and word fluency had pulled the lower-functioning spouses up to their level.

Hold hands whenever possible. In addition to creating feelings of warmth and closeness, holding hands can help inoculate you from stress. One study using brain scans found that when married women were told they were about to receive an electric shock, just holding their husbands' hands minimized their brains' response to the threat. Women in the closest relationships experienced the greatest decrease in stress-related brain activity.

Kiss at least once a day. This intimate touch triggers the release of the bonding hormone oxytocin and lowers levels of the stress hormone cortisol—but that's not all. Researchers say that when we kiss, we activate nearly half of the cranial nerves that affect cerebral function. All of the sensory information of a kiss—the smell and warmth of your partner's skin, the taste and feel of soft lips—shoots into your brain, delighting your neurons and forging new connections.

Put pictures of your honey on your desk. Brain scans show that looking at a photo of your beloved, especially in the early stages of your relationship, activates a part of the brain associated with pleasure and reward as well as focused attention and motivation. This same area is triggered when a cocaine addict gets a fix—so you could literally get a healthy "high" from looking at a picture of your new love. When you're in the throes of new love, your prefrontal cortex also gets into the action, anticipating more time together and planning future events.

Just be together. One study found that average blood pressure was lower when a person spent time with his or her spouse than when they spent time alone or with other people. Even if you don't talk, just spend time in the same room, reading, watching TV, surfing the web, or doing crossword puzzles.

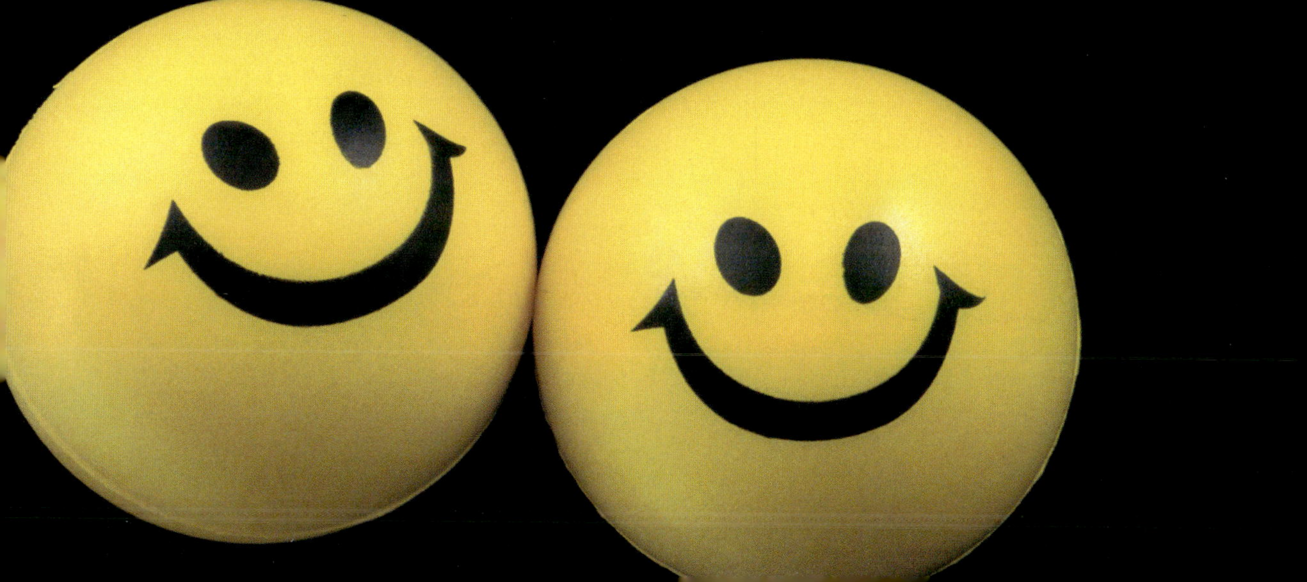

4-year study of Spanish men and women over age 65 found that those who had a high frequency of visual contact with loved ones had a lower risk of cognitive decline.

Throw one party every season. Connecting your friends to one another isn't just fun, it may help your brain, too. One study found that people at the center of their network clusters—in other words, who had a lot of friends—were the most likely to be happy, especially when their friends also had a lot of friends.

Force yourself to attend that cocktail party or church social. Shy people or those unused to socializing can find a million reasons not to go to social events. Instead of thinking of these social "obligations" as chores, think of them as opportunities to grow your brain. Bonus: Just as every personal interaction increases your brain power, they also strengthen your social skills. As those skills increase, you'll feel more comfortable spending time with others. Voilà! A positive brain feedback loop.

Make a point to reach out to at least one person every week, if you're not very social, or once a day if you are.

Say "Hi" to everyone. The simplest possible way to get yourself in a more social frame of mind is to say hello to everyone you meet. Make small talk—any small talk at all—with the cashier at the grocery store while you're checking out or the down-the-block neighbor who passes you while walking his dog. Get coffee at the same café every day, and learn the barista's name. You may be surprised at the positive greeting you get the next time you go.

Get back out there. If you've been widowed or divorced, it can be hard to start dating again. But your brain would love for you to love again. One study presented at the International Conference on Alzheimer's Disease and Related Disorders meeting followed Finnish adults for more than 20 years and found that those who lived with their spouses or partners after age 50 had half the incidence of dementia than people who lived alone during that time. Singles had twice the incidence of married people, but those who'd been divorced and didn't remarry had three times the incidence. People who had been widowed before middle age, but didn't marry again, had six times the incidence of dementia.

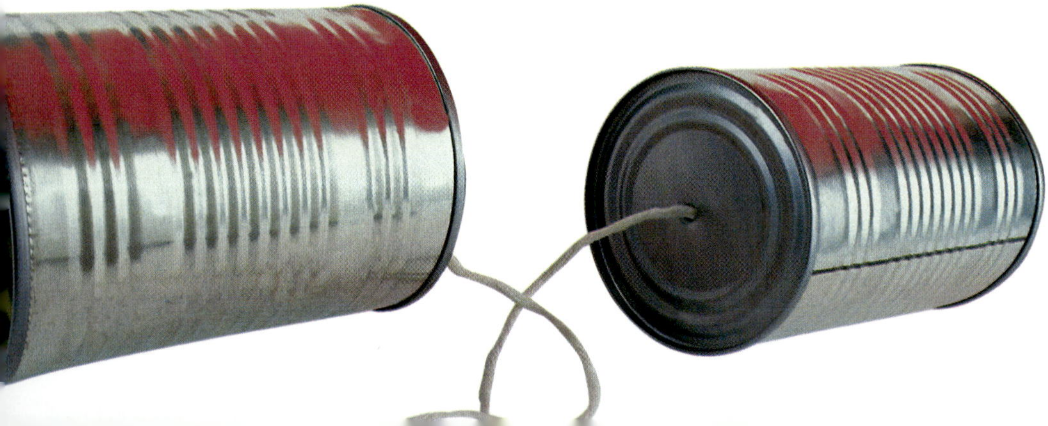

Not sure how to get out there again? Check out online sites like www.match.com or www.eharmony.com. (Choose a public place for your first meeting.) Screen carefully, but don't worry about finding only freaks or misfits—online dating has become an efficient and socially acceptable way to meet nice people with common interests. Investigate www.reunion.com; who knows, you might reconnect with your long-lost high school flame.

If you prefer to meet your dates the old-fashioned way, get yourself to any place that like minds frequent: Attend mixers at your church, community center, or senior center; volunteer at a music festival or your local art museum; sign up for trips to see plays or attend cultural events in nearby cities. And, yes, get ready for that high school or college reunion; you never know who's been pining for you all these years.

PRETEND YOU'RE A KID: SOCIALIZE IN GROUPS

Form a movie gang. Gather a group of six people with diverse interests and take turns selecting a movie to see each month. Make sure to include movies that at least two of you wouldn't normally consider. Go to dinner after the movie, rather than before, so you can review the film together and discuss the high and low points. Why not select the restaurant based on the movie's setting? If the movie is based in India or Thailand, go to an Indian or Thai restaurant; if it's based in Victorian England, go to a teahouse.

Start a cooking club. Get together with four or five other friends to share cooking once a month. Ask each person to bring a new recipe centered around a certain theme, such as Italian food, or a vegetable in season, such as asparagus or tomatoes. Join together to create a meal for everyone to bring home, or have everyone bring one course (appetizer, soup, salad, entrée, or dessert) and enjoy the meal together.

Trade tasks you don't like. Maybe you love to rake, and your friend loves to sew. Why not trade those tasks and relieve each of you of the thing you most hate? Studies have shown that those people who ask for and accept help from others can slow their cognitive decline in later years. Learn from societies with a more communal approach to life, such as many in Asia: Having more help with household tasks keeps people independent longer, increases their time spent with others, and decreases brain-damaging stress.

ADOPT THE RIGHT ATTITUDE

Start a "happiness virus" in your neighborhood. Happiness truly is contagious. Harvard University researchers found, when looking at a group of 5,000 people over a period of 20 years, that even a total stranger's happiness can make you happy for up to 1 year afterward. When you become happy, your next-door neighbor has a 34 percent greater chance of becoming happy, and your friend who lives within a mile has a 25 percent greater chance.

The tradition of bringing a pie or a plant to a new neighbor is an excellent "virus-starter." Encourage neighbors to share good news, even if it's about people you don't know. Host an annual block party. Create a map of all the houses around yours, and note people's names as soon as you learn them—the reminder will come in handy in the spring, when you haven't seen them for a few winter months. When you're out on the front lawn, smile and wave at anyone who walks or drives down your street—who cares if they think you're crazy? You're starting a brain-building epidemic here!

Try to assume the best. Simply imagining that someone has rejected you socially can negatively affect your performance on lab tests designed to assess cognitive function. When you experience social rejection, your brain registers it in an area of the brain that records physical pain. You're also less likely to be able to empathize with the person who "rejected" you or to see things from his or her perspective—high-level cognitive functions associated with what we call wisdom.

If you're an anxious person who tends toward fear or suspicion, try to work on trusting others. Before you react to a neighbor "ignoring" you on the street, ask yourself, "Is this really happening? What evidence do I have? Could I be imagining it?" Give people the benefit of the doubt by presuming the best in their intentions—and approach them with the best of intentions yourself.

Refrain from judging. In one study, people who were concerned about being judged, or who were judgmental themselves, had a more difficult time concentrating and ignoring outside stimuli during a mental task.

Ditch the whiners and the critics. Every happy friend increases your chances of being happy by 9 percent, but every unhappy friend decreases those chances by 7 percent. High-maintenance friendships or interpersonal conflicts also make people do worse on standardized tests.

Make it a habit to check your feelings after visits with friends. Do you feel energized or depleted? Confident or insecure? Steer yourself toward people who make you feel good and minimize time with people who make you feel lousy.

GET INVOLVED

Referee. If you're in good shape and have good eyesight, you can enjoy sports from the field rather than the stands, especially if you used to play a sport in your younger years. Many youth sports teams are desperate for referees; some even offer a modest stipend. You could also organize the rosters, order uniforms, or volunteer

Community Brain-Builders

Joining a group of people who share common interests or values brings countless benefits to your brain. Not only does the activity itself let you challenge yourself mentally or physically but also the supportive environment makes it far easier to form bonds and to receive and give help—both ends of an equation that benefits the brain.

Consider this list of groups you might join:

- Alumni association
- Book club
- Bus trips to cities or casinos
- Choir
- Church committees
- Co-op food bank
- Farmer's market association
- Health club
- Nationality or ethnic social club
- Nonprofit action group
- Political campaign
- Town council
- Walker's club

at the snack bar of your local youth organization. Usually, those programs are manned by the already overstretched parents of participating kids—and they would likely be grateful for your help.

Pitch in at the church nursery. You've had years in the pews; now let the young moms and dads listen to the sermon while you watch their kids in the nursery. Playing with young children creates an entirely different set of stimuli for your gray matter. Further boost your brain by reading a Bible story aloud or indulge your arts and crafts bug while devising fun projects for the kids to do. Break out the construction paper and glue and feel like a kid again.

Usher at concerts, events, and lectures. Get on the list by calling your local theater. Many places have a list of people they call all the time—stick with it and, over time, you can become part of the theater's community. You'll help a theater that can't afford to pay their staff and get to see the event for free.

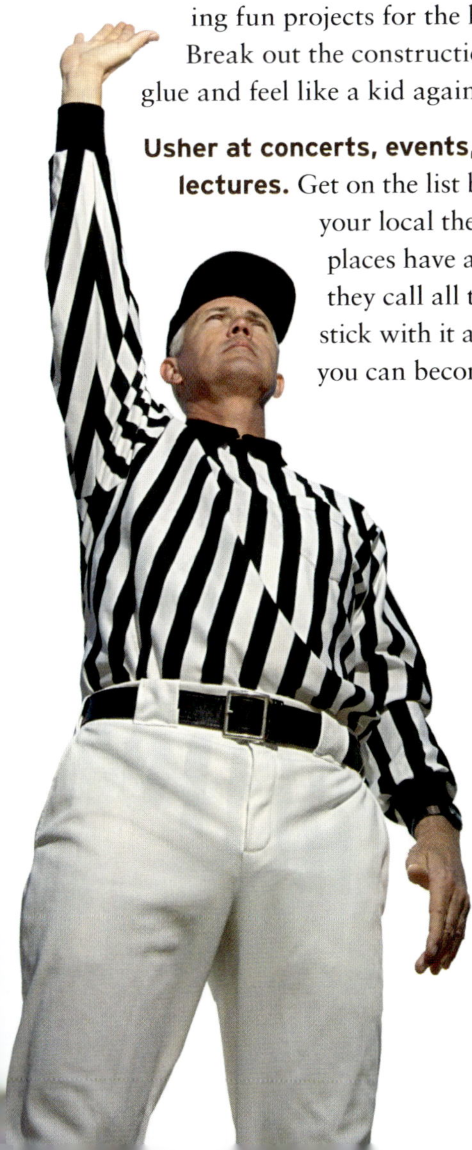

Volunteer for a soup kitchen or Meals on Wheels on the same day every week. If you keep the same schedule or route, you'll create mini-relationships with each person you feed, and those connections help both of you equally. You'll also bond with fellow volunteers and may even find more interests in common with them than with friends you've had for years.

Help out your adult children. They are likely in one of the most challenging periods of their lives: stressful but rewarding work combined with the exhaustion of parenting. By helping them with child care, shopping, or other household tasks, you'll help yourself as well—and maybe even lengthen your life. Research shows that strong emotional bonds between parents and adult children predict longer parental survival.

Bond with the grandkids. Never underestimate the power of time spent with grandchildren to keep a brain young. Depending on their ages, read them Harry Potter and try to keep track of the characters; ask them to show you how to play Nintendo Wii; find out what book they're studying at college and consider reading it yourself so you'll have a new topic of conversation. The opportunities never end.

Whether you referee, usher, babysit, or serve soup, you're serving your brain as well.

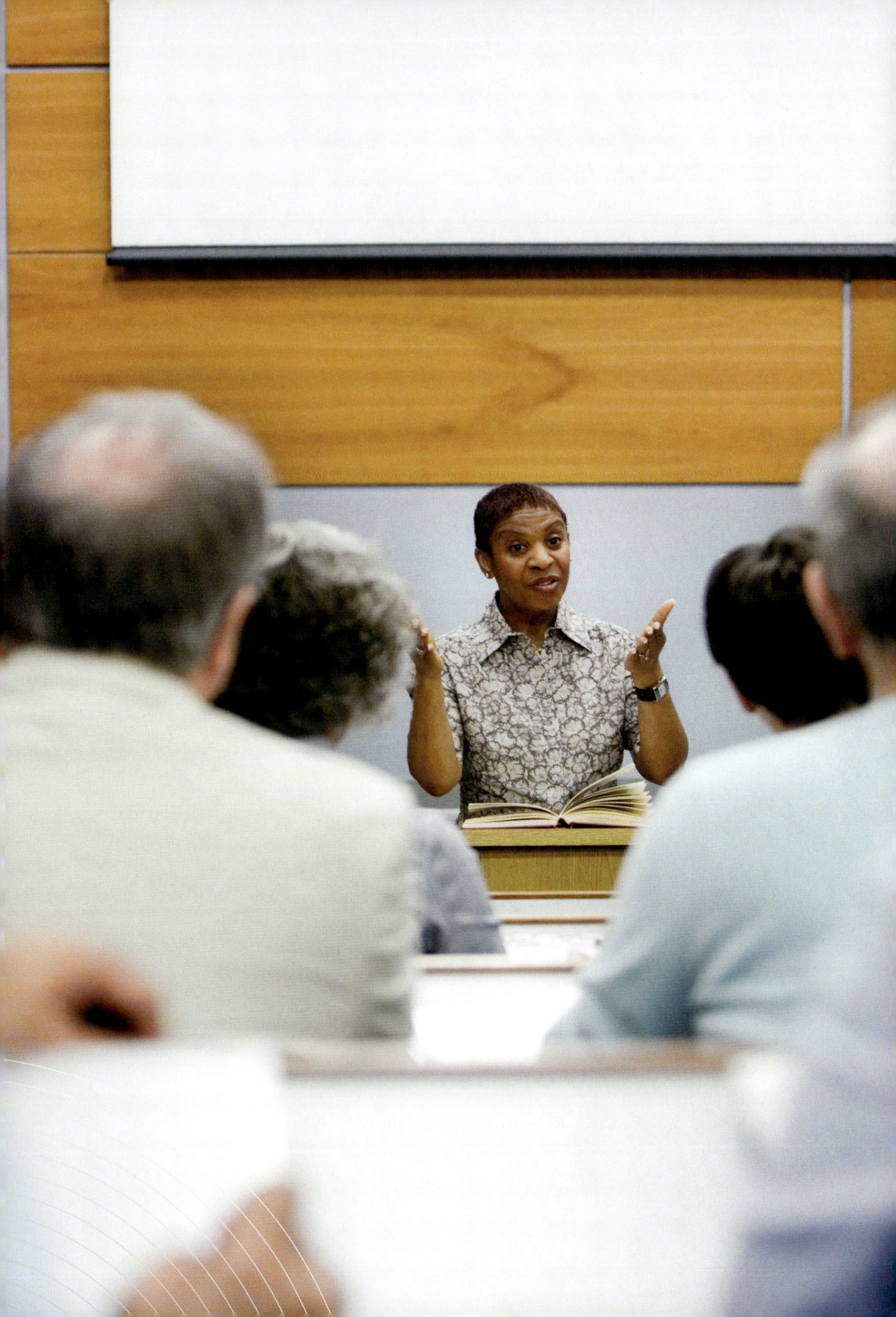

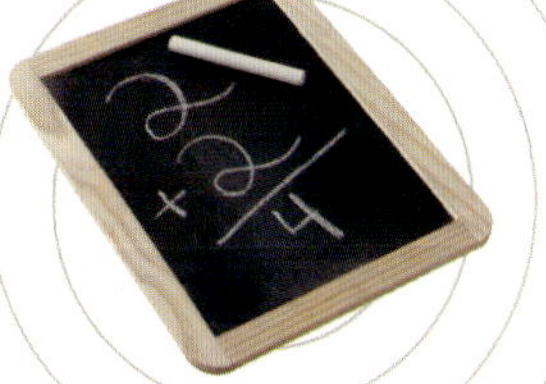

VACCINE #5
learning

Human beings are creatures of habit. We eat the same breakfast every morning, drive the same route to work, watch the same TV shows at night. All of this sameness makes it easy for our brains to operate on autopilot, which has its benefits—but growing new neural connections and protecting the brain from decline aren't among them.

When it comes to brain health, the old cliché of "Use it or lose it" couldn't be more true. When you learn, you grow new neurons as well as new and bigger connections between those neurons, creating more storage space for memories. Recall that long-term memories (including facts and information) are stored in vast networks of nerve cell pathways. The richer those pathways, the more permanent—and accessible—the information in your brain.

Remember the story from Part 1 about the London cab drivers? When some of the drivers, who spent their careers learning to navigate the crazy London streets, underwent MRI scans of their brains, they were found to have an unusually large hippocampus, an area that plays a major role in memory formation, particularly spatial memory. You don't need to study maps of London, but studying something—*anything*—will make your brain bigger, stronger, and better able to resist age-related changes that can slow you down.

Challenging your brain is perhaps the best thing you can do to keep it young. One study looked at the degree of cognitive stimulation a group of older folks experienced over a period of 5 years. Those who experienced the most had 35 percent less decline in their cognitive abilities than those who experienced the least.

Learning may do even more than stave off cognitive decline; it may reverse it. In a review of almost 200 studies on brain aging, mostly in animals, scientists found that with cognitive training and brain-challenging environments, almost every physical manifestation of cognitive decline can be reversed: rate of cell death can be slowed, gray matter can be thickened, amyloid plaques (associated with Alzheimer's disease) can be reduced. Mental challenges may even restore the fatty coating around neural fibers that protects them from age-related damage, a loss previously believed to be irreversible.

WHAT COUNTS AS LEARNING?

"Learning" comes in many forms. Sure, challenging your brain with books, crossword puzzles, card games, and classes is important. But so is brain stimulation of almost any sort. Any new experience you have, especially when it is very different from your normal routine, is a learning experience. Some of the most effective experiences are those that involve your senses.

Imagine walking through a botanical garden, surrounded by colors of every shade and hue, a gentle breeze on your face, and suddenly the smell of lavender transports you back to playing in the park as a young child. Or you attend a wine

You get the biggest cognitive boost when you pick up a new skill: Start with the basics, then practice, practice, practice.

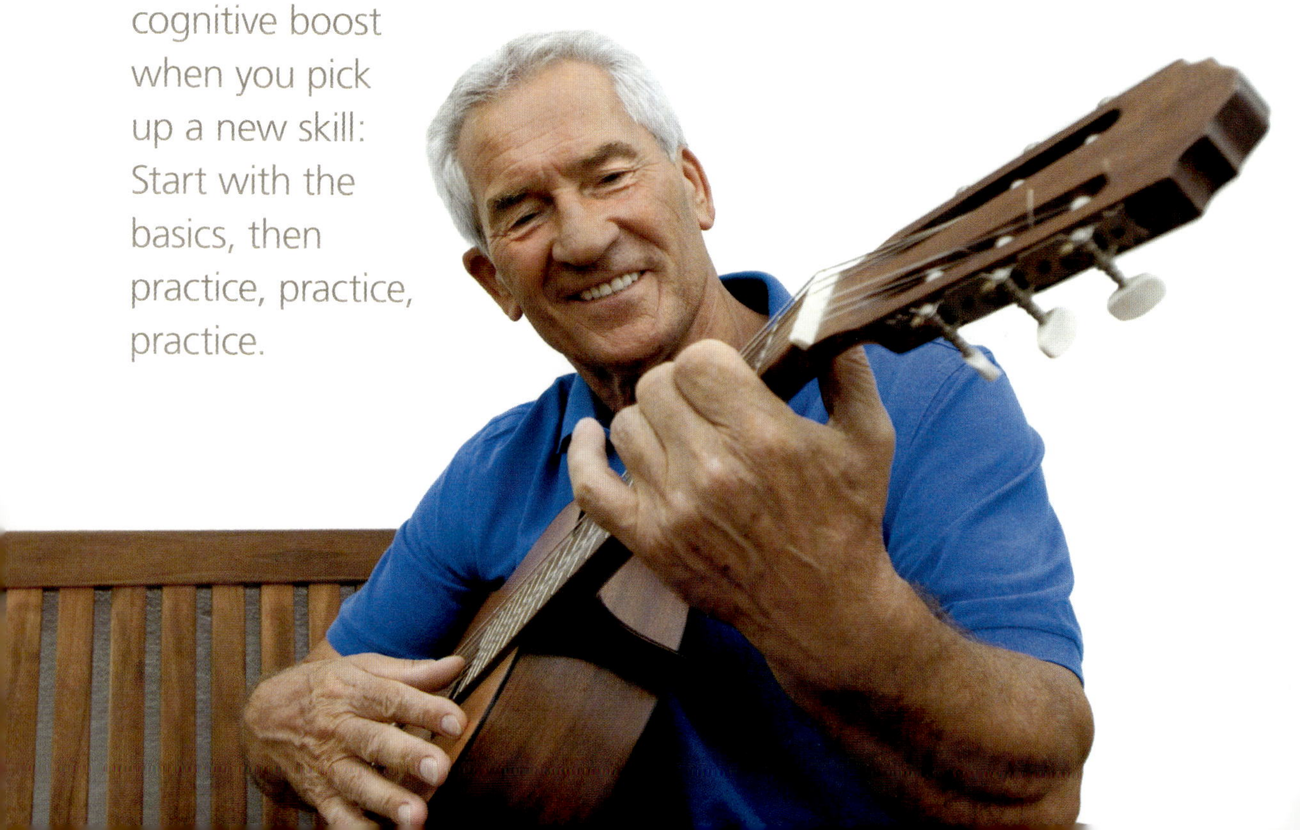

tasting in a villa in Sonoma, and you gaze at your husband or wife in the fading sunlight as you drink a glass of amazing pinot noir and think about the first time you shared a bottle of wine together. Your brain is on alert, absorbing and analyzing the new sensory information and processing it together with stored memories to consider all this data in the new context. And most of this happens just by remaining in the moment and noticing details around you.

Surprise Your Brain

To challenge your brain, you don't have to memorize the periodic table of elements or calculate pi out to a thousand digits. All you really need to do is, well, anything other than what you've been doing. The best way to start is to think of a few things you've always wanted to try, and jump in! Here are a few suggestions to get your brain in gear.

Develop your alter ego. When we like something, we tend to do a lot of it. Readers read; quilters quilt; programmers program. From now on, the old Monty Python line is your personal mantra: "And now for something completely different!" During your down time, do whatever you perceive to be the complete opposite of what you normally do. If you're a carpenter, join a reading group. If you're a book editor, take a kayaking class. If you're an information technology expert, take up watercolor painting.

Change up your environment. If you spend 8 hours a day staring at a computer screen, ban all screens (computers, Blackberries, TVs) from one day of the weekend and head somewhere green instead. If you spend your days tending to others' needs—as a nurse, a volunteer, a teacher, a caregiver—switch to total self-indulgence: Head to a spa and get a massage or pedicure, or see a double feature with a friend. If you tend to spend quiet evenings at home, show up at a sports bar. Anytime you experience new, radically different sensations, your brain is shocked out of its stupor and undergoes a change that builds new connections, associations, and memories—the exact process involved in learning. Your brain will not only thrive on the change of pace, you'll reduce stress (another brain drain), and be refreshed and ready to go on Monday.

Education: Your Brain's Rainy Day Fund

Intellectual experiences throughout your entire life, no matter when they happen, build your brain reserve. Think of this reserve as cognitive cash in the bank, it's the "money" that will cushion you against any shortfalls and delay "bankruptcy" should you run into trouble. Research from the National Institute on Aging on more than 7,000 people found that those who graduated from high school were less likely to develop cognitive impairment in their later years than those who didn't. If a high school grad did experience cognitive decline, he or she experienced it 3 years later than nongrads. The bigger your cognitive reserve, the better your brain is able to tolerate age-related changes and resist dementia, even if you have dementia risk factors such as plaques or tangles in your brain.

Choose an activity you have to practice to master. Most of us reach a point of competency in our jobs and hobbies, and then coast on that competency. But in some ways, being a novice is better for your brain than being an expert. You get the biggest cognitive boost when you pick up a new skill: Start with the basics, then practice, practice, practice until you master it. That thrill of mastery, and even tiny victories along the way, creates a flush of pleasure chemicals that reinforce learning and motivate you to continue.

If you're just learning to cast your rod, practice in the backyard kiddie pool until you feel confident, then take it to a riverbank. Or read up on the card game bridge, then play it online until you feel ready to join a real live bridge game. Progressive learning like this causes specific brain cells to specialize for the demands of your new task. Just like strengthening your abdominal muscles helps improve your posture, as these individual regions of your brain get stronger, they fortify the brain as a whole.

Learn piano—from a Suzuki teacher. Playing an instrument physically strengthens the brain. One Canadian study found that kids who took music lessons experienced a seven point boost in their IQs. Another study showed that drumming helped adults reduce cortisol levels (high levels are toxic to brain cells). Still other studies have shown that mastering an instrument leads to a better facility with numbers and an enhanced sense of spatial relations. At higher levels, music training may help

The Power of Positive Thinking

The doddering old widow. The lonely, forgetful neighbor. Turns out these negative perceptions of old age can be self-fulfilling prophecies. Yale researchers checked on the mortality rates of more than 600 people who answered survey questions some 20 years earlier, when they were age 50 and older. The researchers discovered that those who'd agreed with such statements as "Things keep getting worse as I get older" and "As you get older, you are less useful" were more likely to die early than those who'd agreed with such statements as "I am as happy now as I was when I was younger." People with a more positive outlook on aging lived an average of 7.5 years longer than the negative bunch.

The more negative the vision of old age people held when they were younger, the more likely they were to later experience the very types of physical and mental decline they envisioned—turning into their own stereotypes.

Other studies have found that when researchers used word prompts like "wise" versus "senile" before older people engaged in specific tasks, that vocabulary alone led to enhancement or decline on a wide array of cognitive and behavioral outcomes, including memory performance, handwriting, and mathematical performance.

The moral? Think young. Any time you find yourself saying "I don't do that," write "that" down on a list—you've just found a great opportunity to learn something new and help protect your brain. Show yourself you can do it, and you'll build your belief in your brain's abilities, a key strategy for prolonging your life and avoiding cognitive decline.

improve our ability to manipulate information in both short- and long-term memory, benefits that can help us in many areas of life.

Not sure how to start? The Suzuki musical training method was created for preschoolers, but it's a great method for any beginner. This progressive approach breaks down critical playing skills of several instruments (such as piano, violin, or guitar) into very small and achievable blocks. Suzuki method helps develop your "ear" for music, partially because listening to music is considered part of the practice. With its emphasis on good form, repetition, and motor skill training, Suzuki helps you learn the baby steps to virtuosity in an entertaining way. Call a local music school to see if they have Suzuki-trained instructors, or look online for private instructors in your area. Most Suzuki teachers have tremendous patience and good humor they've developed from working with preschoolers!

Launch, or continue, a career. Fewer and fewer people plan to stop working entirely when they retire. Continuing to work, even on a freelance or part-time basis, is an excellent way to line your pockets and protect your brain. It can even prevent the brain-draining depression that often results from having too much idle time. Need a little help? Career centers for baby boomers are beginning to crop up. For instance, St. Anthony Central Hospital in Denver recently launched a Boomer Career Center in conjunction with a free wellness membership program. Boomers can visit the center for assistance with transitioning to a different career. Online, you can check out 50 Best Employers for Workers over 50 at www.aarp.org and find specific job opportunities at www.retirementjobs.com.

Stay productive. You don't have to keep your job to produce, say experts—you could also pitch in at the food bank, knit hats for babies at the hospital, teach your grandkids how to read, or tend the community garden. While surveys have found that paid work drops sharply after age 55, volunteer work peaks then. And informal help to friends and family peaks thereafter (between 55 and 64) and can continue until 74 or later.

When older people continue to stay productive, they are not considered old by their families or friends, or by themselves—and apparently, their brains agree. A study of more than a thousand Chinese adults age 55 and older found that productive activities, such as painting, gardening, preparing meals, and even shopping, lowered the risk of dementia, presumably because those activities demanded complex thought and planning.

Go back to school. Jobs are tough to find these days, especially for older folks. But with a few years of training, you could become a nurse, health-care technician, or health-care administrator—three in-demand careers.

Volunteer for the Red Cross. Or Habitat for Humanity. Or a local food bank or community garden. You'll be around a whole new set of people handling a unique set of challenges, and probably develop brand-new skills along the way. And you'll be invigorated by the idea of doing good.

TURN CHORES INTO BRAIN-BOOSTERS

Learn a new, useful skill. Choose learning opportunities that help you in real life. Having trouble keeping your banking and investments straight? Take a financial planning course, or learn how to use money-management software like Quicken. Bills and savings fall into line, decreasing the stress that can sap motivation and atrophy your brain. These activities tap into a well of deeper attention because the "saliency"—the degree to which the info matters to you personally—is so high. Best of all, you'll break negative thinking patterns such as, "I can't manage my money" that can actually accelerate cognitive loss.

Trade chores. One survey of more than 20,000 Scottish men and women found that just 20 minutes of weekly housework or gardening was enough to markedly increase their mental health. But here's the twist: Switch jobs. Let your husband pay the bills or send out birthday cards while you whack weeds, change light bulbs, or walk the dog. Trading chores not only challenges your brain in new ways but also helps you see things from your partner's perspective—a higher-level thinking process that exercises multiple parts of your brain at once. Bonus: Your relationship can only improve the more you appreciate each other's contributions.

Time your task. If you're going to sit down and tackle a difficult cognitive challenge, such as reviewing changes in your medical benefits plan, set a timer for 20 minutes and really focus. The combination of committed attention and a focused time period stimulates the nucleus basalis, two small regions in the forebrain vulnerable to Alzheimer's disease. Once you're done, reward yourself—spend a few minutes watching a video bloopers show, throw the Frisbee for your dog, or just sit quietly on the patio and let the sun warm your face. Any of these activities will stimulate your brain's reward system, reinforce the benefits of the effort you just made, and help motivate you to repeat the experience.

Learn, Don't Memorize

Don't bother to remember names—just tell yourself to learn them. One study found that when people were told to "learn" statements from a list, they did much better than when they were told to "remember" them. In fact, when adults between age 60 and 75 were told to "learn," they did as well as young adults between 17 and 24! If you, consciously or unconsciously, believe that a person's memory gets worse with age, anxiety over remembering names and facts can prevent you from remembering them. Think in terms of learning instead and perhaps you can bunny hop over your own self-doubts.

STIMULATE YOUR SENSES

Go to a rock concert or an amusement park. Have you ever gone to an event and thought, "I'm too old for this?" That's exactly where you need to be—at least for a little while. You needn't be a regular at rock concerts, video arcades, or disco night at the bowling alley, but occasional visits could do you a world of good. These experiences assault your brain with new sights, sounds, smells, and sensations

9 Fun, Easy Ways to Learn Something New

1

Buy a word-a-day calendar and try to use the word in conversation at least once the day you learn it.

2

Go to the zoo and actually stop to read all the signs to learn about the animals.

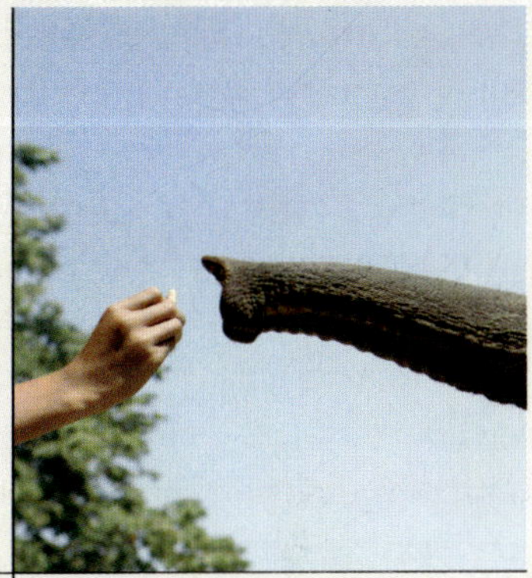

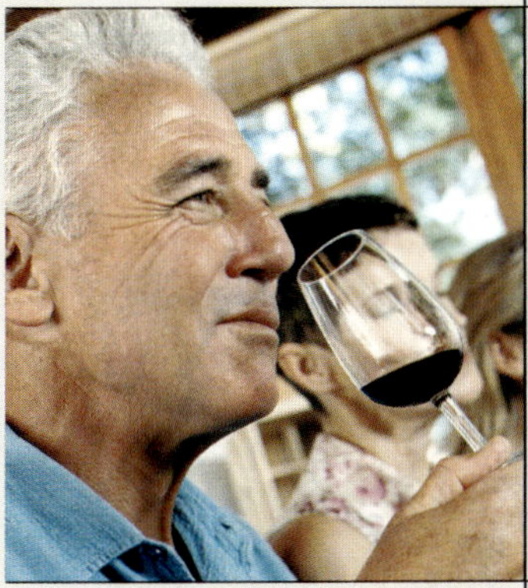

3

Check out Very Short List: Science (www.veryshortlist.com), a free daily e-mail with links to new and fascinating advances in science.

4

Take a 1-day first-aid class.

5

Go to a beginner's wine tasting (free at many wine stores) and learn how to smell, taste, and spit wine like a pro.

6

Pick a random topic—how to grow tomatoes, improve your gas mileage, open a flower shop—Google it, and follow the links for 20 minutes and see where they take you.

7

Read a different genre of book—if you're a mystery reader, try a memoir or biography; if you're a novel reader, try a thriller.

8

Learn to say "hello," "please," and "thank you" in a new language every week.

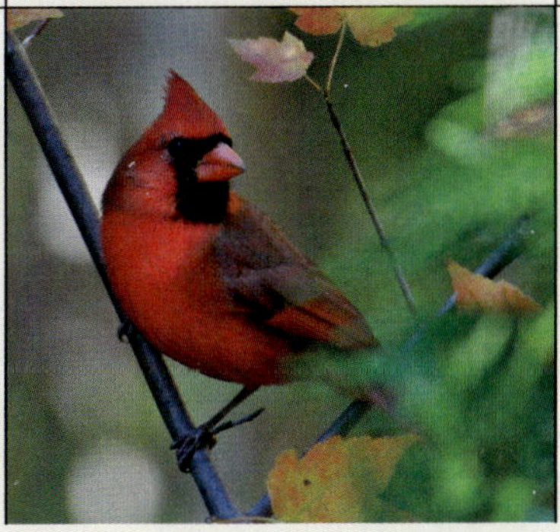

9

Hang a bird feeder by your window and keep a field guide to birds handy to identify visitors.

and nudge you out of your comfort zone, reawakening your senses.

Indulge in small thrills. Another reason fresh experiences benefit the brain is because they stimulate the release of dopamine, a neurotransmitter associated with attention and planning. Older brains release less dopamine, which may in part explain dwindling attention spans as we age. Here's the fun part: You get dopamine surges from lots of very enjoyable things—eating chocolate (make it dark chocolate for its antioxidants), getting a foot massage, having sex. Not too hard to take, right?

Watch foreign movies. Reading the subtitles while simultaneously watching the actors challenges you to keep up. You won't be able to kick back and vegetate on the couch; you'll be actively involved in watching the movie.

CONNECT WITH FELLOW ARTISTS, ACTIVISTS, AND BRAINIACS

Volunteer at the library. Sign up to read books to toddlers, man the sign-out desk, or reshelve books. You'll keep great tabs on the hip books of the moment and get to know the regulars. Plus, what's more inspiring than rows and rows of books containing the accumulated knowledge of centuries of smart thinkers?

Bone up on a cause you care about. There's a lot wrong with the world, and a lot you can do to help set it right. Choose a cause that interests you and learn all you can about it. Maybe it's an upcoming election, an environmental issue (such as recycling), the plight of small farmers in your state, or something larger, like the atrocities in Darfur. Many people find that getting involved in a cause they believe in helps them tap into a reserve of energy and excitement they didn't realize they had. If there's an issue you feel particularly passionate about—like helping feed and school low-income children—go online to search for a local group that's working in your community (try www.volunteermatch.org) or inquire at your church or synagogue.

Develop your art. If you have an interest such as cooking or playing tennis, kick it up a notch. Sign up for a cooking course with a local chef who teaches about how to use local, fresh ingredients.

Creative projects can help manage anxiety and decrease blood pressure, protecting your brain from degenerative stresses.

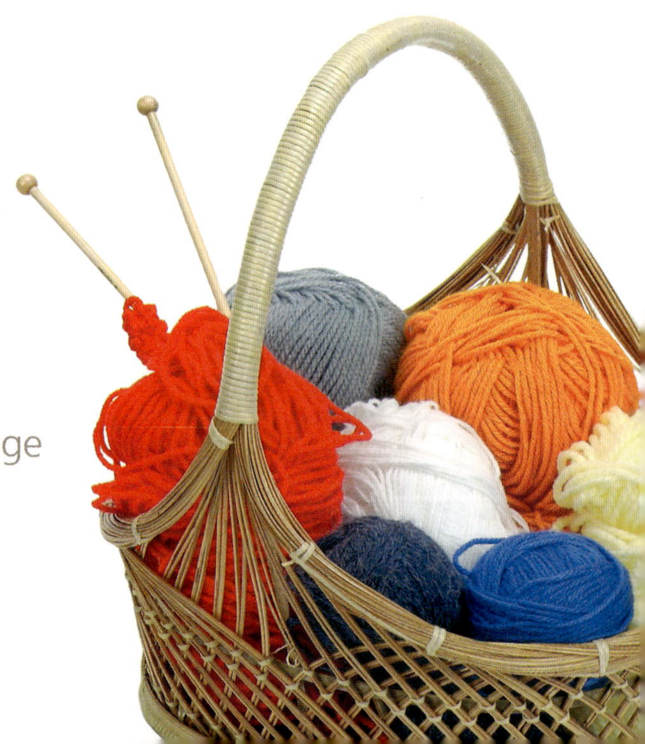

Or, if you're a backyard griller, take a sushi-making class. Like to create holiday crafts? Take a sculpting course. Dabble in the garden? Investigate landscape-design programs in your area. Jump out of your comfort zone into a level two notches above where you currently stand. If you have to struggle to keep up, all the better.

Hit the stage. If you've harbored a secret dream to be an actor, you owe it to yourself to head to your local theater and see if you can audition, even for a nonspeaking part, in their next production. Or help create sets or sew costumes, other creative tasks that will tickle your brain. Research from the University of California found that because we tend to delight in the experience of making art, doing it can help strengthen our ability to pay attention. Actors also employ clever tricks to learn their lines, which can help hone your memory skills.

Walk and talk. You know that exercise and social connections—Vaccines #2 and #4—help sharpen the brain. Combine them with mental stimulation and you'll reap maximum rewards. One study followed 776 Swedish adults over 75 years old for 6 years and found that those who combined at least two of these types of experiences slashed their risk of dementia in half, 10 to 20 percent more than exercising, socializing, or doing mentally challenging activities alone. Try these tactics:

- Walk with a friend and discuss politics or a book you both read
- Learn to waltz, tango, or swing dance—you'll be memorizing the steps, socializing with other dancing students, and moving your body across the dance floor
- Bike to your Bingo game or to a friend's house to play Scrabble.

WORK TOWARD A FINISHED PRODUCT

Alternate difficult and easy craft projects. Don't just knit a bunch of mono-color, one-stitch scarves while staring at TV—really work at creating something you've never done before. Challenge yourself to learn new patterns. Try intricate work that requires careful attention, counting, and memory (how many stitches did I just purl again?). Alternate these brain-intensive projects with more "mindless" scarves, the creation of which can help manage anxiety and decrease blood pressure, protecting your brain from degenerative stresses.

Help your parents organize photos and memorabilia. Or sit down and do it for yourself! Most of us have boxes of photos we never look through because they aren't in albums. Or we have electronic photos scattered on several different photo-sharing websites. (Need help organizing photos online? Look for a continuing education course on using the internet that covers photo management.)

If you sit down with your mom or dad and their boxes of photos, take time to reminisce. Recall of pleasant memories engages your nucleus accumbens, a part of the brain involved in memory consolidation that's also awash in dopamine, a brain chemical associated with pleasure and reward. A bonus: As you help your parents get memorabilia organized, you'll strengthen your own ability to classify and organize, skills that can falter somewhat with age.

Create an audio scrapbook. If your budget allows, buy an electronic voice recorder and voice-recognition software. The combination allows you to turn conversations into digital files that you can copy to CDs and share with the rest of the family, or turn into text. Go to a self-publishing website (like www.lulu.com), turn your text into a book, and order copies for everyone in the family. This multi-stage process might be a big challenge, but certainly one that will increase your brainpower and give you a tremendously valuable skill you can share with other family and friends.

Take a class on using the internet. You'll learn how to do everything from filing taxes electronically (faster returns!) to shopping, balancing your checkbook, even paying bills online. There really is no limit to what you could learn—the internet holds an infinite amount of information on any topic you'd ever want to learn about or experience. TV makes you a passive receptacle; the Web puts you in control of what you watch, read, and learn about.

GO BACK TO SCHOOL–AS STUDENT OR TEACHER

Take a class. Have you always wanted to get your bachelor's degree but never had a chance to finish? Maybe you'd like to sink deeper into art history or French—something you previously thought impractical. If you live near a university, request their community class schedule, but also check into auditing an actual for-credit university class. The rigor of a class, in which students have more than a passing interest, will be infectious. You'll also be able to gauge your smarts against those of younger kids, and you may find that your wisdom gives you a certain edge.

Head back to school–on your kitchen table. If you'd like to experience the rigor of academia from the comfort of your kitchen or couch, check out some of the thousands of online distance-learning programs available from accredited universities around the country (and the world!). Typically, you'll interact with your professor by e-mail and chat rooms (more practice on the computer!). Some programs also have one on-campus weekend requisite, another experience guaranteed to stretch your mind.

Finally learn Spanish. Think kids are the only ones who can learn a new language? Hardly. Adults understand how grammar rules typically work, and we can draw on our vast vocabularies for raw material. Take an intro class in Spanish, and start a happy hour after class with your fellow students right away. (You can all practice with the lip-loosening effects of a margarita.) Supplement with the Destinos video series (available at many online retailers including www.amazon.com), soap operas designed to help you learn Spanish by getting wrapped up in the drama. If, after a few months, you find you love it, consider jumping in with both feet: Take an immersion class in Mexico or Spain for a month. You'll help your brain connect real-world experience to each word, something you just won't get in a classroom.

Let your ears fill up your brain. Always loved school but don't want to go to class? Listen to college lectures while you work on your needlepoint or fly-tying.

The Great Courses program from the Teaching Company collects lectures from the greatest professors in the world on subjects ranging from Albert Einstein to Zen Buddhism. Rediscover what made college such a heady experience. Pop the CDs into your portable player and take them out into the garden, or listen to them on long drives in the car.

Consider computer games for the brain. A handful of computer programs purport to help strengthen your brain and your memory (see "Can Playing Computer Games Make You Smarter?" on page 235). One of them, the Posit Science's Brain Fitness Program, was studied in a randomized, controlled, double-blind trial of 524 healthy adults age 65. Half the group in the study used the program, the other half, a generic computer-based educational training program. Those who used the Posit Science program showed improvements in their speed of processing and other standardized clinical measures of memory gains equal to turning back the clock approximately 10 years. Participants also felt much better about their ability to remember and more confident in their power to remember names and phone numbers. Insurance company Humana was so impressed with the Posit Science results that they've begun to offer the program to their Medicare enrollees. The software isn't cheap though; expect to pay $400 or more.

Another less expensive option is eyeQ, designed to enhance cognitive function and reading speed in 7-minute sessions. Find it at www.eyeqadvantage.com.

Offer your expertise. Sometimes the best way to learn is to teach. If you have a special talent or skill—a flair for decorating or woodworking, for example—design a course for your local community center or public library. When you teach someone something, you have to break it down to its core elements and explain things step-by-step, while also tailoring your message to the audience. This process taps your planning, memory, and perspective-taking centers simultaneously, forcing you to recall the past, project into the future, and put yourself in your students' place all at once. These kinds of multi-center brain demands are like triathlons for your brain.

Another approach: If you have a background in education, or even a college degree, you can apply for a job as a teaching assistant or aid at a primary school. Kids never cease to amaze and challenge us.

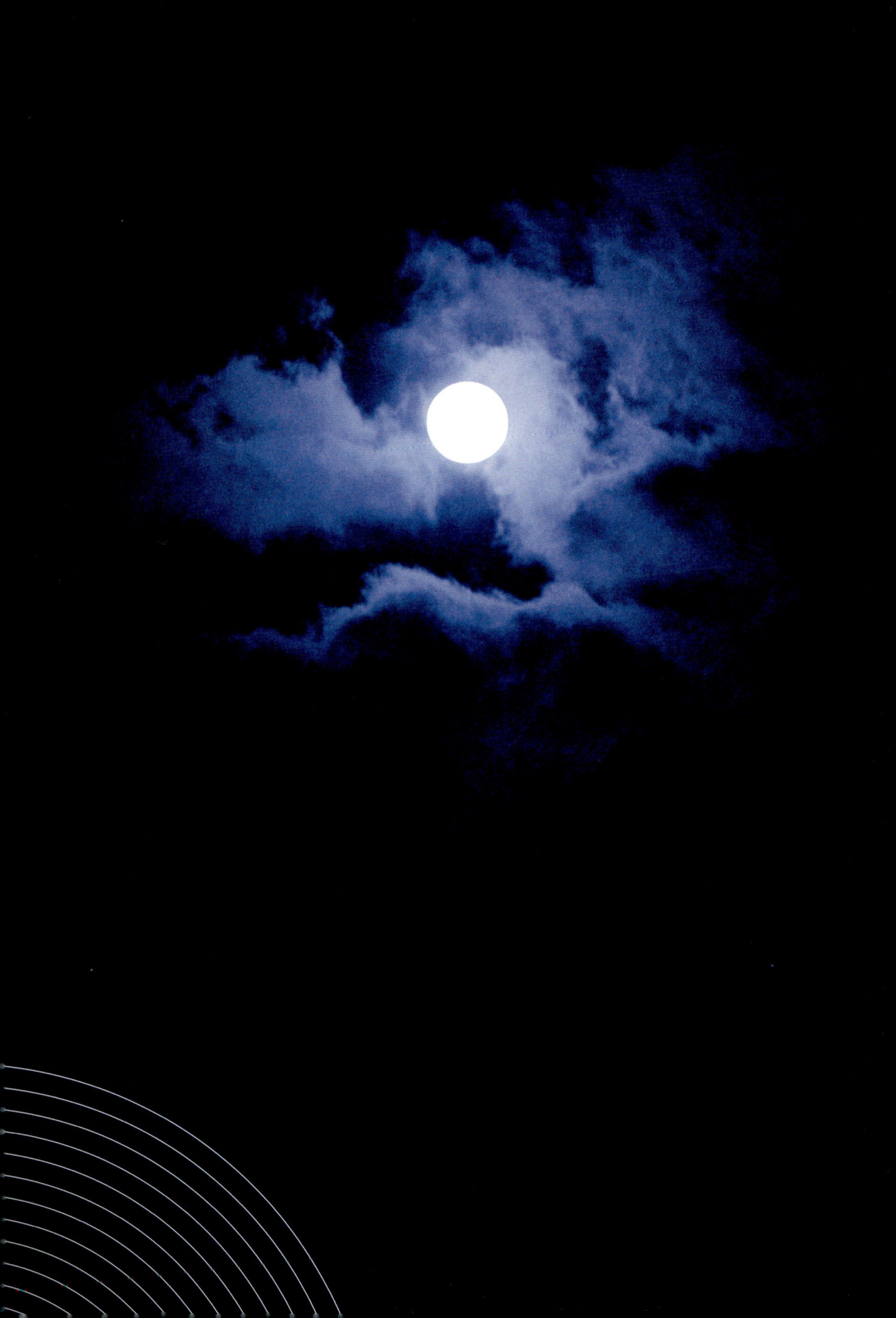

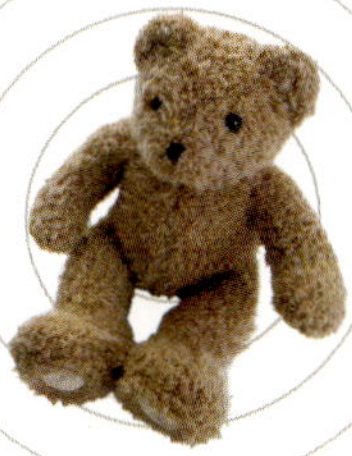

VACCINE #6

sleep

Some Brain Drain vaccines require a bit of work on your part—tweaking your diet and exercise habits, taking a class, making an effort to get out and see people. But vaccine #6 is defined by doing nothing at all. Zero. Zip. To reap its tremendous brain benefits, simply pull back the sheets on your bed, slide in, and allow yourself to drop off to sleep.

While you sleep, your body may be still, but your brain is busy. It sweeps out all the detritus left behind by daily brain cell activities—biochemical clutter that can interfere with normal brain functioning. It also repairs and regenerates tissues critical to memory and other cognitive processes. Indeed, high-quality sleep improves your ability to make plans, solve problems, concentrate, and remember things. Want to get smarter overnight? Catch 40 winks. A person's IQ is actually higher when he or she is well-rested.

Sleep takes the brain "offline," which allows it to do all of its filing and other routine maintenance. During the first hour-and-a-half after you fall asleep, you drift into the first of several nightly cycles of slow-wave Stage 3 and 4 sleep, the deepest forms. This dreamless slumber helps you solidify long-term retention of declarative memories—the facts you have learned or situations you have experienced during the day. In order to reach this state, your levels of the stress hormone cortisol must be very low, a big reason why relaxation is key to a good night's rest—and a good memory. (When levels of cortisol are too high, storage of memories in the hippocampus suffers. Over time, the cortisol slowly erodes this critical memory center, and brain cells in the hippocampus waste away, considerably slowing your access to facts and memories.)

Toward the early morning, cortisol levels naturally rise, preparing to wake you up. Before you are thoroughly awake, you'll cycle through several stages of rapid-eye-movement, or REM, sleep. This dream-filled sleep allows your brain to rehearse skills you learned during the day, such as notes you played on the piano, a new dance step you finally got down, or a new technique for kneading bread dough that made it rise just right.

This rehearsal, which activates the same neural circuits as actually performing the activity, helps the brain store these "procedural" memories for good. "If the old saying was 'Practice makes perfect,' the new saying should be 'Practice with a night of sleep makes perfect,'" according to Matthew Walker, PhD, director of the sleep and neuroscience lab at University of California, Berkeley, in a televised interview.

During REM sleep, you also process and sort emotional memories. High levels of cortisol can hurt here, too: While excess cortisol degrades long-term memory stored in the hippocampus, it actually enhances the storage of disturbing emotional memories in the amygdala, the seat of our most primal emotions.

If getting an adequate amount of sleep benefits your brain, getting extra on occasion can do even more good. Just 1 or 2 extra hours of additional sleep on top of your normal amount can help you perform much better on tasks that require sustained focus. And remember,

What Happens When You Sleep

- Brain cells are repaired
- Experiences are processed into memories
- Memories are solidified and put in places where they can be accessed more quickly
- Health-promoting growth hormone is released
- Connections between nerve cells multiply, increasing your brain's "plasticity"
- Decision-making skills, reaction time, and hand-eye coordination are sharpened

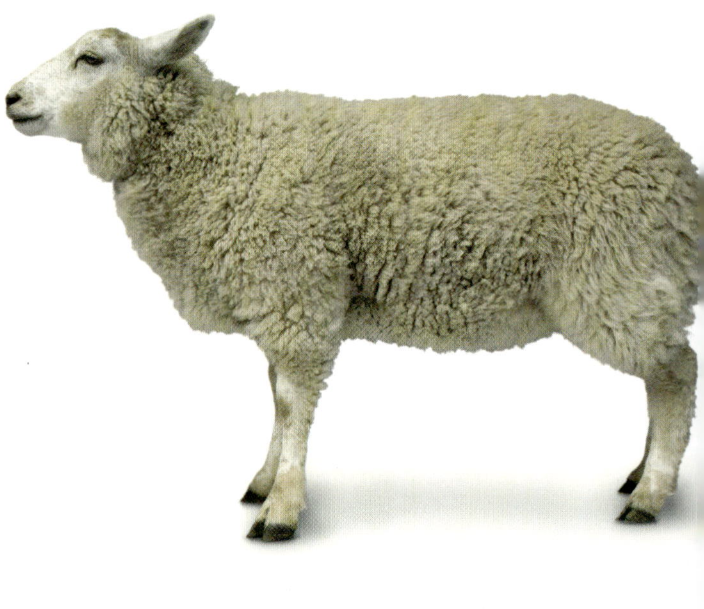

paying better attention is the first step to remembering better. Sleep can even help your brain shuffle newly developed ideas together and solve problems more creatively. And let's face it, you just feel better and happier when you've had a full night's worth.

Many of us don't get enough shut-eye, and that's too bad, especially considering that sleep deprivation increases brain inflammation, which can prevent the formation of new brain cells. Researchers at the University of Chicago have even found that chronic sleep deprivation ages the brain at an accelerated rate, setting us up for early cognitive decline. Yet we often don't realize that we're sleep deprived. A study published in the journal *Epidemiology* found that when more than 650 adults were asked how much they slept, they regularly overestimated their sleep hours (researchers had tracked how much they actually slept).

But don't we need less sleep as we age? No, say the experts, though it may seem that way because of a natural process called sleep phase shift. Basically, as we get older, we tend to go to sleep earlier or nap during the day and wake up earlier. Even if we're logging our sleep hours at different times, though, we still need as many hours as ever.

"Depressionsomnia"

Can't sleep? Insomnia is often the first sign of depression, which is covered in more depth starting on page 153. It's surprisingly common, especially among older folks. Instead of drifting off when your head hits the pillow, you might get stuck ruminating on losses of one sort or another: lost savings, lost opportunities, or simply lost youth. If this sounds like you, ask your doctor to screen you for depression. Meanwhile, think about keeping a journal. Studies have shown that journaling can help people heal after traumatic events, reduce medical visits, and perform better at work. Writing not only helps you just get your emotions out, it also helps you figure out strategies for solving your problems.

Surefire Steps to Better Sleep

Getting more sleep is perhaps as simple as going to bed earlier. It also helps to perfect what sleep experts call your sleep hygiene, that is, your sleep habits. What doesn't help much? Sleeping pills. People who take them don't get as much extra sleep as they think—sometimes only a few minutes more. And once you start taking sleep aids, including over-the-counter products, you could become trapped in an addictive cycle for a while. Even "natural" remedies like supplemental melatonin have not been conclusively proven to work, and melatonin supplements may even hamper your own natural melatonin release. Stick to these strategies.

COMBAT STRESS HORMONES

Hit the gym. One of the best ways to get a good night's sleep is to exercise. Most researchers think exercise reduces insomnia because of its effects on stress hormones. People with insomnia tend to have abnormally high levels of stress hormones, or release the hormones with very little provocation. Exercise initially

Are You Sleep Deprived?

If you feel drowsy during the day, you probably didn't get enough sleep the night before. The Epworth Sleepiness Scale, developed by Dr. Murray Johns of Epworth Hospital in Melbourne, Australia, is a test used by sleep specialists to judge a person's level of daytime sleepiness. To find out your level, ask yourself what the chances are that you'd doze off in the situations below, and give yourself the appropriate number of points.

Sitting and reading

__ 0 None
__ 1 Slight
__ 2 Moderate
__ 3 High

Watching TV

__ 0 None
__ 1 Slight
__ 2 Moderate
__ 3 High

Sitting inactively in a public place, such as a theater or a meeting

__ 0 None
__ 1 Slight
__ 2 Moderate
__ 3 High

As a passenger in a car for an hour without a break

__ 0 None
__ 1 Slight
__ 2 Moderate
__ 3 High

Lying down to rest in the afternoon

__ 0 None
__ 1 Slight
__ 2 Moderate
__ 3 High

Sitting and talking to someone

__ 0 None
__ 1 Slight
__ 2 Moderate
__ 3 High

Sitting quietly after lunch (without alcohol)

__ 0 None
__ 1 Slight
__ 2 Moderate
__ 3 High

In a car while stopped for a few minutes in traffic

__ 0 None
__ 1 Slight
__ 2 Moderate
__ 3 High

YOUR SCORE

Less than 8 points: You're in good shape. You probably get enough sleep.

8–11 points: You're getting a little less sleep than you need; your brain probably isn't quite as fast or sharp as it would be with more sleep.

12–15 points: You clearly aren't getting enough sleep. This is an issue you need to address.

16–24 points: You get so little sleep that you shouldn't be behind the wheel of a car, balancing your checkbook, or figuring out your income tax.

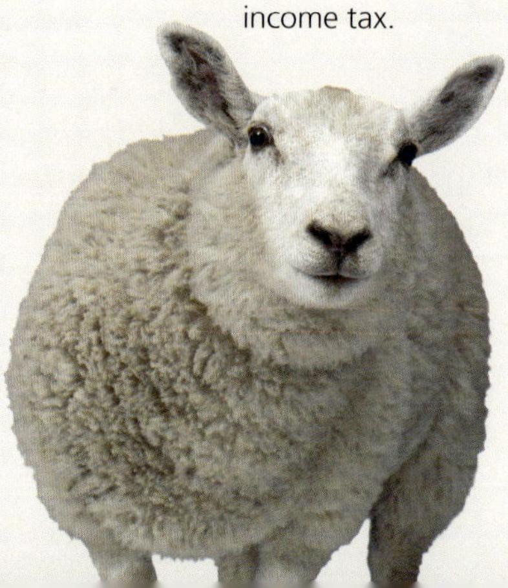

increases stress hormones, but then a few hours later, seeking to return to balance, your body sends out signals to reduce them. That's why you shouldn't exercise in the evening. Try to get in your workout at least 6 hours before bed.

Read—don't watch—your news, and only in the morning. Make it a habit to consume your news before noon, either in the form of a newspaper or online website. Television news often sensationalizes stories about child abductions and other crimes and makes them seem more common than they are. If you read your news instead of passively watching it, you are in control of what type of stories you consume.

Wean yourself from afternoon coffee. A morning cup of coffee is very good for your brain indeed—caffeine increases brain activity in your hippocampus, and it may also increase levels of a key neurotransmitter. But make sure that you've finished your last cup of the day by lunchtime, since it can take as many as 10 hours for caffeine to leave your system. Until then, caffeine keeps your cortisol levels elevated, which can interfere with your ability to fall asleep.

Snooze to Remember

Concerned that you'll blank on names at tomorrow's wedding or reunion? Study the guest list the night before and then get a good night's rest. During sleep, new memories are strengthened within their own neural circuits and are also distributed throughout the brain to be filed in and among pre-existing long-term memories. This makes the information more solid and easier to access. Also plan to get a good night's sleep after the event. If you go to bed remembering Mary's name but you don't sleep enough, studies suggest that you're likely to falsely remember the name the next day. You might call Mary "Martha" at breakfast.

STAY TRUE TO YOUR BODY CLOCK

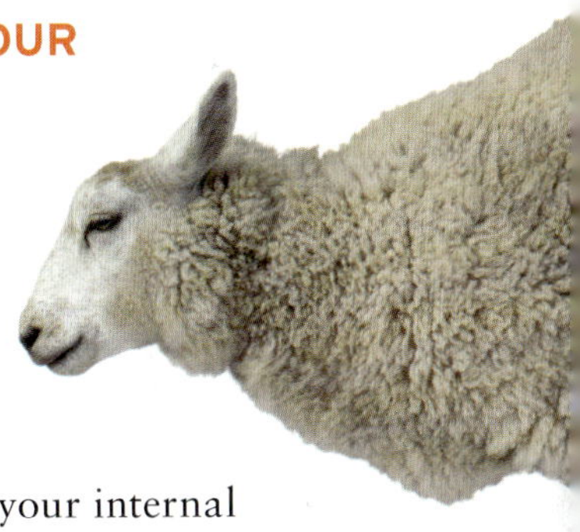

Get some bright light and outdoor sun during the day. If you expose your eyes to bright light in the morning, you'll help reset your internal clock, making it easier for you to sleep at night. Light enters your eyes and triggers your suprachiasmatic nucleus—your brain's "circadian pacemaker"—which regulates several biological rhythms during the day and night. One of these rhythms is the rise and fall of melatonin, a hormone that makes you more sleepy and less mentally sharp. Bright light depresses melatonin, and the lower your melatonin during the day, the higher it tends to climb at night, which allows you to fall into a deeper sleep.

The day-to-night shift in melatonin levels is extreme when we're young but much less dramatic as we age. One reason is that our eyes become less able to transmit light to the pineal gland (which produces melatonin) as we age. Less rise and fall in melatonin can result in more fatigue and decreased speed of thinking during the day, while also making it difficult to sleep at night. To combat this phenomenon, expose yourself to as much daylight as possible—the intensity of light is measured in lux, the amount of light you receive at a specific distance from the light source.

- Walk the dog in the early morning (400 lux)
- Use a light therapy box for 15 minutes to 2 hours a day (2,500 to 10,000 lux)
- Take a stroll at noon or sit outside with the bright sun on your face (50,000 to 100,000 lux)
- Keep all the lights on in your workspace or sitting area during the day (500 lux)

Keep lights low in the evening. Even a slight bit of light can disrupt melatonin release, so put dimmers on your switches and keep your lights lower after sunset. Shoot to have just one small bedside lamp on for the half-hour before you go to sleep. Install blackout shades to guard against any exterior light entering your bedroom during the night. This is especially important if you have blue, green, or light brown eyes—one study found that, compared with people with dark brown eyes, those with light-colored eyes experienced 20 percent lower melatonin when exposed to light at night.

Establish a strict bedtime and wake-up time. When it comes to sleep, the body loves routine. Going to bed and getting up at the same time every day, even on weekends, is one of the surest, most proven ways to help yourself fall asleep at night. Working backward from when you need to be up in the morning, choose a bedtime—such as 11 p.m.—and make sure that you're in bed with the lights off when the clock hits that time. Work backward from there to create your set prebed routine, such as:

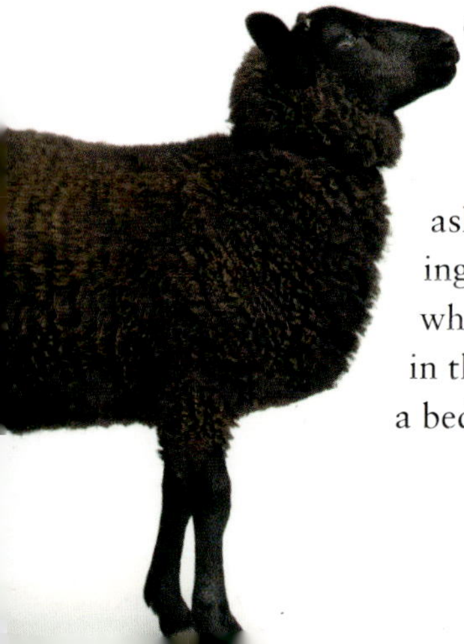

10:25 – Shower and brush teeth

10:35 – Slip into pajamas, soft robe, and socks

10:40 – Read something relaxing or write in journal

11:00 – Lights out!

At 7 a.m., it's time to wake up. Having a routine and keeping regular sleep hours minimizes circadian rhythm disturbances, which can become more prevalent as we get older. In Alzheimer's disease, such disturbances are so severe that they may contribute to mental decline. Some experts believe that lower nighttime melatonin levels might serve as an early marker of the first stages of Alzheimer's; they're not sure if it's a cause or a symptom.

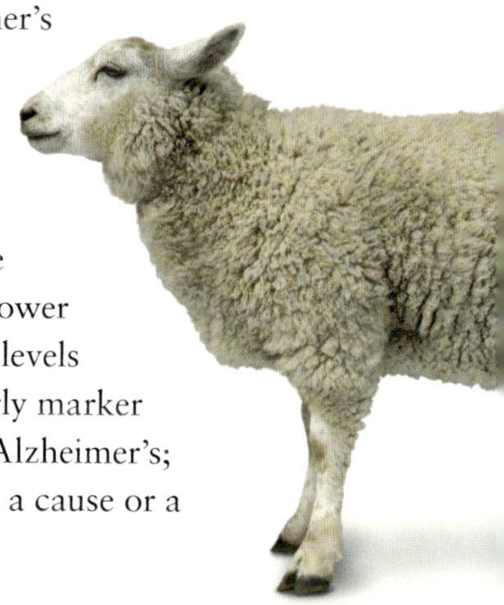

Go to bed 15 minutes earlier every week. Do this until you're getting the amount of sleep you need, then set your new bedtime in stone. A recent study found that 1 additional hour of sleep a night can lower your risk for developing calcified coronary artery plaque—hardened calcium deposits in the arteries of your heart—by up to 33 percent, the equivalent of lowering your systolic blood pressure by 16.5 points. The result? Better blood flow throughout your entire body, including your brain.

Coffee or Nap?

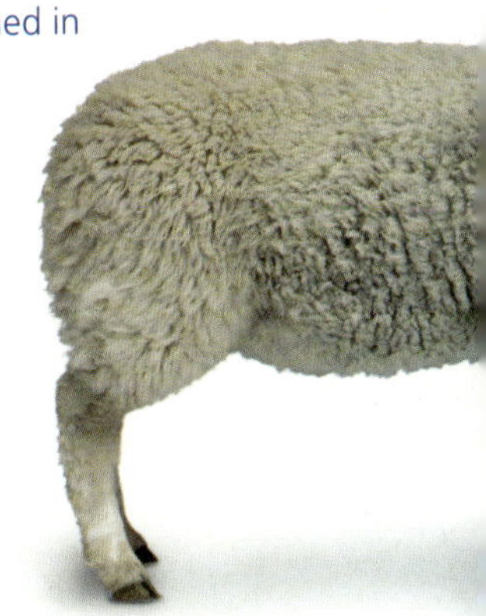

Take the nap. A study published in the journal *Behavioural Brain Research* looked at the performance of three groups of people: one group that napped from 1 to 3 p.m.; one group that got the caffeine equivalent of 2 cups of coffee at 3 p.m.; and one group that took placebo pills. The caffeinated group thought themselves the least sleepy but, in fact, they performed the same as the placebo group, or worse, on several cognitive tests. The nappers did the best, outscoring the other two groups significantly on the sensory and verbal tests.

Buy an electronic enforcer. If you're having trouble holding yourself to a bedtime, buy a timer for the switch to your TV and all the lights in your living room. Set it to turn off at 10:45 p.m. or earlier. Turning them back on will be a hassle, and you'll find it much easier to just get to bed. Or set an alarm clock to ring at 10:30 p.m.—an alert that time is almost up. If you tend to surf the web at night, program a reminder into your computer schedule software to alert you: "10:45—bedtime!"

MAKE BEDTIME A PLEASURE

Buy some high-thread-count sheets. Then change them regularly, at least once a week, so they're always soft and fresh. And why not splurge for a down pillow? There's nothing like an inviting bed to lure you away from the television at night.

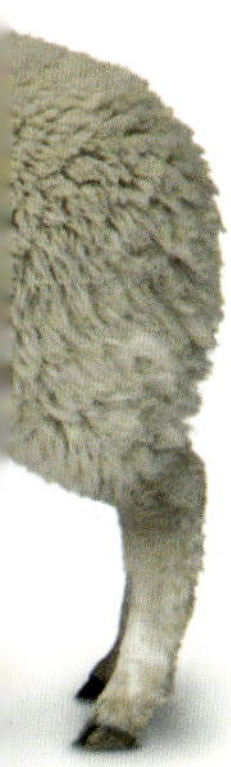

Add a white-noise machine. Or a fan, air-conditioner, or earplugs—anything to block out noise and help you stay asleep longer. The longer you sleep (up to a maximum of 8 or 9 hours), the more cycles of restorative Stage 3 and 4 sleep you'll have. Your body doesn't get to REM sleep until you've gone through several cycles of Stage 3 and 4, but REM is essential for creating new neurons in the areas of the brain associated with long-term memory.

Keep it cool. When it's time to sleep, your body temperature drops, usually starting 60 and 90 minutes before you fall asleep and hitting bottom about 2 hours before you wake up. Help it along by turning down your thermostat before you go to bed, especially if you have trouble sleeping. Researchers at the University of South Australia have found that insomniacs have a higher core body temperature than people who sleep soundly.

PERFECT YOUR BEFORE-BED ROUTINE

Skip the bedtime snack. The hunger hormone ghrelin must be high in order to help your body easily slip into Stage 3 (or deeper) sleep. Eating before bed makes ghrelin levels decrease. Shoot to have all your eating done by 9 p.m. Make sure that your last meal or snack of the day is high in protein and fiber; sugary snacks can cause insulin spikes, which can disturb sleep.

Also skip the nightcap. You might think that alcohol helps you sleep, but you'd be wrong. It may help you fall

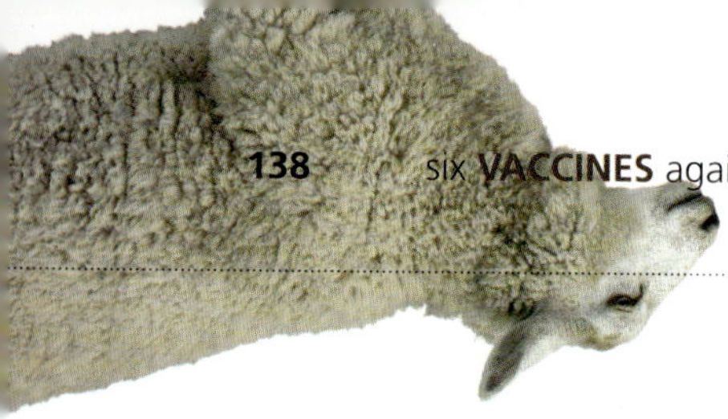

asleep—if you don't drink very regularly, that is—but as the effects wear off, you may wake up again.

Comedies only at night. If you must watch murder or crime shows, tape them and watch them early in the evening. One dream study found that people who watched more coverage of the terrorist attacks on the United States on September 11, 2001, experienced a dramatic change in the features of their dreams, even when they lived nowhere near Ground Zero or the Pentagon. Researchers said these results proved a direct association between watching images of violence on television and increased stress and trauma. Remember that high levels of stress hormones rob us of deep sleep. And as we get older, our bodies become even more vulnerable to stress hormones.

Turn off the TV before you nod off. Many people keep the TV on at night, especially if they live alone, to keep them company. But you may squander the important Stage 3 and 4 sleep that comes within the first hour-and-a-half by dozing off and waking with a start to gunshots or news bulletins. Several studies on children have found that television and computer before bed decreases their quality and length of sleep and increases overall tiredness. It also causes kids to perform worse on tests of verbal and cognitive skills. If TV can impact resilient little brains of kids this way, why would we be any different?

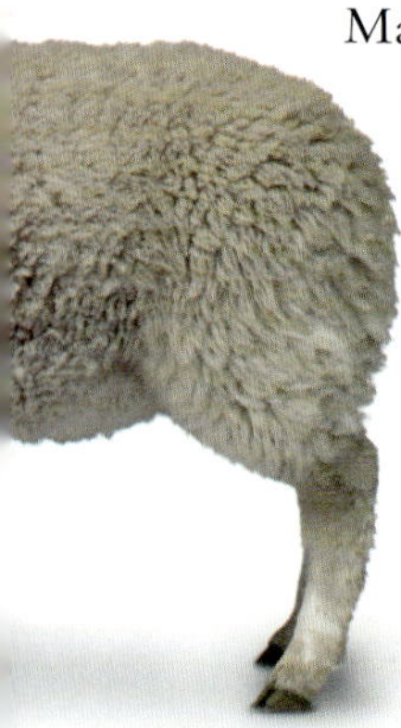

After you put down the remote, pick up a pen. A pilot study of people who had trouble falling asleep found that those who wrote about their problems for 20 minutes before bed nodded off almost 25 percent faster than those who didn't. And the benefits of journaling seemed to snowball. Before the study, each group averaged 40 minutes before they fell asleep. The first night, the writing group cut that in half, falling asleep after 20 minutes. The second night, they fell asleep after 15 minutes. By the third night, they'd cut their lie-awake time by 75 percent, falling asleep in a mere 10 minutes. (In contrast, the control group stayed awake for 35 minutes.)

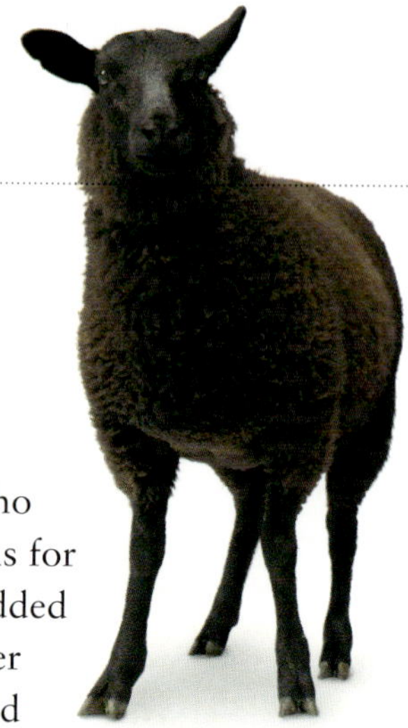

Keep a journal next to your bed and, each night, write down what you need to do the next day. Then take a moment to "declutter" any angry, worried, or otherwise negative thoughts by simply getting them out on the page. End your writing on a positive note: "The thing that made me happiest today was ____ because ____."

Read a boring book. One study found that books were the only media that actually helped people fall asleep, rather than prevent sleep. Keep one not-terribly-exciting book on your nightstand, and dip into it for a few pages a night. The second you feel yourself nodding off, close the book and turn off the light.

Tired? Go immediately to bed. If you ignore your first wave of sleepiness, your body may think you need to stay awake to fight some kind of threat and will

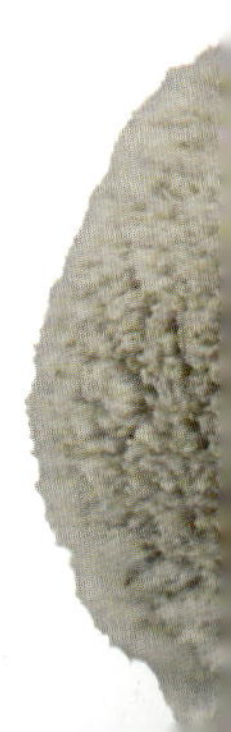

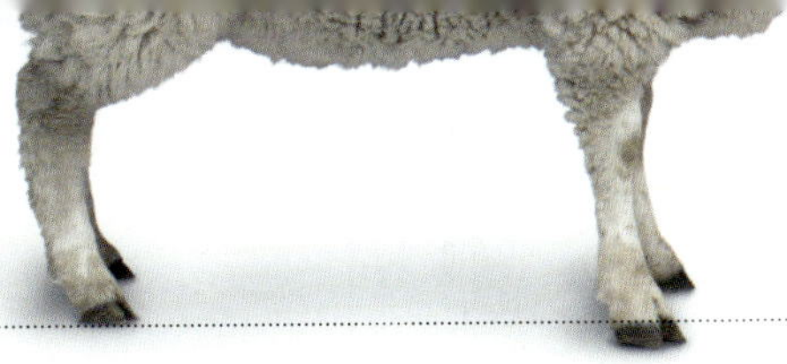

compensate with an extra burst of adrenaline, giving you a second wind. That adrenaline might last several hours in your bloodstream and can interfere with subsequent attempts to fall asleep.

WHEN SLEEP WON'T COME

Get out of bed. When insomniacs limit their nonsleeping time in bed, they actually increase their desire to sleep. If you lie awake in your bed for more than 20 minutes, get out of bed and do something else, such as read or knit. (Don't watch TV!) Designate a comfortable warm spot where you can go for this quiet time. Put your lamp on a dimmer, to keep lights low. Buy a meditation or relaxation CD, and have your portable CD player and headphones ready. As soon as you feel ready to sleep again, head back to bed.

Play musical beds. In order to break a cycle of insomnia, some people find it helps to sleep in another bed. If you've had several nights of poor sleep, make up the guest room bed or the couch. As soon as you've been awake for 20 minutes in your own bed, move there. Often the change of environment will help you break the cycle of repetitive thoughts and anxiety about falling asleep that have kept you awake in your own bed.

Talk to your doctor. As we get older, some of us may have trouble sleeping due to health conditions that cause pain or discomfort, such as arthritis, heartburn, or chronic obstructive pulmonary disease (COPD). Talk to your doctor about how you can best manage your condition and preserve healthful sleep at the same time. If you're taking a prescription drug, check with your pharmacist to find out if sleeplessness or insomnia is a common side effect. He or she may be able to suggest less sleep-disrupting alternatives—or possibly just a change in timing or dosage—that you can discuss with your doctor. Common culprits include antidepressants, decongestants, some asthma medicines, and some blood–pressure–lowering drugs.

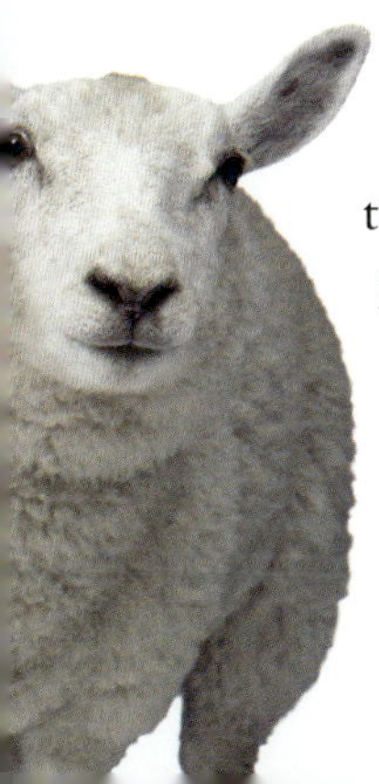

Enlist your partner in a bit of presleep relaxation therapy, a.k.a. sex! In both men and women, orgasm floods the system with endorphins, opiate-like chemicals released from the pituitary gland that reduce pain and increase feelings of well-being, and oxytocin, the bonding hormone that induces a sense of contented relaxation—both absolutely perfect for sleep.

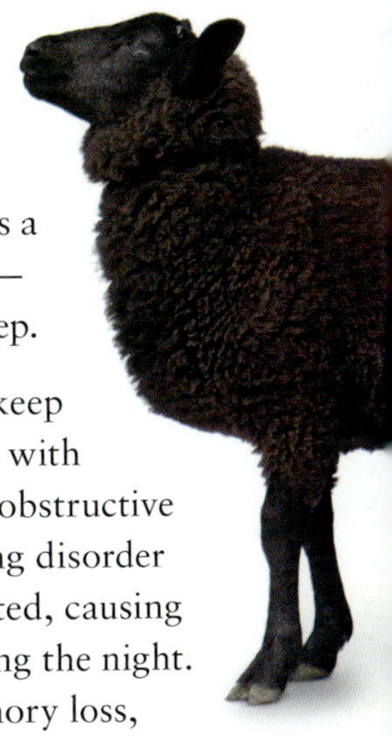

Lose a few pounds. If you keep your husband or wife awake with your snoring, you may have obstructive sleep apnea, a serious sleeping disorder in which breathing is disrupted, causing you to wake repeatedly during the night. Sleep apnea can lead to memory loss, high blood pressure, or even stroke. If you are regularly tired during the day and a loved one has told you that you snore, make an appointment with your doctor or with a sleep specialist. He or she may suggest that you use a continuous positive air pressure (CPAP) device to keep your airways open at night. For some people, surgery will help, too. But for people who carry excess pounds, losing just 10 percent of their weight can help reduce sleep apnea.

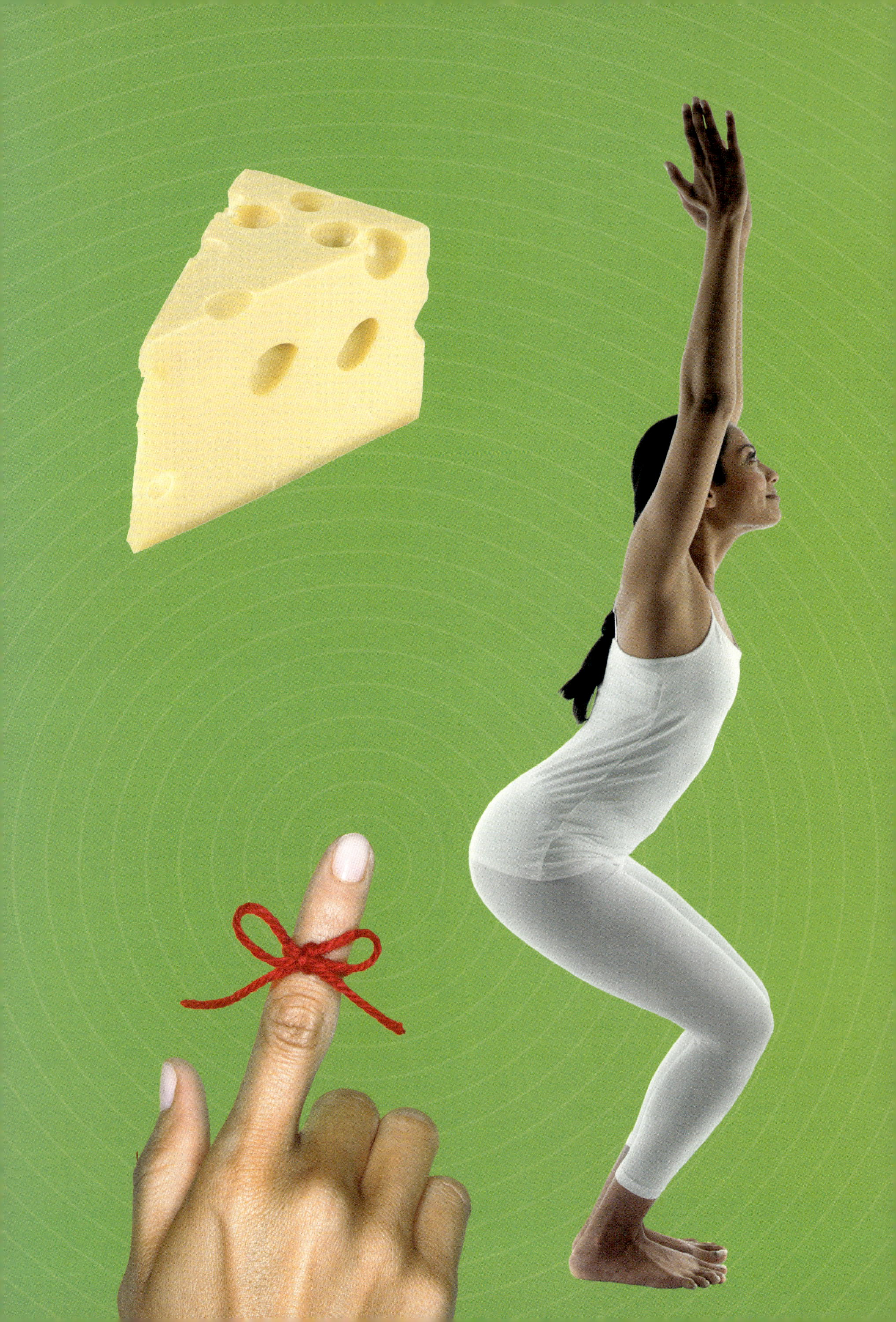

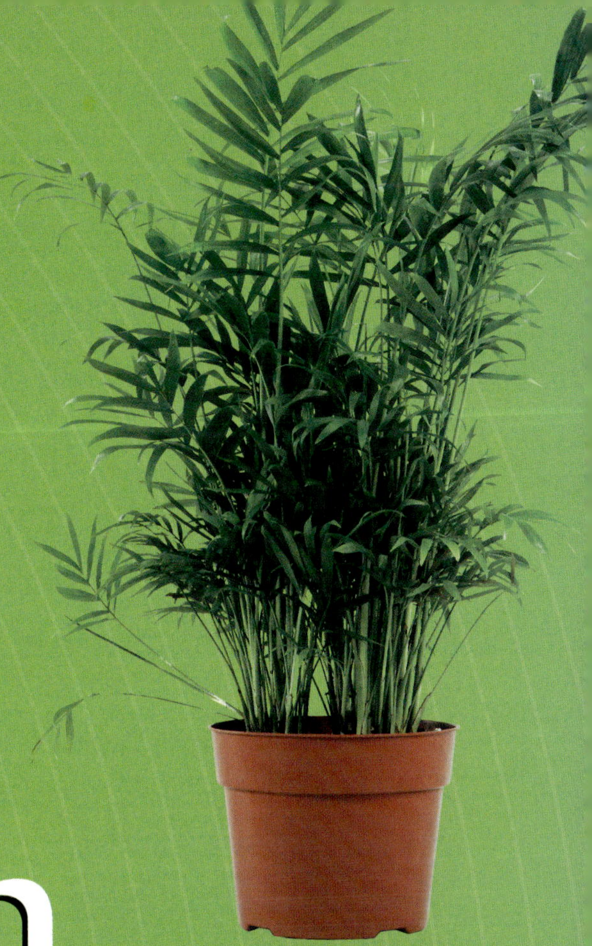

PART THREE

six brain drains and how to plug them

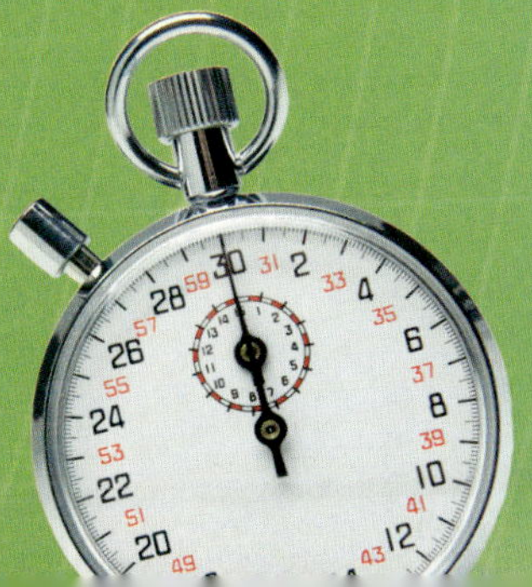

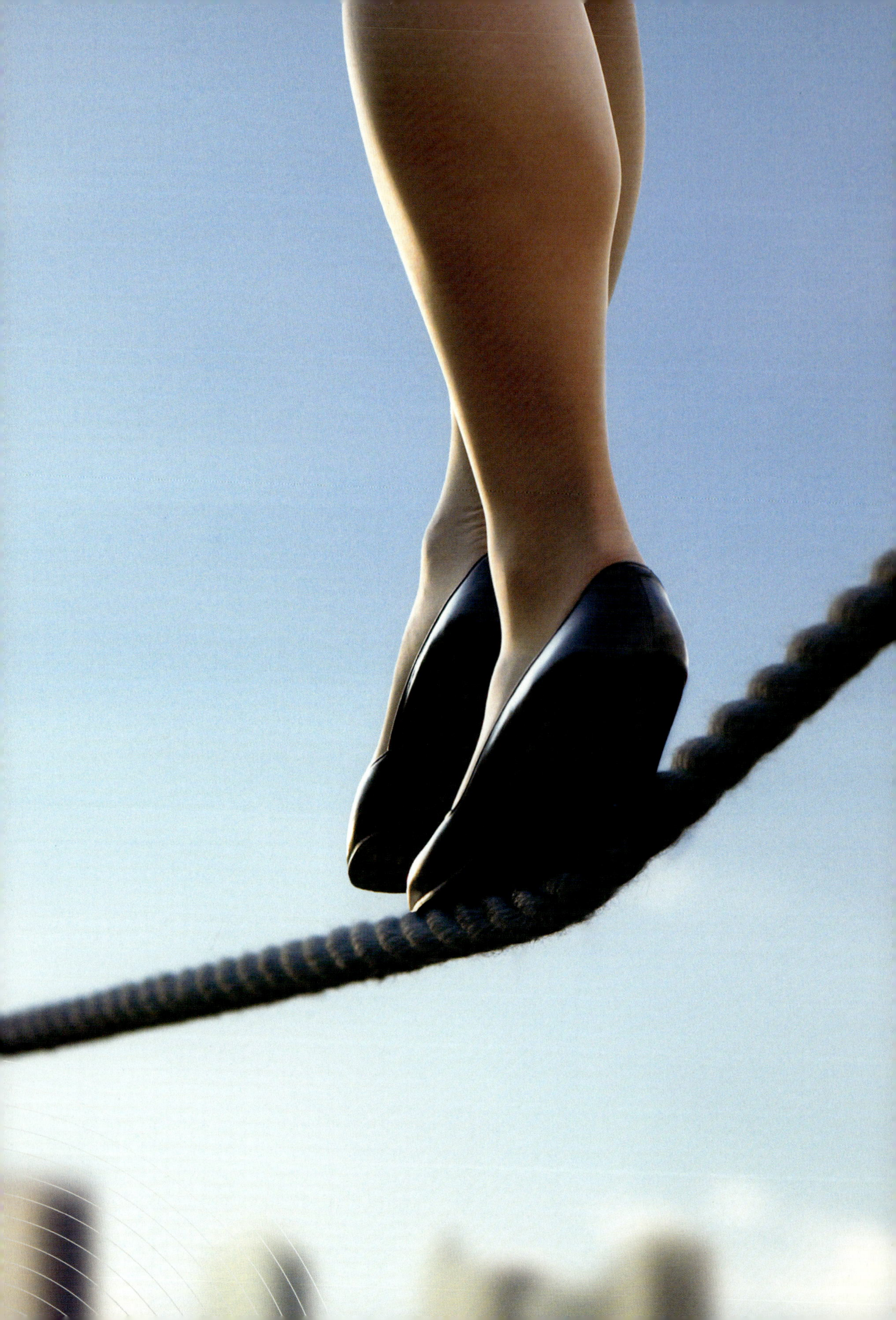

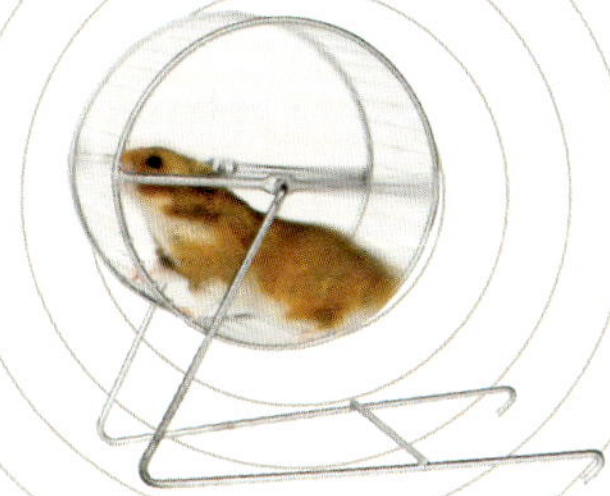

DRAIN #1

stress and anxiety

Layoffs and unemployment up! The economy in decline! The planet in jeopardy! Add in family squabbles, health problems, and, for some people, a never-ending to-do list, and a person can begin to feel like a rat on a 24/7 stress wheel.

As the primary organ of stress, the brain alone decides what is stressful and what is merely exciting. Some stress is good for you—it keeps life interesting, challenges you to develop your skills, and prepares you to deal with whatever gets thrown your way. Short bursts of stress excite neurons in the hippocampus and make you more alert. Especially in early adulthood, small increases in the stress hormone cortisol can increase the activity in your prefrontal cortex, help you make memories, and even help you retrieve them.

The problem? Not all stressors are exciting or short-lived; some are just, well, stressful. Too many of us worry, fret, and wring our hands as a matter of course over broken lifestyles or ongoing issues that don't seem to get resolved, leaving us keyed up most of the time. The toxic effects of chronic stress can contribute to diseases such as heart disease and diabetes, as well as brain drain.

While small cortisol spikes can improve young adults' mental performance, in older adults, an excess of cortisol makes it more difficult to form new memories or to recall them later. The more cortisol in the blood, the less the right middle frontal gyrus, an area of the brain that records memories of events, will be activated. Ongoing stress can even shrink key areas of the brain.

One study found that the hippocampi of people who'd experienced 5 years of high cortisol levels were 14 percent smaller when compared with the brains of more easygoing people the same age.

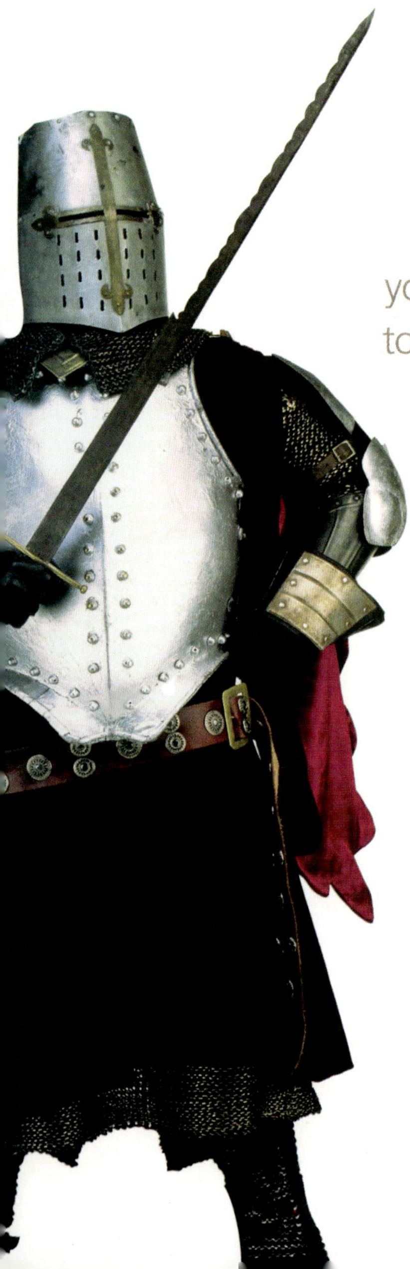

One way to improve your response to challenging situations is to work on believing that you are equal to the task.

(Depression also shrinks the hippocampus.) Once the hippocampus starts to shrink, it's less and less able to control stress, creating a vicious cycle. Stress hormones can even alter the function of the hippocampus, changing the way it handles memories.

Stress: Ditch the Bad, Embrace the Good

If stress is so bad for us, why can't we just learn to relax? Easier said than done, especially for some people.

The stress response is different for every brain and every body. One person may look at a challenge and feel a burst of norepinephrine, the "fight" hormone. That person might seize the moment, meet the challenge, and attack the situation head-on. Another person might sense the situation is getting out of his control and after the initial burst of norepinephrine, the "flight/anxiety" hormone epinephrine will surge higher. He might decide to flee or otherwise manage his anxiety, but not to fight back (or tackle the challenge head-on). A third person might undergo the same initial reaction, but instead of fighting or fleeing, he might give up and see the entire situation as hopeless. This person's belief that he is not equipped to handle the task will trigger an extra release of cortisol from the adrenal glands.

What we all need is a happy medium—enough challenge to make life interesting and mentally stimulating, but not so much that the brain drowns in neuron-killing cortisol. In other words, to be stressed but not stressed out. You may never be able to totally control the outside stresses that come in (though taking a hard look at your lifestyle is a good start), but you can control how you respond to them.

One of the very best ways to improve your response to challenging situations is to work on believing that you are equal to the task and that you have the resources necessary to meet the challenge and succeed. That one single shift in attitude can make the difference between a thrilling, engaging life and a constant slog of never-ending torture—not to mention the difference between a healthy brain and a weak one. By shoring up your self-confidence as well as your coping mechanisms, you can go out and tackle the world and whatever it throws at you.

DE-STRESS YOUR THOUGHTS

Imagine the worst-case scenario. Sometimes forcing yourself to think of the worst thing can be the best thing for an anxious brain. If you find yourself trapped in "what-ifs," a common state of mind for people with chronic anxiety, face your fears head-on: "If the stock market doesn't recover, I won't recover my lost savings and I'll be forced to live on the street." When you say it out loud, doesn't it seem a little far-fetched? What's more likely to happen?

Imagining worst-case scenarios accomplishes two things: It helps you see how unlikely the fear really is, and it helps you confront the fear head-on so you can prepare at least a tentative plan for recovery.

Create a personal mantra. If you're going through a stressful period or you tend toward anxious thoughts, a personal mantra can help you refocus your mind on positive thoughts. To create yours, make a list of the three things that matter to you most. Then think of one word that represents each. Choose positive, powerful words that resonate deeply with you. Let's say your top three things are a close family, good health, and your religion. Your mantra could become, "Love, strength, God." Whenever you are presented with a challenging situation, recite your mantra in your head. Speak the words to yourself as you walk down the street, head into a meeting, or work in your garden, timing them with each step or arm movement.

Label the feeling. One of the cornerstone teachings of mindfulness meditation is to learn to recognize stress and other emotions without giving into them. Here's how it works: You remember that your performance review at work is next week, and you're not sure what your boss is going to say. Your heart starts to pound or your mind starts spinning with possible scenarios. Rather than try to talk yourself out of the stress or pretend it's not there, you simply look inward and label how you're feeling. You might say "nervous" or "anxious," objectifying the emotion as a scientist would. With practice, this technique has been shown to help people head off the cascade of negative emotions that comes from stress.

Functional MRI scans of people's brains, taken while they matched facial expressions to appropriate emotional labels, have shown that labeling emotions activates the prefrontal cortex, the seat of logical thinking and emotional control, and reduces activity in the amygdala, the seat of reactive, primal emotion such as fear.

Create a worry book. Worriers need a place to deposit their negative thoughts. Keep a small memo pad handy, and whenever you feel yourself starting to worry about something, open it and do a "brain dump"—write down everything that's concerning you, without thinking about how you're saying it or whether you've said it a thousand times before. Putting thoughts on paper can help break a repetitive cycle of worry, which can deplete your capacity for performing other cognitive tasks.

One British study found that hand-wringers performed worse on a cognitive test when they were thinking about a current worry, suggesting that chronic fretters have less working memory capacity when worrying than when thinking about other topics. Just getting it out of your head and down on paper will help.

Keep a gratitude journal. If your worry book is a strictly functional memo pad, make your gratitude journal a beautiful, hardbound book with luscious paper—an object you love to look at and feel in your hands. Write in this journal for 5 minutes a day, jotting down the top three things you are grateful for that day. Make them detailed and specific. Instead of writing "I'm grateful for my family," write "I'm grateful that my granddaughters came for dinner tonight. I love to watch them learn how to use proper manners. I'm grateful they live nearby so I can watch them grow up." Over time, doing this routinely will help you start to notice the beauty and grace of each day as it happens.

Listen to hypnosis CDs. Hypnosis may sound like quack medicine, but some research shows that it can be tremendously useful. One Yale University study found that hypnosis cut presurgery anxiety in patients entering the operating room by more than half. Other research

Is It Just Stress—or Chronic Anxiety?

If you've experienced excessive worry or tension regularly for more than 6 months, you've likely gone beyond standard stress; you may have Generalized Anxiety Disorder (GAD). People with GAD often expect disaster to strike. They seem overly concerned about health issues, money, family problems, or difficulties at work. Even when they know they don't have reason to worry, people with GAD still fret about things longer than other people. They may experience physical symptoms, such as sweating, nausea, fatigue, headaches, muscle tension, twitching, light-headedness, or a constant need to go to the bathroom.

If this sounds like you, take heart; you have many options. Often just talking with a counselor can help you start to feel better. The best therapists for people with anxiety are often practitioners of cognitive behavioral therapy, in which people are taught new techniques that help them break negative thought patterns and react differently to everyday situations. Some doctors will prescribe a short course of anti-anxiety medication for patients to use while they learn these techniques.

Exercise, plenty of sleep, and meditation are also proven balms for the raw nerves of chronic anxiety. Each of these methods not only soothes in the short run but also helps reshape and grow the brain in ways that counteract the detrimental effects of chronic anxiety.

suggests that hypnosis may be even more helpful at relieving anxiety than cognitive behavioral therapy. To find a licensed psychologist certified in hypnosis, go to the referral tool on the American Society of Clinical Hypnosis web site, www.asch.net/referrals.asp. Avoid "hypnotists" or "hypnotherapists," as they don't necessarily have adequate training. You might also consider investing in a hypnosis CD from The Hypnosis Network.

Learn to focus and calm your thoughts. To quiet down the chatter in your mind, simply close your eyes and focus on your breath, "watching" it flow in and out of your nostrils. If thoughts pop up about the groceries, the bills, or the state of the economy, notice them and then redirect your attention to your breath. Keep doing this for 5 minutes. At first you might spend 20 seconds truly focused on your breath and 4 minutes and 40 seconds redirecting your thoughts away from your worries, but that ratio should improve with practice.

This little 5-minute exercise—which, by the way, is mediation, though you don't have to think of it that way—has been shown to lower heart rate, respiration, blood pressure, anxiety, pain, insomnia, and the production of cortisol—pretty much a one-stop shop for stress reduction.

Want better focus? Especially in older people, regular meditation can actually thicken the prefrontal cortex, which tends to thin with age, making it more difficult to pay sustained attention.

Clear clutter. Oftentimes, chronic stress and indecision go hand in hand. What's the connection with clutter? People who accumulate clutter tend to have trouble deciding what to do with their stuff ("I'll keep this catalog/insurance form/magazine article until I can find the time to deal with it"). In one study, when compulsive hoarders and nonhoarders were asked to make decisions about whether to keep or discard an item, MRI scans showed much more activity in brain areas that regulate decision making, attention, and controlling emotions in the hoarders. In other words, they had a much harder time deciding.

Keep a handle on your clutter and you'll likely discover a greater sense of control over your life. Start with one small area. For example, make it a solemn rule to completely clean off the kitchen counter every single night, even if that means piling the junk on another surface. Wipe it down with cleanser so it really shines. Savor the sight of a clean surface to reinforce your progress. Then add another rule: Completely clean off the table. And another: Clean out the sink. Continue until you can maintain several areas of your home without clutter.

Conquering clutter is a constant battle with no finish line—you must continue to make those decisions, and not put them off, if you want to stay on top of things. Make it easier by getting rid of stuff you don't need. Try putting items up for sale on the free want-ad site www.craigslist.org—freedom from clutter is its own reward, but a few extra dollars never hurt either.

CARVE OUT TIME FOR R & R

"Punch out" even if you don't have a time card. When you're done with work, be sure you're really done. A large study of more than 2,600 American workers found that the more control people have over their schedules, the more likely they are to bring work home or receive contact from colleagues during family hours. If you're never "off the clock," your body (and brain) will never get a chance to recover.

Staying late doesn't always help you accomplish more, so make a deal with yourself to leave at a specific time every night. Doing so will force you to stay efficient and productive until the minute you leave. Switch on your out-of-office e-mail notification every Friday night. Not only will this help you mentally disengage, but people who try to reach you will appreciate understanding exactly when you'll get back to them.

If you absolutely must stay connected, decide in advance on one designated time every day to check your voicemail and e-mail; give yourself a half-hour to scan through and respond to only the most critical items. Then disconnect for the rest of the day.

Prescribe yourself at least two vacations a year. Vacations are sometimes the only complete break from stress our bodies get, but one in three Americans doesn't take the allotted vacation time. Those who shun vacations are at increased risk for heart disease and are 20 percent more likely to die of any cause in a given year. Don't be one of them! Consider your vacations doctor's orders. Make one to your favorite haunt (even if it's a bed-and-breakfast nearby), the other one to a new place. The anticipation of visiting the old familiar place will help decrease stress, while the novelty of the new will stimulate new brain connections.

Let a movie crack you up. Laughing is one of the best ways to reduce stress and boost immunity, and watching funny movies is a cheap, easy way to do more of it. Researchers at Loma Linda University found that just looking forward to seeing a funny movie had a profound stress-relief effect, decreasing cortisol 39 percent, decreasing adrenaline 70 percent, and increasing feel-good endorphins by 27 percent

Everyone's taste is different, but the American Film Institute's list of the top 100 funniest American movies includes gems like *Annie Hall, Blazing Saddles, The Apartment, Tootsie,* and *There's Something about Mary.* Make a list of funny movies you want to see and add them to the queue of movies you get delivered to your home with a service like Netflix. You'll get a double benefit from looking forward to its arrival in the mail and actually watching it.

DE-STRESS YOUR SOCIAL CIRCLE

Stay away from competitive people. If you find yourself around someone who makes you feel uncomfortable or with whom you have to compete, try to minimize your time with that person. Research shows that competition is one of the most potent stressors among any animal, humans included.

Competitive people make you feel like you need to defend yourself or get another word in during conversations. In contrast, noncompetitive friends love and accept you as you are; when you're with them, you'll never have the impulse to prove yourself. You'll walk away feeling appreciated, not insulted. Those friends can reduce cortisol and epinephrine and increase oxytocin and endorphins, all positive changes in your brain chemistry.

Hug someone you love. Your husband or wife, brother or sister, child or good friend. Hugs are proven stress-relievers. One study found that the more hugs a woman got from her partner, the higher her oxytocin (the "cuddle hormone") levels and the lower her blood pressure and cortisol levels. Oxytocin helps bond people together. No wonder happier couples hug more often!

DE-STRESS YOUR BODY

Break a sweat. Perhaps the most effective stress-buster of all is the activation of your own sweat glands. Regular exercise helps your body—your heart, your muscles, your nervous system—practice a positive response to stress. Over time, it reduces cortisol levels and raises levels of norepinephrine, helping increase activity in a part of the brain that controls many aspects of your emotional reactions and stress levels.

If you haven't gotten moving yet, start with 10 minutes of walking, and be sure to do it every day—establishing the habit is the hardest part. If you can commit to a friend or even a dog, these "workout partners" will make you less likely to renege. Once you've built that time into your day, expand it by 5 minutes a week until you're walking 25 minutes a day. Add in some sit-ups, modified push-ups, and lunges on two or more days a week, and you have a stress-busting program that will keep your brain and your body strong for years to come.

Do some deep breathing. At least once a day, sit in a chair with your feet flat on

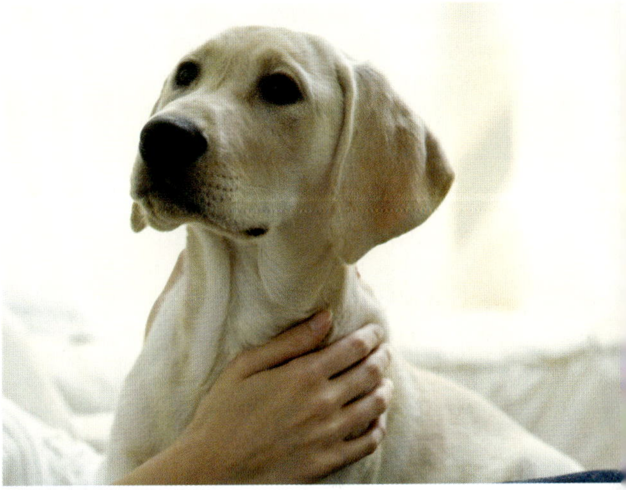

15 Wonderful Stress-Busters

1. Bake cookies and take them to your neighbor.
2. Call a friend to vent, then give each other a coaching session—limit it to 10 minutes each.
3. Cancel one item from your schedule.
4. Go to bed at 9 p.m. tonight.
5. Have sex.
6. Smile for no reason.
7. Listen to your favorite album.
8. Pet your dog or someone else's.
9. Cut out pictures from magazines of a travel destination you want to visit.
10. Make funny shapes with your grandchildren's Play-Doh.
11. Write a to-do list, and do the easiest thing on it.
12. Walk to the nearest green space and spend 10 minutes looking at the leaves and smelling the air.
13. Sit in a silent church.
14. Read the comics.
15. Watch a funny www.youtube.com video (search for "baby laughs" or "cute puppies").

the floor and take a slow, deep breath through your nose, expanding your belly (not your chest), then slowly release your breath through pursed lips. Repeat for several minutes. You'll get more oxygen to your blood—and to your brain—and melt away tension in your body.

Get a weekly massage. Don't wait for massage to be a reward for getting through a rough patch—use it as a technique to build up your reserves. Numerous studies have found that massage decreases anxiety, stress, and pain. It releases enkephalins, proteins that act like morphine in your brain, giving you a natural high, and increases dopamine and serotonin, neurotransmitters that enhance mood. Some forward-thinking health insurance programs have begun to cover massage therapy. If yours doesn't, consider taking a couples massage course with your partner, so you can give each other effective massages. Or call a massage therapy school in your area. Many offer significantly reduced rates for massages from students.

Try a yoga class. In one German study, a group of women who considered themselves emotionally distressed signed up for a 3-month yoga program. The researchers split them into two groups. One would participate in the program right away; the second were told they were on the waiting list. During the 3-month study period, the first group attended two 90-minute yoga classes each week. After 3 months, when compared with the women on the waiting list, the women who did yoga demonstrated significant improvements in perceived stress, anxiety, fatigue, and depression. Those who'd previously suffered from headaches or back pain reported marked pain relief, and their cortisol levels plummeted.

Women who did yoga twice a week were less stressed, anxious, and fatigued.

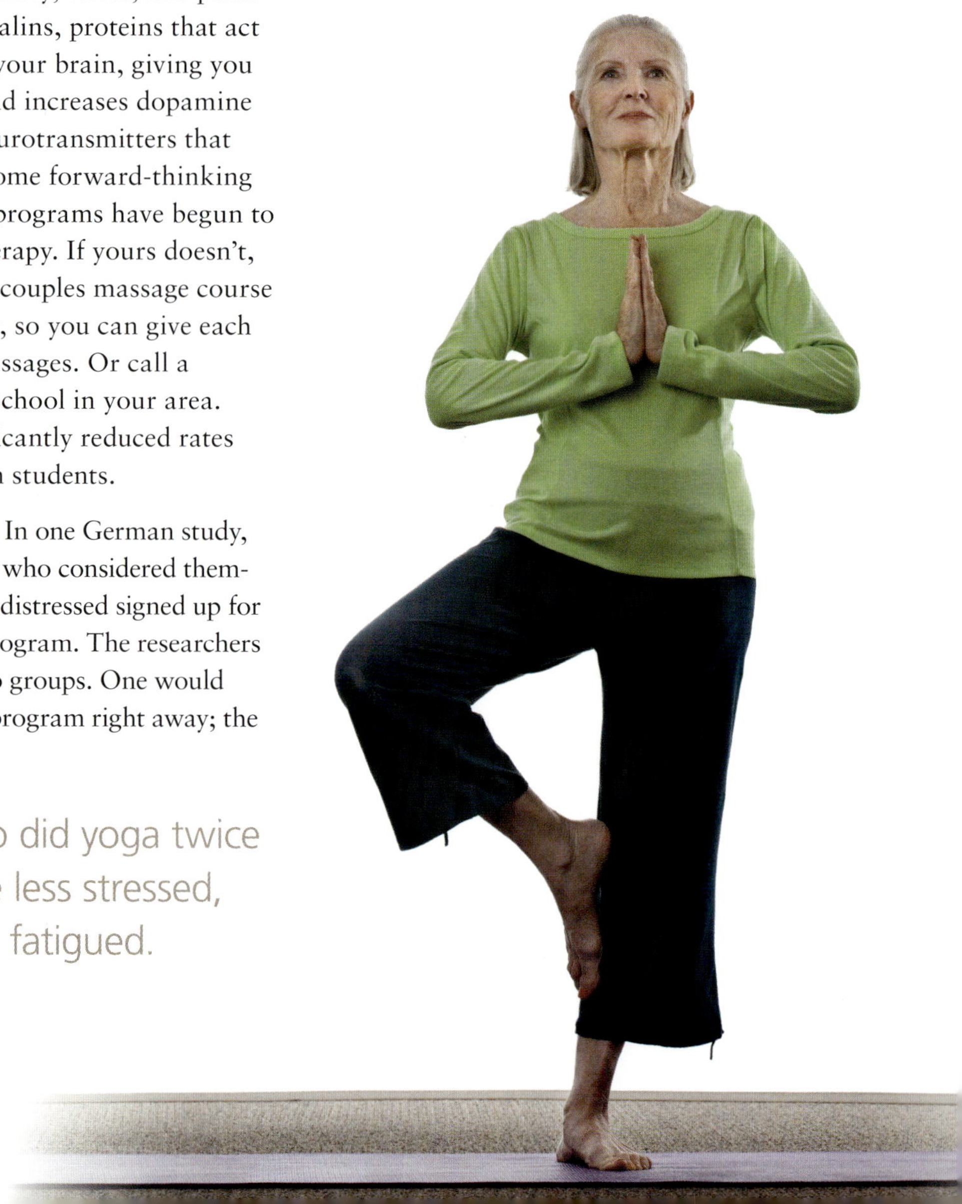

The best way to safely learn yoga is from an instructor, not a video. Find a class for beginners, and bring a friend if you feel intimidated.

Supplement with fish oil. You already read our recommendation on fish oil in the form of DHA in Vaccine #1: Diet beginning on page 64. Here's another good reason to take it: A French study suggests that fish oil may help your body manage stress better. Researchers measured stress hormone levels in a small group of volunteers before and after they gave them an intense cognitive challenge. After taking fish oil for 3 weeks, the group was given a similar challenge and this time, their stress hormone levels were significantly lower after the fact. The researchers believed the fish oil might influence the adrenal glands to produce fewer hormones in response to stress.

Study participants were taking more than 7 grams of fish oil a day, more than doctors typically recommend. Check with your doctor for advice.

Steer yourself toward safer snacks. Stress increases appetite for fat and sugar. How do you outsmart your cravings? The truth is, if you're a stress-eater, you've probably spent much of your life running toward food when times get tough—and those neural grooves are pretty deep. Your brain has grown accustomed to the satisfying dopamine and calming serotonin release that you get when you eat under stressful conditions. If you must turn to food to help manage your stress, crunch on carrots or celery; eat a hard-boiled egg; spoon up a bowl of low-fat yogurt or cottage cheese. Just don't dip into the cookie jar. You'll find that the less you eat sugary, carb-loaded foods, the less you'll crave them.

Cut the coffee. Caffeine keeps cortisol and adrenaline levels higher than they already are. If you're the stressed-out type, it's best to give up coffee altogether. If you can't or won't, hold yourself to no more than 2 cups a day, no matter what, and drink them in the morning so your body has plenty of time to fully metabolize the caffeine before bed.

Quit smoking—with two friends. Many smokers think that cigarettes help them manage stress, but surveys indicate that smokers are actually more stressed than nonsmokers. Nicotine withdrawal can temporarily increase stress, but within a few weeks of quitting, once your body is used to being nicotine-free, chances are your stress levels will decrease and continue to drop over time. By quitting, you'll also reduce your risk of cognitive decline and stroke.

Quitting with friends helps you all improve your chances of success. One recent study found that people tend to do best when whole clusters of friends and relatives quit at the same time, usually in groups of three or more. The group momentum encourages everyone.

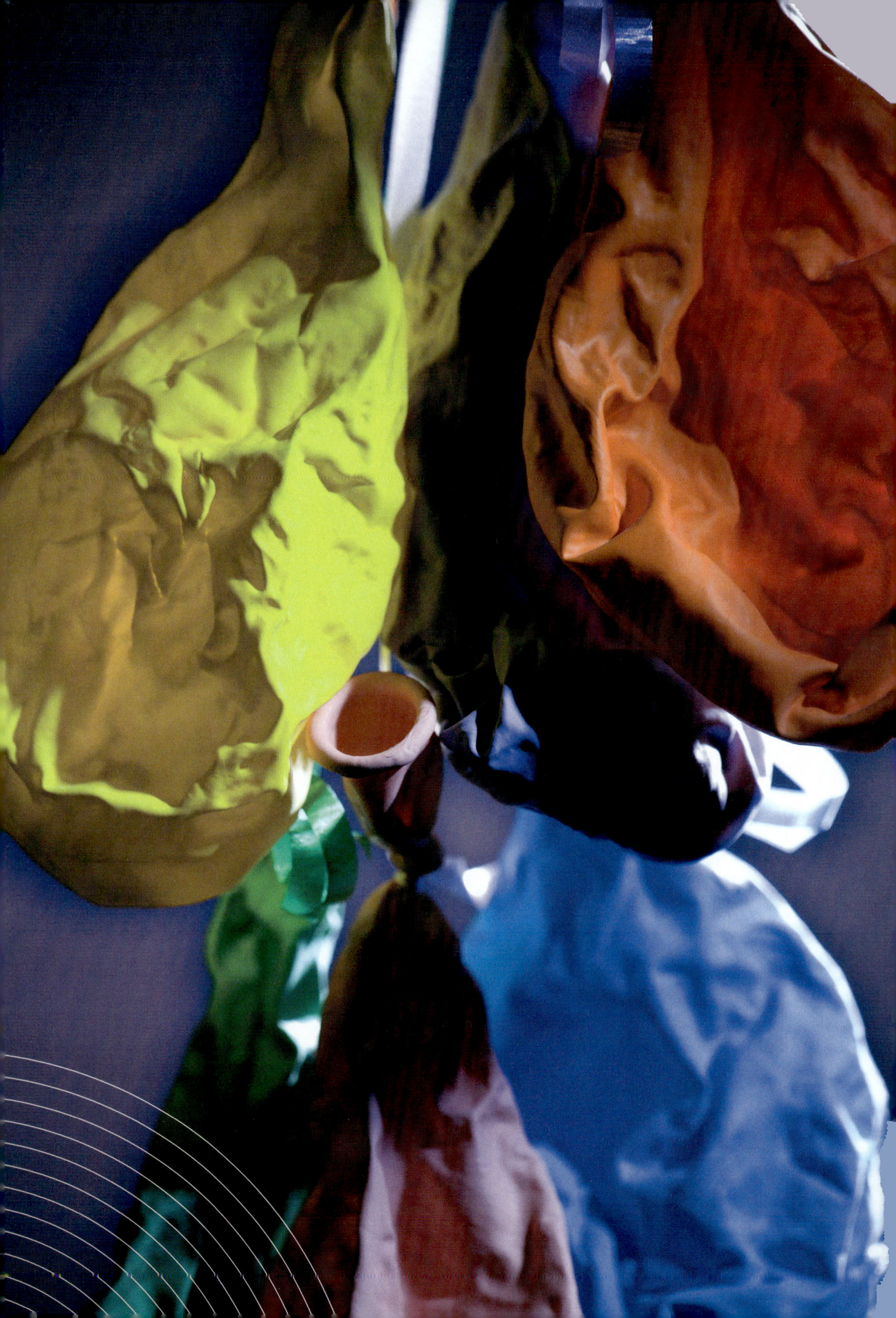

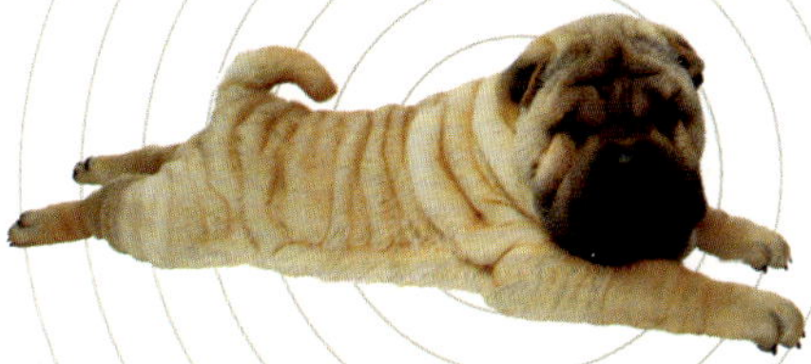

DRAIN #2
depression

Your mood and energy have been laid low, and your thoughts are as murky as an underwater ocean view after a storm. Coincidence? No. Depression has real, measurable effects on memory and cognitive function. The good news: Treating it can help bring back days of mental clarity, not to mention sunnier moods.

If you've ever been depressed, you've experienced firsthand the slow-motion thinking, difficulty making decisions, and trouble remembering everyday things that come along with this illness. Depression slows your brain's ability to process information, robs you of the ability to concentrate, and causes real memory problems, all thanks to changes that take place in the brain.

When Washington University School of Medicine researchers scanned the brains of 38 women with long-standing depression, they saw something shocking. Study volunteers who had suffered from untreated depression the longest—in some cases, for more than a decade—had up to 30 percent shrinkage of the hippocampus, the brain area responsible for many kinds of memory and learning. In addition to killing existing brain cells, depression also reduces the birth of new ones. And it shrinks the connections between neurons that allow thought signals to zip along from one cell to another.

The result? Difficulty forming and retrieving memories. Depression interferes with everything from locating your car keys to remembering words and names. One fascinating study has even found that depression hobbles your ability to remember where things are. When British researchers used a virtual reality game to test spatial memory in 49 people, they found that those who were depressed performed significantly worse than those who weren't. Volunteers were told to navigate through a virtual city in search of landmarks such as a movie theater and a pool hall. Depressed people found one-third fewer of the sites than mentally healthy people.

The longer depression goes untreated, the greater the damage—and the bigger memory problems can be, conclude the authors of a large study on people with depression, published in the *American Journal of Psychiatry*. Depression also makes taking the steps proven to keep your brain sharp—such as exercising, learning new things, having new experiences, spending time with friends and family—difficult. Instead, you retreat and isolate yourself, a surefire recipe for dulled thinking, all by itself. Depression also makes caring for your health more difficult, leaving the door open for untreated medical problems that raise the risk for dementia, such as high blood pressure, diabetes, and high cholesterol.

Are You Depressed?

It can be surprisingly easy to explain away warning signs of depression. And while experts recommend that family doctors screen for it, many do not. That means it's up to you to monitor your mood and recognize red flags.

If you have experienced even one of the following symptoms in the past 2 weeks, talk to your family doctor or a mental health professional about depression and what you can do to lift it.

- A persistently sad, empty, or anxious mood
- Persistent physical symptoms that don't respond to treatment, such as headaches, pain, or digestive disorders
- Sleeping too little or sleeping too much
- Reduced appetite and weight loss or increased appetite and weight gain
- Loss of interest in activities once enjoyed, including sex
- Feeling guilty, hopeless, or worthless
- Having thoughts of suicide or death

IS IT DEPRESSION, DEMENTIA, OR BOTH?

For older people, depression can mimic dementia, and vice versa. This could make identifying and fixing mood and memory problems tricky for you, your family, and your doctor.

People with a history of depression before age 60 are four times more likely to develop Alzheimer's disease than those who were never depressed. But it's not clear that depression actually causes dementia...or that treating depression lowers the risk for late-life dementia. And sometimes, a diagnosis of Alzheimer's disease can trigger depression—deep sadness over the loss of memories, thinking skills, and a big piece of a person's identity.

What you need to know about this puzzle: If you or a loved one is experiencing mood and thinking problems later in life (age 60 or older), many doctors will suggest a short course of antidepressants to see whether they help. Sometimes, that's all that's needed to restore alertness, memory, and thinking skills. Other times, cognitive problems persist, a clue that dementia may be involved, too. If you or your doctor suspects Alzheimer's disease, it's important to get a referral to a physician experienced in diagnosing the disease. An early diagnosis raises the chances that medication, such as donepezil (Aricept) and rivastigmine (Exelon), can improve cognition and possibly slow the course of the disease.

About one in four people with Alzheimer's disease also has depression. Studies show that certain antidepressants can make daily life easier for them, even though these drugs won't improve their thinking problems.

Feeling Good Again

When you're depressed, the most difficult job in the world is finding the motivation to fight back. But your brain—and your heart, and the rest of your body—depends on it. Help is out there. Your best first step is to call your regular doctor and make an appointment expressly to talk about your mood. Don't be embarrassed; depression is a medical condition like any other, and needs to be treated like any other. It may be up to you to bring up the problem with your doctor, but once you do, it's up to him or her to evaluate you and suggest the next step.

With treatment—whether it's an antidepressant or talk therapy—most depression improves in 8 to 12 weeks. Without treatment, it could take months or even years, time that allows this illness to eat away at your brain, your life, and your health.

Ask your doctor about an antidepressant. Many people find relief on these drugs, especially if they also get therapy. There are several different types of antidepressants; you may need to work with your doctor to find the right drug at the right dose for you. Aside from boosting your mood, antidepressants also seem to shield your brain from the effects of stress, as well as jump-start the growth of new brain cells. As a result, memory improves and you can think more clearly. When researchers in North Carolina tested memory, thinking skills, and mental processing speed in 138 people with depression, they found that those who were taking antidepressants performed significantly better than those who were not.

Be persistent...and patient. You may have to try several antidepressants to find the one that's best for you. That's what happened in a landmark study of 3,700 people with depression. Seventy percent eventually felt like their old selves again, but only 37 percent got relief with the first medication they tried. The rest test-drove up to four different therapies before finding the right one for them.

Keys to success: Plan to try a treatment for 8 to 12 weeks to see if it's working, stay in close contact with your doctor, and expect a big improvement. A successful treatment will allow you to feel like yourself again and enable you to do

12 Short Paths to Joy

Happiness can help you live longer, stay married longer, even earn a higher income, experts say. And while about 50 percent of your outlook is encoded in your genes, you can teach yourself to feel more joy. What works:

1 **Keep a gratitude journal.** Feeling thankful isn't just for Thanksgiving. It can boost your mood and your energy. Jotting down what you're grateful for five times a week works better than three times a week, one study found.

2 **Perform five acts of kindness this week.** Bring flowers from your garden to a friend or a help an elderly neighbor with her groceries. Altruistic acts are genuine mood-lifters.

3 **Listen to the music you love best**. It triggers joy by unleashing feel-good brain chemicals called endorphins.

4 **Cuddle...and more.** Physical affection and sex release endorphins as well as the "cuddle chemical" oxytocin, which strengthens your relationship with your main squeeze.

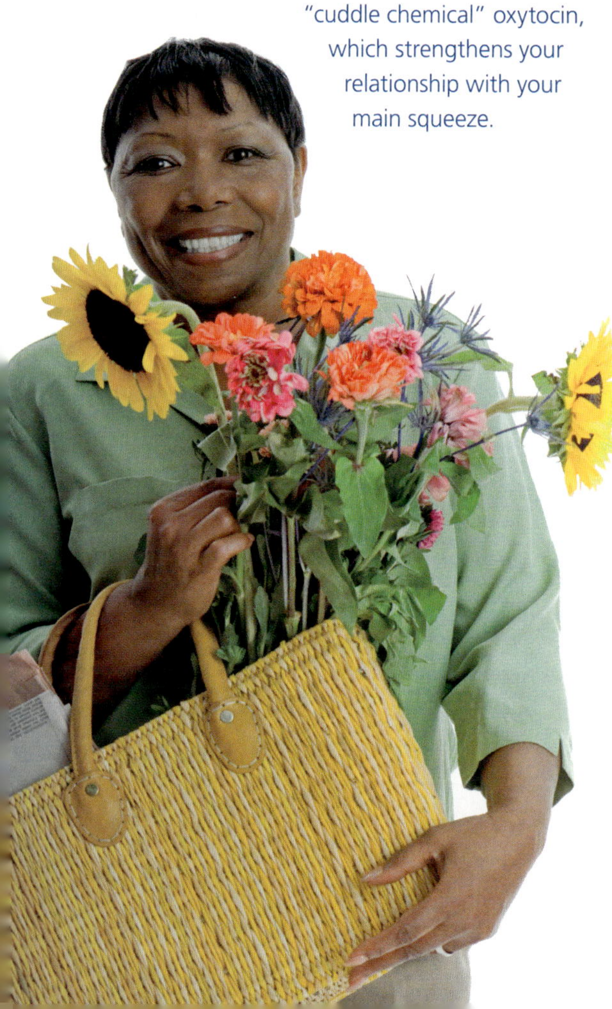

5 **Live your faith.** Strong religious beliefs bolster happiness, perhaps by giving you a sense of purpose as well as a church home—a place in a community of accepting, like-minded people.

6 **Yuk it up.** Watch a funny movie, tell a joke, or ask your friends and family to share jokes and funny stories. A good giggle or guffaw raises levels of feel-good brain chemicals.

7 **Adopt a happy posture.** Square your shoulders, stand up straight, and when you walk, take big, quick steps. That's the body language of a happy person—and studies show that acting happy can help you feel happier.

8 **Do something new.** Then do something else new. Trying new things turbo charges positive emotions.

9 **Set up clear work/home boundaries.** Turn off the cell phone or Blackberry and shut down the laptop when you get home. This can reduce stress at home and help you feel closer to your mate, kids, and grandkids.

10 **Appreciate "good enough."** You didn't lose 3 pounds this week...but did you lose 1 pound? That's a victory, not a defeat. In large population studies, people with more realistic expectations come out ahead, happiness-wise, of those looking for perfection.

11 **Unleash your inner Matisse.** Create a greeting card, decorate a cake, plant an herb garden, do a craft. Creative endeavors allow us to enter a timeless, worry-free state called flow that's both absorbing and thrilling.

12 **Imagine that you're already happy.** Shut your eyes and see yourself doing something that makes your heart sing. Experts say this "thought experiment" boosts confidence and helps make happiness a habit.

all the things you used to do. Once you find the right treatment, stick with it. You may need your medication for 6 to 12 months, the usual length of a bout of depression, or longer if you've had depressive periods in the past.

Try cognitive behavioral therapy. This practical, solutions-oriented kind of therapy is the most effective form of talk therapy and can help up to 75 percent of people with depression to get better. And studies show that it may be a good way to protect your brain from future bouts of depression. Cognitive behavioral therapy usually comprises 8 to 16 sessions and is aimed at changing thoughts and feelings that may lead to depression. One British study of 123 people with depression found that it cut the chance of a relapse in half. Ask your doctor for a referral to a psychologist specifically trained in this type of therapy.

Reach out to a friend. Talking over the day, in person or by phone or e-mail, helps us emphasize the good stuff and process the not-so-good stuff so that we're not turning it over and over in our minds, research suggests. In a British study, when 86 depressed women were paired with a volunteer friend, 65 percent of the women felt better. In fact, regular social contact worked as effectively as antidepressant medication and psychotherapy. Regular social contact with a close friend may boost self-confidence and encourage you to make other positive changes that will help lift depression, such as starting an exercise program.

Add a 10-minute walk two to three times a day. Walking has been proven to lift mild to moderate depression—plus you get a dose of mood-boosting sunshine. One study of older adults found that 10 weeks of regular exercise was 20 percent more effective at reducing depression symptoms than medication. However, because depression may make you want to do anything but exercise, many physicians recommend combining the two treatments.

Garden...or just get outdoors. Too many of us spend our days in a man-made environment, shut away from the sun, the earth, green plants, and the blue sky. Get back to our original home—it's as close as walking out your front door.

Let more light in. Bright light therapy can ease seasonal affective disorder, a type of depression some people experience during the winter months when sunlight is in short supply. It may also ease other types of depression as well. The therapy involves sitting in front of a special light box for 20 minutes to an hour shortly after waking each morning. You can purchase a light box for home use from a variety of companies, including SunBox, Northern Lights, and Apollo. They range in price from $200 to $400.

Take fish-oil supplements. There is some evidence that taking fish oil can help relieve mild to moderate depression. And you know from Vaccine #1: Diet, beginning on page 64, that these supplements—especially in the form of DHA—can benefit your brain in other ways. For depression, talk to your doctor about taking a dose as high as 4 grams a day.

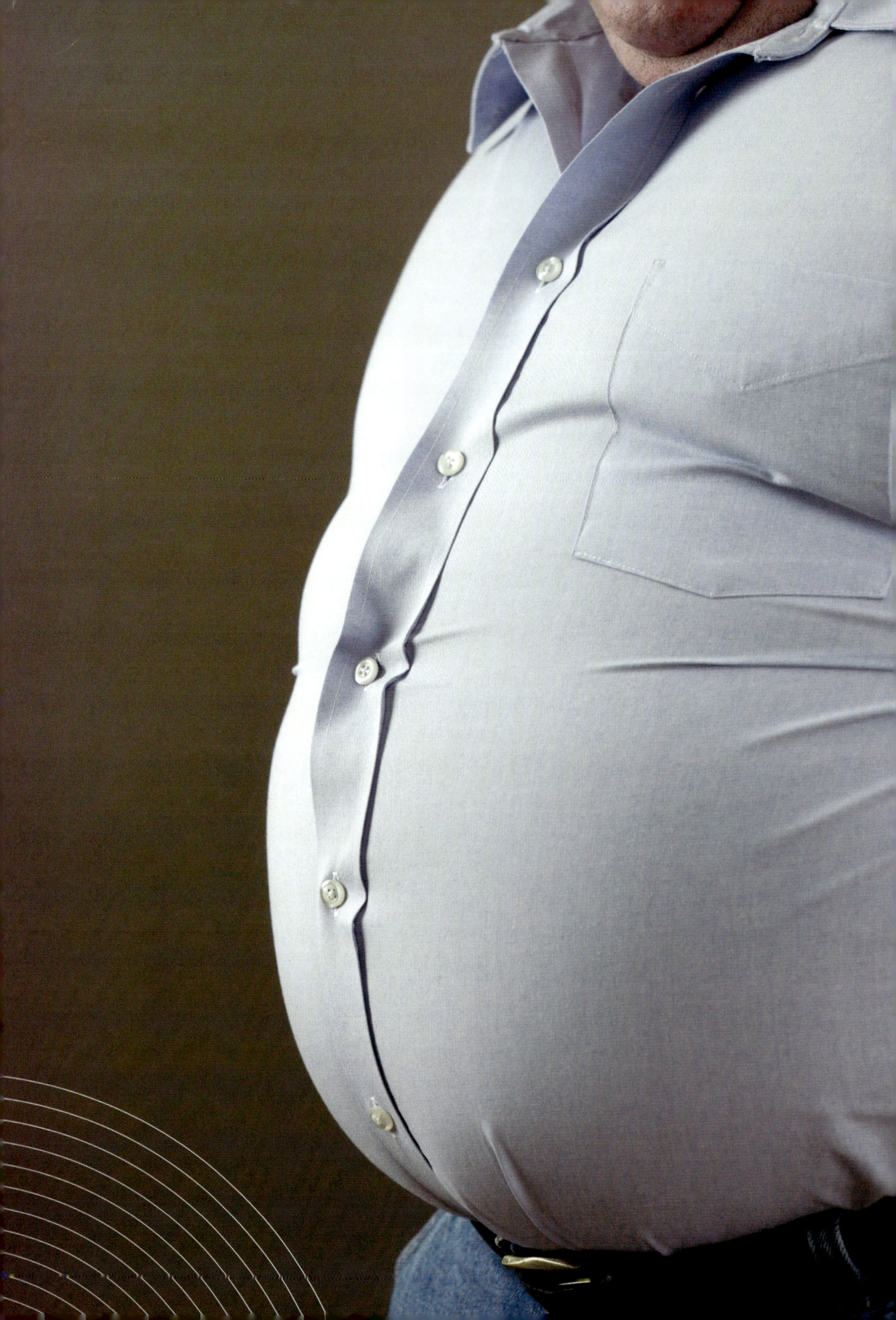

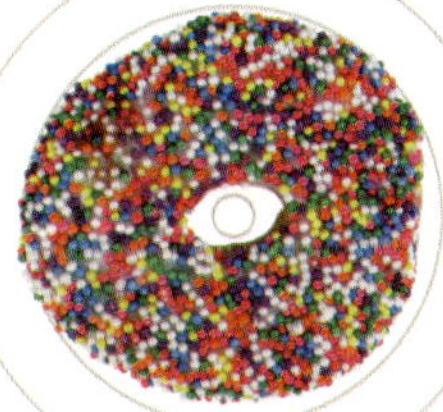

DRAIN #3

visceral fat

You've heard of "gut instinct," that certain inkling that tells you when someone's being less than truthful or that points you toward the right path when you have to make a snap decision. Of course, that instinct doesn't actually stem from your gut, which afterall, has nothing to do with your brain…or does it?

In fact it does—but not in a good way. Trouble begins when fat accumulates in your gut, invading and surrounding your internal organs like butter overtaking the nooks and crannies of an English muffin. Doctors have known for years that this type of fat, known as visceral fat, increases the risk for heart disease, diabetes, and cancer. Now they're beginning to recognize the dangerous role it plays when it comes to your brain. Bottom line: If your waistline increases, over time you can expect your brain power to decrease.

Read on to discover whether your waistline is putting you at risk for brain drain as well as simple strategies to send this hidden fat packing.

Incredible Brain-Shrinking Belly Fat

The fat in your gut isn't like the stuff that causes bottoms to jiggle or thighs to thunder. It's an active organ, secreting chemicals and hormones that affect your health, including your ability to remember where you parked the car or the name of your second cousin, not to mention balance your checkbook without tearing out your hair. Even if no one would accuse you of having a beer belly, you still might have too much of this fat. (See "Risky Waistlines" below.) Here's how it wreaks its havoc.

It shrinks your "memory center." That's your hippocampus, a horseshoe-shaped group of neurons that plays a major role in the formation and recall of memories. Researchers at the University of California used MRIs of the brain to show that a big waist and a smaller hippocampus go hand in hand. Studies have even shown a direct correlation between a big waist and a reduced ability to memorize words.

It creates "brain rust." Your brain cells communicate with each other via a superhighway of connections—think of them as information cables—called axons. Brain scans of people with wide waistlines show areas of damage to these cables. Doctors sometimes call these areas brain rust, which is typically seen in people with dementia. But some experts think this "rust" may drain memory and thinking power even in people who don't develop dementia.

It fuels metabolic syndrome. Visceral fat is the number one risk factor for metabolic syndrome, a group of health problems that includes slightly high blood pressure, cholesterol, and triglycerides (and sometimes blood sugar), plus slightly low levels of "good" HDL cholesterol. Metabolic syndrome paves a path to diabetes and heart disease. Now it has also been linked with sludgy thinking. In one Dutch study, people with metabolic syndrome scored about 10 percent lower on tests of mental processing speed and about 6 percent lower on memory tests than people without it.

It raises blood sugar. Visceral fat churns out chemicals that make the body less sensitive to insulin, the hormone that lets blood sugar into cells. When that happens, insulin levels rise and, ultimately, so do blood sugar levels. The combo is bad for your brain. In fact, researchers suspect it's one reason that people with Type 2

Risky Waistlines

Check out the numbers below for a sense of the risk your waistline poses to your overall health. Note that experts recommend lower waist sizes for people of Asian descent because of a greater inherited risk for diabetes and cardiovascular disease.

	HEALTHY WAIST RANGE	AT-RISK WAIST RANGE	HIGH-RISK WAIST RANGE
Men	Below 37 inches	37–40 inches	Above 40 inches
Women	Below 32 inches	32–35 inches	Above 35 inches
Asian Men	Below 30 inches	30–35 1/2 inches	Above 35 1/2 inches
Asian Women	Below 28 inches	28–31 1/2 inches	Above 31 1/2 inches

diabetes score lower on memory tests than people without diabetes.

It heats up inflammation. Inflammation is a tough concept to grasp, but think of it as your body's response to injuries of all sorts, even at the microscopic level. Visceral fat increases inflammation, which appears to affect the brain. In one study published in the *Journal of the American Medical Association,* inflammation raised the risk for cognitive decline by 66 percent. On one standard test for cognitive decline, which looks at skills such as concentration, language use, and immediate and delayed recall, volunteers with chronic, low-level inflammation scored at least five points lower than volunteers without chronic inflammation. That's enough of a difference in cognitive function for you or your family to notice.

ARE YOU AT RISK?

To find out, measure your waist on bare skin. Use a soft, flexible measuring tape (the kind used for sewing). Don't wrap it around the smallest part of your waist and don't use your belly button as a landmark. Instead, align the bottom of the tape measure just above the top of your hip bones. This ensures that you're measuring the part of your abdomen where visceral fat is thickest. Make sure the tape is straight, not twisted, and don't pull it too tight. Take your measurement at the end of a normal exhalation of breath (don't suck your tummy in!).

What do the results mean? According to the National Institutes of Health, health risks begin at 35 inches or greater for women and 40 inches or greater for men. But some experts warn that trouble begins at waist sizes 3 inches smaller than that. See "Risky Waistlines" on the opposite page for more details. About one in two adults has dangerous levels of visceral fat, and that percentage continues to grow as the obesity epidemic intensifies.

Not overweight? Don't assume you can safely ignore the threat; there's a convincing body of evidence that even some relatively thin people have too much belly fat hiding inside. When British researchers took MRI images of the torsos of more than 700 women and men, they made a sobering discovery: Forty-five percent of the thin women and 65 percent of the thin men had enough visceral fat to raise their risk for health problems. The scientists concluded that these TOFI (Thin on the Outside, Fat on the Inside) people were actually pre-overweight—they didn't exercise much and ate diets packed with high-fat, high-sugar foods.

The take-home lesson: Track your waist measurement even if the number on the bathroom scale is in the healthy range.

Whittle Your Middle to Save Your Brain

Everyone has some visceral fat, but if you're overweight, you might be hauling around 5 to 10 pounds of it. The good news: It's easier to lose than the stubborn fat on your hips, thighs, and butt. A little effort yields big rewards. When 173 women walked briskly for just 50 minutes, three times a week in a Yale School of Medicine study, they dropped an average of 2 inches from their waists—and said good-bye to 13 percent of their visceral fat. Here's how to vanquish it.

Hit the pavement, the pool, or the pedals of your exercise bike. Aerobic exercise—the kind that gets your muscles moving in a steady rhythm and your heart pumping—is your first line of defense against visceral fat. In one study of overweight men, those who exercised for an hour three times a week at a moderately brisk pace (can hold a conversation, but not able to sing "Happy Birthday") lost a significant percentage of the visceral fat packed around their hearts, Japanese researchers report. (Visceral fat can occur anywhere in the torso, including the heart.)

Several studies suggest that weight-loss programs that include physical activity are far more effective than diets alone for trimming this brain-dulling flab. When Syracuse University researchers put 33 women on an exercise plan, a low-calorie diet, or a combination of the two for 14 weeks, everyone lost weight and overall body fat. But the diet-plus-exercise group lost the most visceral fat.

If you choose *not* to exercise, you're allowing this stuff to continue to grow. When 175 overweight, sedentary women and men volunteered for an exercise study at Duke University, those who got the most vigorous routines—equivalent to jogging 20 miles a week—saw visceral fat levels fall by 7 to 20 percent, while those in the no-exercise control group saw visceral fat levels increase by 9 percent to 17 percent in just 8 months!

Add strength-training. Sit-ups and crunches may make your tummy look tighter, but you can't spot-reduce deep ab fat. What does work: A whole-body strength-training routine (one that works all the muscles, including the legs, arms, abdominals, and back). In one University of Pennsylvania study of overweight and obese women, those who strength-trained twice a week lost almost 4 percent of their body fat and were more successful at keeping off visceral fat than those who didn't.

Strength-training increases your metabolism by building muscle mass, which means your body will burn more calories around-the-clock. More muscle also means you'll burn more fat and calories during aerobic exercise, supercharging your fat-fighting efforts.

Banish the "bad" fats. Ice cream, fatty meats, full-fat milk, cheese, yogurt, and the half-and-half for your coffee are all loaded with saturated fat—the dietary fat that one Johns Hopkins University study showed raises your odds for packing on more visceral fat. Other research suggests that the human body may also store more trans fatty acids—the processed fat in commercial fried foods, bakery treats, and snack items—in deep abdominal fat.

Welcome the "good" fats. A growing stack of research studies suggests that putting more monounsaturated fats on your plate discourages the accumulation of visceral fat and may even help you shed it more easily. When Spanish researchers studied the impact of three diets—one packed with monounsaturated fats, one with saturated fats, and one with carbohydrates—they discovered that the "good fat" diet helped slash visceral fat. The others didn't.

To get more of these good-guy fats, snack on a small handful of nuts instead of pretzels or chips, use olive and canola oil in place of butter or other vegetable oils, have avocado slices on your sandwich in place of cheese, and go for all sorts of nut butters on your toast, in your sandwich, and at snack time. You'll love peanut butter and banana sandwiches, almond butter on whole-grain raisin bread at breakfast, and sliced apples or baby carrots dunked in a tablespoon of cashew butter as a mid-afternoon pick-me-up.

Eat more fiber and fewer refined carbohydrates. Eating whole-grain bread and whole-wheat pasta instead of the white stuff, and high-fiber cereal instead of, say, rice or corn cereal, can help your brain not only by preventing blood-sugar spikes, which are toxic to brain cells, but also by fighting visceral fat. People whose diets boost blood sugar the most tend to have more body fat, especially around the abdomen. Eating fiber-packed foods, on the other hand, helps you to shed this fat. In one Pennsylvania State University study of 50 obese people, those who followed a weight-loss diet packed with five daily servings of whole grains lost two-and-a-half times more abdominal fat than those whose diets had virtually none.

Whole fruits and vegetables are also great sources of fiber. A Harvard School of Public Health study of 486 women found that those who ate the most fruit and vegetables—equivalent to 1 1/2 apples, a cup of cooked green beans, and a handful of baby carrots a day—were 20 percent less likely to have a dangerously large waist.

Put it all together. People who exercised for 30 minutes at least five times a week, cut saturated fat, increased fiber, and lost 7 percent of their body weight (that's 10 pounds if you weigh 150) saw their visceral fat trimmed by a very significant 18 to 22 percent in a landmark study.

Soothe stress. High levels of the stress hormone cortisol prompt your body to send more fat into storage in your abdomen. Researchers suspect that this is an ancient survival mechanism, intended to maintain reserves of fat in emergencies. It was an ingenious lifesaver way back in Fred Flintstone's day, but today, stress is a near constant, which means cortisol sends fat into your torso 24/7. Fight back by de-stressing daily in any way that works for you. For some great stress solutions, see Drain #1: Stress and Anxiety, beginning on page 142.

Belly Fat Bombshells

The belly fat–brain drain connection isn't just a theory; unfortunately, it's real, and so are the consequences.

Researchers at Kaiser Permanente in Oakland, California, tracked the health of more than 6,000 adults for 30 years and found that those who had the biggest waists in middle age were 65 percent more likely to develop dementia 30 years later than those with the trimmest waists.

- When University of Michigan scientists studied 1,351 people, they found that those with the thickest middles were 90 percent more likely to have mental-processing slowdowns and memory gaps than those with the slimmest torsos.
- French researchers gave word recall tests to 2,223 women and men in their thirties through their early sixties, and then repeated the test a decade later. People with wide waistlines performed 35 percent worse than those who were svelte.

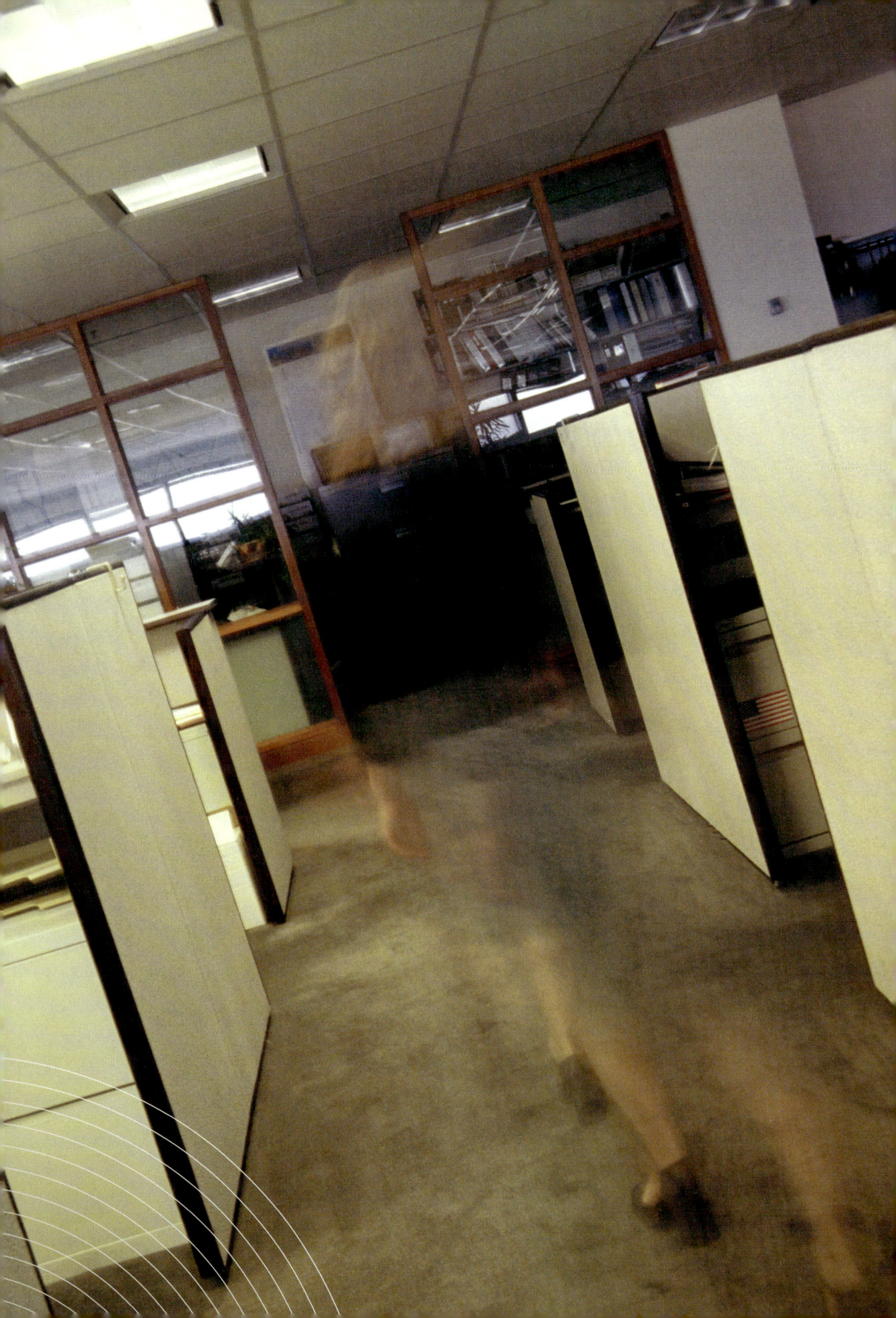

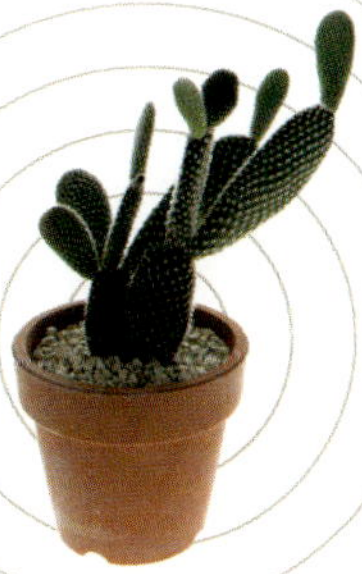

DRAIN #4

environment

When was the last time you walked through the woods, felt the wind in your hair, or got mud on your shoes? If it's been awhile, your brain may be paying the price. Experts estimate that adults today spend at least 90 percent of their time indoors, caught up in modern man-made environments that pose subtle threats to mental clarity.

What's so bad about life inside? For starters, there's the lack of alertness-inducing natural light; the shortage of fresh, oxygen-rich air; and, if you live with a smoker, the exposure to brain-draining secondhand smoke. And let's face it, living in our offices and living rooms simply can't deliver the deeply restoring experience of being in nature—a quality so connected to better brain power that some doctors are beginning to prescribe outdoor time to patients who are so stressed out they can no longer think straight.

Here, then, are five ways in which you can make your environment more brain-friendly. You won't find alarmist warnings about disproven brain threats here—we've weeded out myths like "metal fillings are bad for your brain" (there's no good evidence to support this claim), "aluminum pans cause Alzheimer's disease" (they don't), and "cell phones cause brain cancer" (so far, the evidence says no). You *will* find ways to minimize real environmental hazards and protect your brain from some of the perils of modern-day life.

CORRECT "NATURE DEFICIT DISORDER"

Adults and children alike report spending more time watching TV and playing with computers, cell phones, and video games than enjoying a walk around the block, an afternoon in the park, or a backyard barbecue. Even visits to national parks and scenic outdoor areas are declining. Experts call this growing disconnection from the outdoors nature deficit disorder, and there's plenty of evidence that if you're not getting outside much, your brain is missing out.

Exposure to green plants and flowers has been shown in numerous studies to boost thinking skills, speed mental processing, and reduce stress. There's even some early evidence that artificial plants have some of the same benefits.

Why do our brains seem to work better when the surrounding scene is green? Perhaps the answer lies in our prehistoric beginnings, when human beings lived, loved, and fought for survival on the African Savanna. Greenery then meant life was good—plenty of water, food, and tall grass for shelter. Scientists speculate that we're hardwired to feel that all's well when we're back in the setting that nurtured us for millions of years.

Trouble is, most of us spend little time in nature—25 percent less today than 20 years ago. These strategies can help you get back in touch.

Take a long walk in the park (not the city). The University of Michigan boasts a lovely, well-maintained arboretum. To test the affects of nature on memory, psychologists at the university had 38 students take a memory challenge—repeating a sequence of numbers backward—before and after strolling through either the arboretum or the town of Ann Arbor for 50 to 55 minutes. The nature group's scores on the "after" test improved significantly; those of urban walkers did not.

The great outdoors can also recharge your cognitive batteries. Spending just 2 hours a week outside helped 74 women newly diagnosed with breast cancer overcome extreme mental fatigue—the kind that makes everyday decisions and activities (like holding a conversation, planning a meal, or balancing a checkbook) nearly impossible.

Petals for Peace of Mind

The sight of cheery flowers on the kitchen table is one of the best happiness-inducers. If you don't want to buy them from a store, it's simple enough to arrange a bouquet from your own garden, especially if you use a few tricks from the experts.

1. Start with a sparkling-clean vase; your flowers will last longer.

2. Remove any thorns or leaves that would fall below the water line in the vase.

3. Cut the bottoms of the stems diagonally to give them a large surface to absorb water. This is best done under water so the vessels of the stems won't be obstructed by air bubbles.

4. To keep flowers from sagging in the vase, crisscross several pieces of transparent tape across the mouth of the vase before putting the flowers in. The flowers will look perky and fresh for a few extra days.

Fill your home with houseplants and your yard with greenery. Green plants foster sharper recall, quicker reactions, and creativity. In one Japanese study, men who could see plants during creative word-association tests scored higher than men who couldn't. In another study, houseplants in the test room were correlated with faster reaction times. And in a third study, people taking the written portion of a driver's license exam got higher scores when there were green plants on the desk.

In your yard, plant greenery and flowers where you can see them from the windows you look out most often, and open your curtains on the pretty view. No yard? Plant a container garden on your apartment patio or balcony. And don't forget the houseplants (in your office, too)!

Consider windowsill herbs. You'll get a double bonus by growing rosemary, in particular; it's not only pretty but its strong, resinous scent will perk up your brain every time you walk by and take a sniff. (In fact, studies show that inhaling either rosemary or basil increases the brain's production of beta waves, which signal heightened awareness.) Rosemary grows well near sunny windows. It's terrific with grilled fish, meats, and Mediterranean-style vegetables.

Surround yourself with images of nature. Simply hanging a photo or painting of a beautiful nature scene in your home or office could help boost your memory. The same University of

Green plants foster sharper recall, quicker reactions, and creativity. Don't forget to keep them in your office, too.

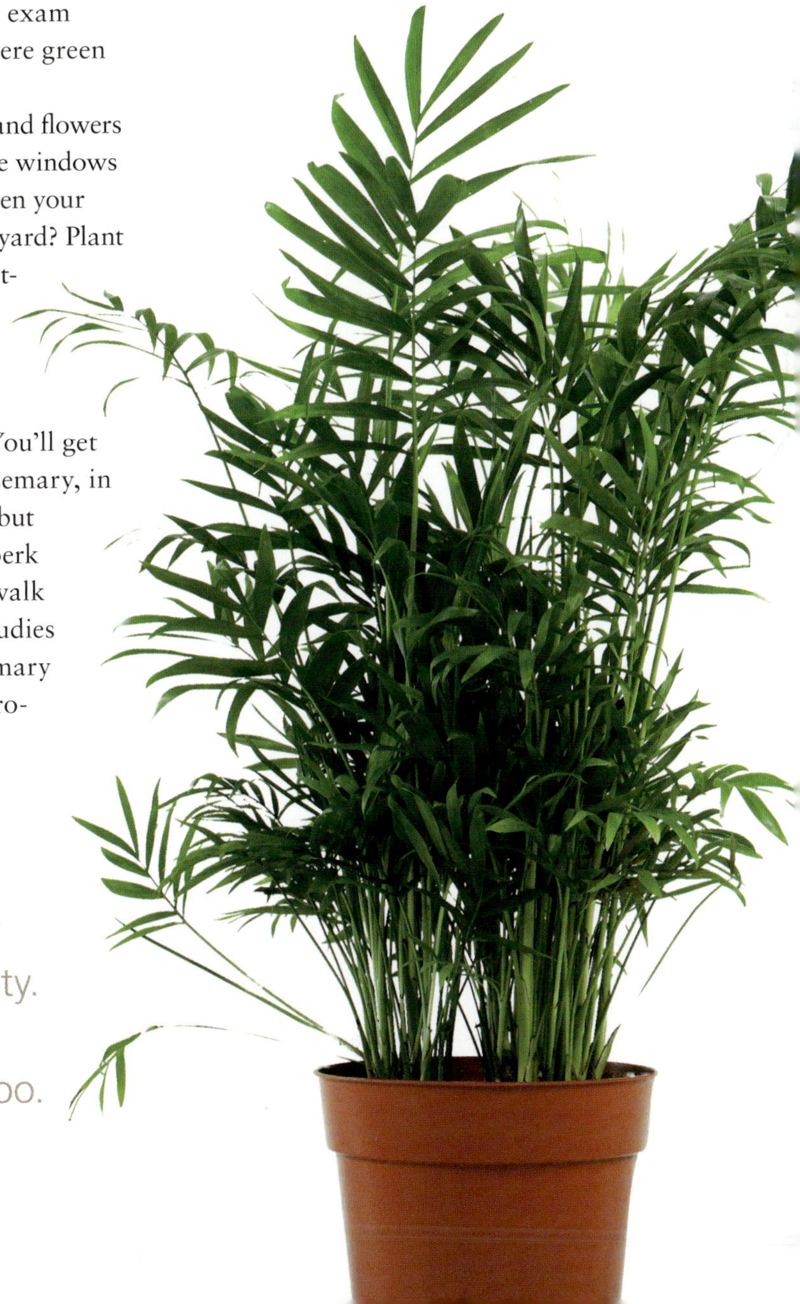

Michigan psychologists mentioned above asked 12 students to view nature photos or photos of city scenes for 10 minutes. The volunteers also took a memory test before and after—and the nature group, again, improved their scores the second time around, while the urban group did not. "These experiments demonstrate the restorative value of nature (for)...cognitive functioning," say the researchers, who add that having natural areas near your home or work is more than a nice amenity—it's vital for tip-top thinking.

Move meals and parties outside. Got a picnic table? You're ready to go. Food in the great outdoors tastes extra-good, and sitting in the yard or on a deck or balcony invites you and your tablemates to linger and enjoy each other's company, not to mention the fresh air.

Explore the night world. Too busy for a daytime nature break? Night's good, too. Stargaze, sign up for a night hike at a local nature center, or simply sit outside listening to the sound of spring peepers, summer cicadas, and autumn crickets.

Take your kids or grandchildren outdoors. Most kids now get just 30 minutes a *week* of unstructured playtime outdoors, according to the nonprofit conservation organization The Nature Conservancy. Instead, they're spending 6 1/2 hours a day with computers, television, video games, and cell phones. Round 'em up and hit the backyard for a game of Frisbee, a search for interesting leaves or bugs, or a silly game of tag. The kids won't be the only ones to benefit.

EMBRACE QUIET

Deep within your inner ear, tiny "hair cells" quiver, quake, and shimmy along to the sounds in your world, from the latest country music hit on the radio to the neighbor's noisy lawn mower to the quiet rustling of trees in the woods. These microscopic bristles convert sound waves into electrical signals that travel to your brain, delivering important information about what's happening around you. But too much noise can mean too much information—overloading brain circuits and leading to that it's-so-loud-I-can't-think-straight feeling.

In studies comparing schools near noisy airports, highways, and railroad lines with those in quiet areas, researchers have found links between noise pollution and problems with memory, concentration, reading ability, and performance on tests. It makes sense that noisy environments would have similar effects for adults learning new things, too, especially since older brains are more distracted by noise.

Noise also ratchets up your blood pressure, which is bad for the brain. When researchers checked the blood pressure levels of 140 adults living near London's Heathrow Airport and three other major European airports, they found that both the top and bottom numbers rose 6 to 7 points whenever there was a "noise event"—such as a plane flying overhead. Traffic noise had a similar effect. Over time, elevated blood pressure increases your risk for dementia and age-related problems with mental processing, memory, and reaction time.

How much noise is too much? That depends on the situation, and on you. You might love the big sound of a loud disc jockey as you dance and socialize at a party, but find that a radio playing in the next room at home makes it nearly impossible to focus on the newspaper you're trying to read. The murmur of traffic outside your window may be just background sound during the day, but could rob you of the deep, restorative sleep your brain needs at night for optimal performance tomorrow.

Turn off the TV and radio when you're trying to concentrate. Subtle changes in brain activity, beginning in middle age, make it more and more difficult for our gray matter to tune out distractions and concentrate on the task at hand, whether it's reading, driving, or writing a report at work. Scientists at the Rotman Research Institute in Toronto scanned the brains of 12 young adults and 12 older adults (average age 70), while they took a memory test, and they found a surprising difference. While the volunteers were looking at pictures they were supposed to commit to memory, the auditory cortex, a brain region that processes sound, lit up in older brains in response to the loud banging noises emitted by the MRI machine. This may help explain why the older folks did worse on the test; their brains simply couldn't block out the noise distraction. In the younger brains, the auditory cortex was quiet.

Shush night noises. A snoring bedmate, the rush of traffic outside your bedroom window, a loud air-conditioner, or noisy neighbors can all disturb your sleep and lead to diminished brain power by reducing the amount of time you spend in phases of deep sleep, when memories are locked in place and the brain restores itself. Earplugs can help, as can moving your sleeping quarters to the quietest part of the house. As for the snorer on the next pillow, ask him or her to roll over or get an evaluation for sleep apnea if earplugs don't block their rasps and rattles. A small Canadian study found that bedmates of snorers suffered hearing loss

Are You "Noise-Sensitive"?

If sounds affect you more profoundly that they do your friends, co-workers, or family members, you may be among the estimated 1 in 13 people who are noise-sensitive. Experts aren't sure whether hyperacusis—the medical term for extreme noise sensitivity—is something you're born with or whether it's the result of early environmental exposures (and it's not clear whether growing up in quiet surroundings or amid noise raises risk more).

But the effects of noise sensitivity on your cranium are real. In one study from Missouri Western State University, noise-sensitive people had greater difficulty concentrating on reading when noise levels were high. In others, highly noise-sensitive people have reported feeling mentally confused and even nauseated when subjected to loud sounds. If noise bothers you, seek quiet—your brain will thank you!

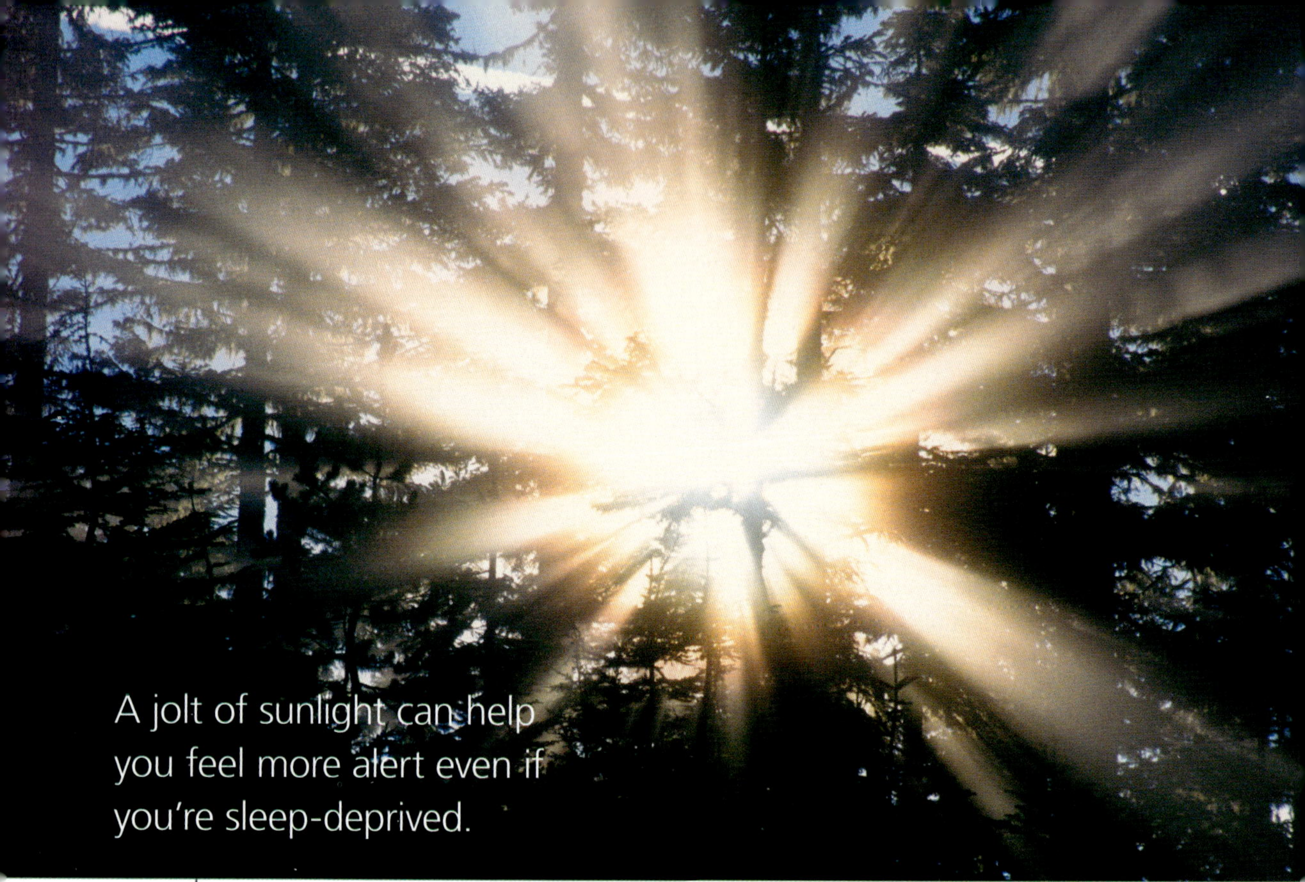

in the ear closest to the person making all that night noise. Snoring can reach 80 decibels—as loud as someone yelling for help—or even 90 decibels—equivalent to truck traffic.

Buy a white noise machine. These generate a consistent, calming sound that covers other noises. They can help you fall asleep and stay asleep till morning.

Invest in double-pane or soundproof windows. When it comes to real estate, it's all about location. If you live in a noisy area, you can't necessarily pick up and move to a quieter one, but you can make sure your windows keep out as much sound as possible.

Boycott loud events and restaurants. If you have to raise your voice to talk to your dining partner, the restaurant is too loud; take your business elsewhere.

Wear earplugs. In one informal review, published in the online magazine *Slate* (www.slate.com), reviewers found that cheap polyurethane earplugs—at about $1 per pair—were more effective, comfortable, and easy to use than pricey customized silicon plugs or extra-fancy plugs that deliver white noise directly into your ears. Keep a pair by your bed, in your purse, and in your briefcase. In one Israeli study of factory-workers, those who started wearing this type of earplug saw noise-related rises in the stress hormone cortisol, toxic to brain cells in excess doses, disappear.

LET THE LIGHT SHINE IN

Millions of years before the first alarm clock was ever invented, Mother Nature devised a surefire wake-up call for the human brain: sunshine. When the dawn's early light strikes the human eye, it sends a signal to brain regions that control alertness. The result: You go from drowsy to mentally bushy-tailed, fast.

We seem to have an intuitive understanding of the connection between light and sharp thinking—just consider the phrases "it dawned on me" and "I've seen the light." Now, science is catching up with this age-old wisdom and shedding new light of its own on the link.

A jolt of sunlight can help you feel more alert even if you're sleep-deprived, studies show. In brain-imaging studies, even a short burst of blue light—a predominant wavelength in natural light—triggered new activity in the brain stem and thalamus, areas that control wakefulness and sleepiness.

When lights in a large British office building were outfitted with experimental "blue-white" bulbs for 4 weeks, alertness, concentration, and work performance improved. Workers even reported that they slept better at night. Researchers suspect that the blue-white light is effective because it mimics energizing natural light.

Bright light may even slow down dementia. When Dutch brain scientists installed extremely bright lights in long-term care centers, people with dementia scored 5 percent better on thinking tests and saw depression drop 19 percent. The lights used in the study aren't available for home use—they were three times brighter than typical home lighting, on par with television studio lighting. But the lead study author says it makes sense for people with or at risk for dementia to live in well-lit environments.

These steps can help you take advantage of the connection between light and alertness.

Pull up the shades first thing in the morning—then get outside. Your eyes and brain may be especially receptive to the energizing effects of natural light first thing in the morning, studies suggest. Take advantage of this window of opportunity by flooding your home with sunshine. Then get outside, either by taking a walk (good for the brain!) or by lingering on your patio with a cup of coffee (also good for the brain!).

When you're inside, sit near a sunny window. In one Japanese study, 16 women reported that they felt more wide awake and performed better on a series of mental-alertness tests after sitting beside a sunny window than after sitting in a dimly lit lab.

Get a booster dose of natural light later in the day. A half-hour of sunshine is all it takes to increase alertness. That's another good reason to devote part of your lunch hour to an outdoor stroll.

Turn on the lights. During the morning and afternoon, make sure the area where you're spending your time is brightly lit. After dinner, dim the lights to signal your body that it's time to wind down.

GET SOME FRESH AIR

Fresh air doesn't just smell good, it supplies the oxygen your brain needs for snappy thinking and all-around alertness. But newer, energy-efficient buildings don't always provide enough of this vital brain fuel. Why? Two reasons: Newer ventilation systems may not exchange indoor and outdoor air as frequently as older, "leaky" buildings do. And even if enough oxygen is coming in, the building's ventilation system may not circulate fresh air effectively, according to the U.S. Environmental Protection Agency.

Airtight rooms are low in oxygen and high in sleepiness- and fatigue-inducing carbon dioxide. Outside air contains about 350 parts per million of carbon dioxide; in some studies, levels in office buildings have risen to 1,000 parts per million or higher—enough to cause drowsiness and foggy thinking.

Another significant danger of life indoors, if you live with a smoker, is secondhand smoke. (We assume the smoke isn't coming from you! If it is, you already know it's time to quit.)

Open the window. If you notice that you feel drowsy, get headaches, or feel low on mental energy and live or work in an energy-efficient building (many structures built after 1970 are energy efficient), you may be breathing recirculated air that's not fully oxygenated. The fix: If possible, open a window or door to the outside. If that's not possible, make extra-sure to get outside for a walk at lunch, and add another short 10-minute outside break in the afternoon.

Ban smoking in the house. Long-term exposure to secondhand smoke raised the risk for dementia by 30 to 250 percent in one University of California study. In another study of more than 5,000 older nonsmoking adults, published in the *British Medical Journal*, Cambridge University researchers found that those with the highest levels of cotinine (a

Multitasking: Bad for Your Brain?

You may be able to walk and chew gum, converse with your spouse while cooking dinner, or even crochet an afghan while watching your favorite TV show. But 21st century–style multitasking feats such as driving while talking on a cell phone or texting while working at your computer may be too much for the brain.

"Despite having these incredibly complex and sophisticated brains, with 100 billion neurons processing information at rates of up to a thousand times a second, human beings have a crippling inability to do two tasks at once," says neuroscientist Rene Marois, PhD, associate professor of psychology at Vanderbilt University. In brain scan studies, Dr. Marois found that the brain region crucial for decision making seems able to process just one task at a time.

Other research shows that asking your brain to switch back and forth between activities actually wastes time—and that doing one thing at a time is often more efficient.

Mental juggling may also make you dumber. Brain imaging studies at Carnegie Mellon University show that when volunteers did two things at the same time, the brainpower available for each job dropped to *less* than half. The result is a kind of mental power shortage or brownout. Researchers also see evidence that stress hormones produced by chronic multitasking inhibit short-term memory.

A better plan: Stick with the old-fashioned one-thing-at-a-time approach when you have something mentally challenging to do.

marker for recent secondhand smoke exposure) were 44 percent more likely to have dementia than those with the lowest levels. The brain drain isn't just a problem for older people; in one study of high-school students, those who breathed secondhand smoke at home decreased the chances that they would pass standardized achievement tests by 30 percent.

CUT DOWN ON CLUTTER

Some people thrive on chaos, but for the rest of us, a messy world just creates stress (see the tip on clutter in Drain #1: Stress and Anxiety beginning on page 142) and distraction. Piles of papers and stacks of stuff remind us of all the things we should be doing (like reading our mail and paying our bills) and simultaneously make it harder to get anything done (where *is* that checkbook, anyway?).

The mess around you could even contribute to poor decision making and fuzzy thinking. According to brain scientists at the Massachusetts Institute of Technology, navigation screens in fighter jets that show too many details (known as visual clutter) interfere with a pilot's ability to find a target. Similarly, web sites with too many extra features on one page keep viewers from locating information that they're seeking.

Of course, clutter is in the eye of the beholder. Some studies suggest a messy desk may actually be more conducive to creativity than a neat one. But if clear thinking and less stress is your goal, it's probably time to clean up.

Do a fast sweep. Choose three surfaces that you see as soon as you walk into a room and do a 5-minute "keep or toss" blitz with each one. If you can return objects to their rightful storage locations, do so. If not, designate a box for items that you'll store later. Toss everything you don't use or need. The idea is to create the feeling of calm.

Dig deeper with the A-B-C method. When you have more time, attack a room with this approach. Start with closets, to make room for other objects that need a home, then tackle piles in the room itself. Place orphan items or those for which there's not enough space into one of three piles: A for "Always used"; B for "Used only occasionally", such as for holidays or seasonally; and C "I haven't used this in over a year." Store A items in easy-to-reach spots in closets, drawers, and cabinets. Place B items on a special shelf or at the back of storage units. Toss C items (if they're valuable, make plans to sell or donate them).

Buy some organizers. You simply can't clear clutter if you don't have a place to store the stuff you want to keep. Retail stores devoted entirely to helping you organize your life, such as The Container Store (www.containerstore.com), are an excellent place to start. Buy a set of accordion file folders for paperwork you need to keep, some under-the-bed storage boxes for housing sweaters, a large straw or wicker basket for keeping current magazines in your living room, back-of-door shoe hangers for overflow shoes, and so on.

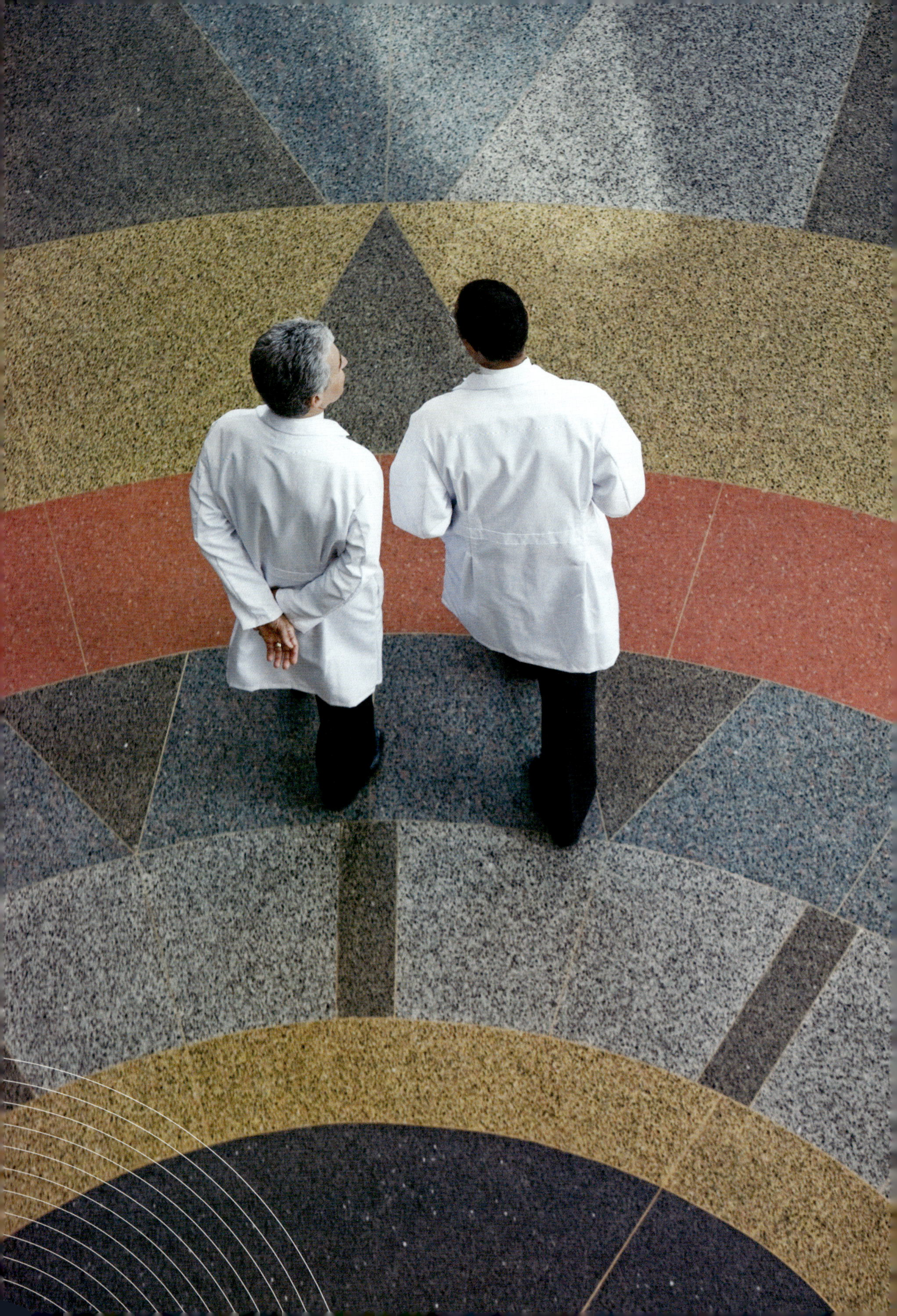

DRAIN #5

medical causes

Don't blame your age or senility for memory slips, cognitive slowdowns, and attention deficits—at least not until you've ruled out common, seemingly unrelated medical problems that can affect your brain. Getting back to your own mental self may be as simple as getting one of these problems such as high blood pressure, high cholesterol, or hearing loss, under control.

PUT A LID ON HIGH BLOOD PRESSURE

Take a brittle, worn-out garden hose, turn the water on full force, and what do you get? Lots of little leaks, and maybe even a blowout. If you have high blood pressure, this messy scenario could unfold deep within your brain as fast-moving blood slams against the walls of fragile blood vessels. You could end up with tiny leaks that damage surrounding brain tissue (blood that escapes blood vessels is toxic to brain cells), plus a big risk for a brain-altering—and life-altering—stroke.

The bottom line: If you want to protect your brain, keeping your blood pressure healthy is one of the single most important steps you can take. In one 10-year study of more than 8,000 older women and men, high blood pressure raised dementia risk by 50 percent. In another, thinking skills declined measurably in people whose high blood pressure levels went unchecked for just 2 years.

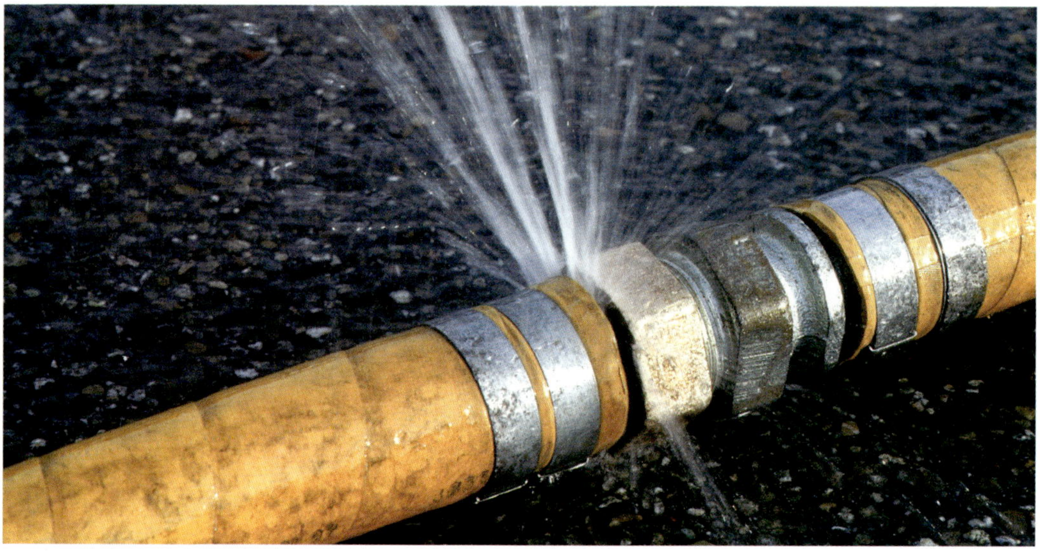

Blood Pressure Blips You Should Never Ignore

Are you—or your doctor—shrugging off early warnings of brewing blood pressure trouble? The answer is yes if any of these "little" problems haven't prompted you to take steps to lower your blood pressure:

It's "high-normal." Thirty percent of American adults have slightly elevated blood pressure levels, between 121/81 and 139/89. But this gray zone is no small problem: It nearly doubles stroke risk. Researchers warn that many family doctors see pre-hypertension as a borderline condition that should be watched, rather than a warning that needs prompt attention.

It's creeping up slowly. In one eye-opening study, women's blood pressures inched upward 8 to 10 points each decade, and men's by 4 to 5 points, between the ages of 35 and 64. That's enough to land you in the pre-hypertensive or even the hypertensive category—and a good reason for you and your doctor to nip rising blood pressure in the bud.

It's only high in the doctor's office. So-called white-coat hypertension—elevated blood pressure readings in the doctor's office but not other places (such as at a health fair, on a home monitor, or from a drugstore blood pressure machine)—isn't a fluke you can ignore. In one Scottish study, people with this sign of raised blood pressure under stress showed early signs of stiff arteries and an overworked heart that could lead to higher blood pressure later on.

High pressure begins to threaten your memory and dull thinking skills far earlier and at lower pressure levels than doctors ever realized in the past. Even slightly high pressure—levels considered normal or near-normal less than a decade ago—eroded memory, focus, and verbal skills in one recent study.

If your levels are healthy now, you're not off the hook; high blood pressure becomes more common with age, and lifetime odds for developing it are as high as 90 percent. It's never too early—or too late—to take some pressure off.

Aim for the right numbers. Experts have lowered the target numbers for blood pressure, reflecting new thinking about what's truly healthy and what's dangerous for your brain and body:

- *Optimal blood pressure:* 115/75 mmHg
- *Healthy blood pressure:* Below 120/80 mmHg
- *Pre-hypertension:* 120–139/80–89 mmHg
- *Hypertension:* 140/90 mmHg and above

Quit smoking. The nicotine in tobacco constricts blood vessels and raises your blood pressure 10 points or more for an hour after you smoke just one cigarette.

Lose weight sooner rather than later. Whittling 8 to 10 pounds can trim 4 to 5 points from the top number (systolic pressure) in your reading and 1 to 2 points from the bottom number (diastolic pressure). The best way to start is to exercise for at least 30 minutes on most days of the week. The sooner you start, the better: Researchers suspect that over time, chemicals churned out by body fat can make artery stiffness—which causes high blood pressure—hard to reverse.

Eat more produce, whole grains, and low-fat dairy. Calcium and other minerals in low-fat milk, yogurt, and other dairy products have pressure-lowering powers. So do the potassium, vitamins, and antioxidants in many fruits and veggies (like bananas, melons, spinach, and sweet potatoes) and the fiber in whole grains and produce.

Minerals That Lower Blood Pressure

Calcium, magnesium, and potassium all play a major role in keeping blood pressure low. Find them in these foods.

Potassium: Baked potato with skin, tomato sauce, lima beans, orange juice, cooked spinach, winter squash, bananas, raisins, and prune juice.

Calcium: Low-fat yogurt, low-fat milk, cooked spinach, turnip greens, and broccoli.

Magnesium: Bulgur, oat bran, barley, beans, cooked spinach, plantains, and pumpkin seeds.

Cut back on high-sodium foods. Cutting your sodium intake by just 300 milligrams (about the amount in two slices of processed cheese) reduces systolic pressure by 2 to 4 points and diastolic pressure by 1 to 2 points. Cut more sodium, and pressure drops even lower. The biggest source of excess sodium in our diets are processed foods such as canned soups, beans, and vegetables; microwavable entrées and side dishes; bottled salad dressings; salty snacks; hot dogs, sausage, and lunch meats; pickles; olives; and cheese.

Move it! Four daily walks of just 10 minutes each cut systolic pressure by 5 points and diastolic pressure by 3 points in an Indiana University study.

Take your blood pressure meds—and be sure they're working. Blood pressure medications can halve the risk for stroke and reduce the odds of developing

Alzheimer's disease by up to 40 percent. But research shows that these meds can't protect your brain if they're not lowering your blood pressure to healthy levels. That's important news for the 6 out of 10 people who don't take their blood pressure drugs as directed, or skip them entirely, and for the others who don't schedule follow-ups with their doctors to be sure their drugs and dosages are working.

GET YOUR CHOLESTEROL NUMBERS IN LINE

Could ordering the grilled salmon instead of the gourmet cheeseburger help you think faster? Could taking a stroll after dinner instead of watching a game show strengthen your memory? Could switching to oatmeal in the morning instead of a fast-food breakfast sharpen your mental clarity? The answer is yes, especially if your cholesterol levels are less than ideal.

Everyone knows by now that unhealthy cholesterol levels—high LDL ("bad" cholesterol) and low HDL ("good" cholesterol)—are dangerous to the heart. They're also dangerous to the brain. Remember that the brain is made up largely of fat. It's actually teeming with "good" HDLs, which seem to protect against blood vessel injury, brain plaques, and inflammation. As far as your brain is concerned, the more HDLs, the better! In one study of 3,673 people, all age 61, those with low HDLs (below 40 mg/dL) were 53 percent more likely to have memory problems than those with high levels (over 60 mg/dL). Those whose HDLs fell the farthest between age 55 and 60 had the most trouble remembering words on a test.

Having high LDLs, the type of cholesterol that clogs arteries, increases the risk for a stroke and also, at very high levels, can triple dementia risk. Here's how to rein in LDLs and bolster HDLs.

Hit the right target. It's not enough to know your total cholesterol number; you need to know your breakdown of HDLs and LDLs. Ask your doctor for those details the next time you have your cholesterol tested. By the way, you should have it checked at least once every 5 years starting at age 30 (earlier if you have a family history of heart disease or if you smoke), every 2 years in your forties, and every year starting at age 50.

Eat for high HDLs and low LDLs. This means serving yourself more fish, nuts, olive and canola oil, oatmeal, barley, beans, and produce. When you eat meat, make sure it's lean. Go easy on cheese and butter, and buy low-fat or fat-free milk and yogurt. This strategy cuts LDL-raising saturated fats from your diet and fills your plate with more good-for-you fats that protect HDL levels. It also gives you more

Cholesterol by the Numbers

LDL Level	Brain Effects
Below 100 mg/dL	Highly protective
100–129 mg/dL	Somewhat protective
130–159 mg/dL	Somewhat dangerous
160 mg/dL and above	Dangerous

HDL Level	Brain Effects
Below 40 mg/dL	Not protective
40–59 mg/dL	Somewhat protective
60 mg/dL and above	Highly protective

soluble fiber, which whisks LDLs out of your body. Including walnuts or pecans may even nudge HDLs up a little.

Have a glass of wine or beer a day. Studies suggest that drinking alcohol in moderation (one drink per day for women and up to two drinks a day for men) lowers LDL while raising HDL.

Achieve a healthier weight. Gradually moving to a healthy weight could raise your HDLs by 1 point for every 6 1/2 pounds you lose.

Walk briskly three times per week. You can raise your HDLs by taking a fast stroll for a half-hour three times a week. Adding strength-training three times a week should lower them even more.

PREVENT A STROKE

Suddenly, without warning, a blood clot closes off an artery. A fragile blood vessel bursts. Your leg, arm, or face goes numb. You can't see straight, or speak, or walk. Your brain is under attack, and it may never be the same again.

Moments after a stroke begins, brain cells die because they're deprived of oxygen-rich blood. If the stroke occurs on the right side of the brain, it may affect speech, short-term memory, emotions, and judgment. A stroke on the left side may lead to disorganized, compulsive, or extremely cautious behavior. A stroke also greatly increases the risk for dementia and Alzheimer's disease down the road.

A stroke happens in no time flat. But the health problems that conspire to unleash a stroke may be years in the making. You can take steps now to make sure you never have one.

The Brain-Healthy Fruit

Avocados are incredibly rich in good-for-you monounsaturated fat. In one study, adults who ate an avocado a day for a week saw their total cholesterol drop by 17 percent. Better still, their "good" cholesterol rose while their "bad" cholesterol fell. Add avocado slices instead of cheese to your sandwich and you'll get a double bonus: more brain-healthy good fat and less artery-clogging saturated fat.

Prevent and control high blood pressure. Sobering fact: Your risk for a stroke begins to rise as soon as blood pressure inches higher than an optimal level of 115/75, according to the landmark Framingham Heart Study. In fact, stroke risk doubles with every increase of 20 points in the top blood pressure number and/or 10 points in the bottom number. If you don't know your blood pressure, write down the numbers at your next doctor visit so you can see which direction they're heading.

Get treatment for off-beat heart rhythms. We mean atrial fibrillation, irregular heartbeats that can hurl clots into blood heading to your brain. Symptoms may include palpitations, chest pain, or fainting.

Keep blood sugar and cholesterol levels healthy. Diabetes doubles or even triples your risk for a stroke; levels of "bad" LDL cholesterol above 130 mg/dL also raise risk for strokes caused by blood clots—notably for repeat strokes in someone who's already had at least one ministroke (more about these shortly). Controlling diabetes cuts stroke risk by 50 percent; lowering LDLs can reduce risk by up to 25 percent.

Know the signs of a stroke–and act fast. Clot-busting drugs can stop and even reverse brain damage caused by the most common form of stroke—an ischemic stroke due to a blood clot—but only if they're administered within 3 hours of the start of a stroke. Too many people hesitate before calling for help and miss this precious window of opportunity. Call 9-1-1 immediately if you or a loved one has these signs:

- Weakness on one side of your body or an inability to move a part or all of one side of your body, such as your face, arm, and leg
- Numbness, tingling, or a feeling of heaviness on one side of your body
- Trouble seeing, such as blurred or double vision, dimness, or a sensation that a shade has been pulled down over your eyes
- Trouble speaking or finding words
- Trouble understanding words
- Unsteadiness, dizziness, clumsiness, fainting; trouble walking; or a sudden loss of strength in your legs
- A sudden, severe headache

Take ministrokes seriously. Days, weeks, or months before having a major stroke, 30 to 40 percent of people get a strange warning sign: a brief ministroke, called a transient ischemic attack, or TIA. The symptoms are the same as those above, just shorter and less intense. They stop as swiftly as they start, but that doesn't mean the danger has passed. The risk for having a full-blown stroke in the next 2 days is 1 in 20; over the next 3 months, it's 1 in 10, unless you take action.

What to do: Call your doctor immediately and explain what happened. He or she may want to put you on medications to prevent blood clots, lower cholesterol, and reduce blood pressure. In a British study, the combination cut the odds for a major stroke after a TIA by 80 percent.

If you think you've had a ministroke in the past, also let your doctor know. Having had one means you may have more in the future. Your doctor will decide whether you are a candidate for a blood thinner or blood pressure medicine.

Have You Had a Stroke and Don't Know It?

An odd, brief dizzy spell. A weird episode of blurred vision. That strange moment when half your face felt numb. A brief, inexplicable inability to think straight. These strange occurrences can all be signs of a transient ischemic attack (TIA), which often goes undiagnosed.

Experts are also uncovering evidence of yet another type of stroke: a "silent" stroke that causes no symptoms at all. Like TIAs, these can block tiny arteries in the brain, diminish brain power, and increase the risk for a major stroke or for more small strokes that can add up to brain drain. As many as one in five adults over age 45 has had at least one silent stroke, yet most never realize it.

KEEP BLOOD SUGAR UNDER CONTROL

High blood sugar is a "major ager" of the human brain. Its not-so-sweet consequences range from memory lapses and fuzzy thinking to dementia and Alzheimer's disease. You don't even have to have diabetes to suffer the consequences. Long before high blood sugar causes diabetes, it can damage blood vessels that bring oxygen and nutrients to the brain, doubling the risk for vascular dementia (the type caused by insufficient blood flow to the brain). It can even shrink the hippocampus, an area that stores memories and facilitates learning. In one University of California study, high blood sugar raised the risk for memory problems fourfold.

High blood sugar not only damages arteries but also it encourages the buildup of artery-clogging plaque. It also seems to increase inflammation in the brain and often goes hand in hand with insulin resistance, a condition in which cells stop responding to the hormone insulin. Insulin resistance in brain cells affects how the cells function, and not for the better.

If you have full-blown diabetes, studies suggest that you are about 50 percent more likely to develop Alzheimer's disease than someone who doesn't. The good news: Taking insulin-sensitizing drugs may offer some protection.

If you have diabetes or pre-diabetes (blood sugar of 100 to 125 mg/dL on a fasting blood sugar test), or you've been told you're at risk for diabetes, work with your doctor to prevent high blood sugar.

new thinking

Is Alzheimer's disease a form of diabetes? Researchers at Northwestern University have discovered that in people with Alzheimer's disease, a toxic protein chops insulin receptors off brain cells. That's a huge problem because, in the brain, the hormone insulin and its receptors not only help usher blood sugar into hungry brain cells but also help nerve cells survive and form memories. Removing a neuron's ability to handle insulin, the scientists speculate, results in a kind of "Type 3 diabetes"—and could be a major factor in the development of Alzheimer's disease. Levels of brain insulin and of insulin receptors are already known to be lower than normal in people with the disease. Now, researchers hope that further studies will show whether diabetes drugs can protect neurons from this memory-robbing damage.

Know your blood sugar levels two ways. If you have diabetes, it's important to perform daily blood sugar tests and keep track of the results as recommended by

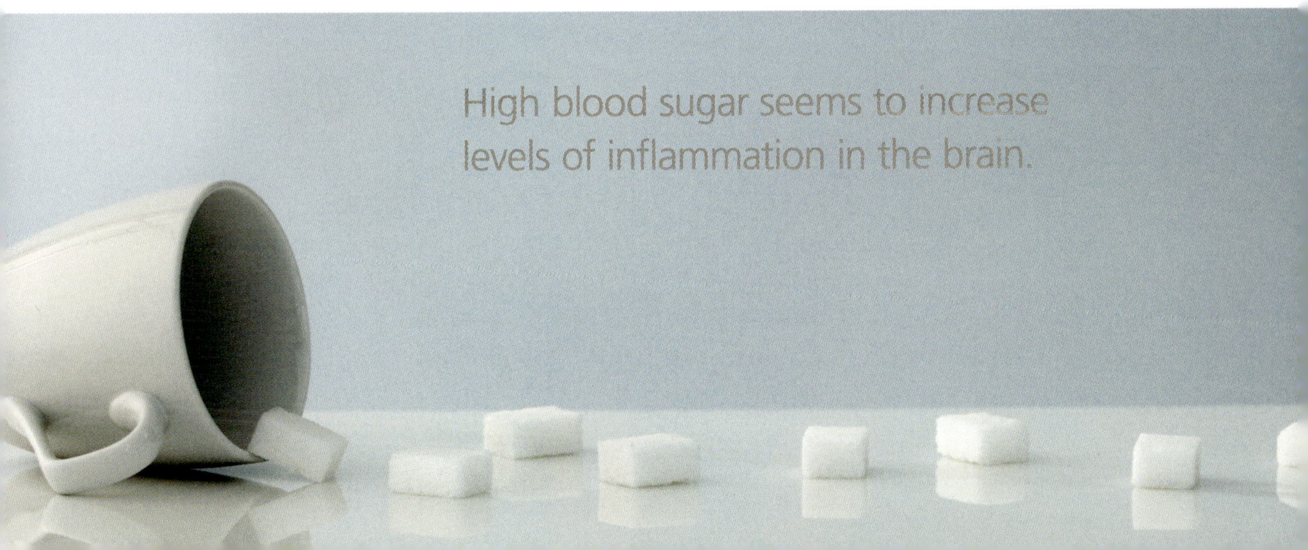

your doctor. But don't stop there: Also get an A1C test at least twice a year. This test tells you how well you've managed your blood sugar over the past 3 months. Shoot for an A1C reading of 6.5 to 7. Every 1-point rise above that range increases your risk for a stroke significantly and also boosts your odds for dementia and mild cognitive impairment.

Be vigilant about blood pressure and cholesterol. About 70 percent of people with diabetes also have high blood pressure and/or high cholesterol, yet surveys reveal that most worry only about their blood sugar. Mistake! Both high blood pressure and high cholesterol are even more dangerous to the brain when combined with high blood sugar. Put these risks on your radar—and take the steps outlined in this chapter to control them.

Get the meds you need. If your blood sugar is creeping higher despite your best efforts, it may be time for diabetes medications or insulin shots or for a change in your medication regimen. Diabetes is a progressive health condition that often requires more intense treatment over time, even if you've done everything right. Don't shy away—your health and your brain are at stake. In one study of 145 people with Type 2 diabetes who were already taking one blood sugar-controlling drug, those who added a second drug for 6 months saw blood sugar levels improve—and after 6 months, their scores on tests of working memory improved by 25 to 31 percent.

EASE YOUR WAY AT MENOPAUSE

If you're approaching menopause, you may be wondering where your mind's gone. Suddenly, your keys are always lost (so is your checkbook, your gardening shears, and, sometimes, your car.) And that new co-worker? What *is* her name?

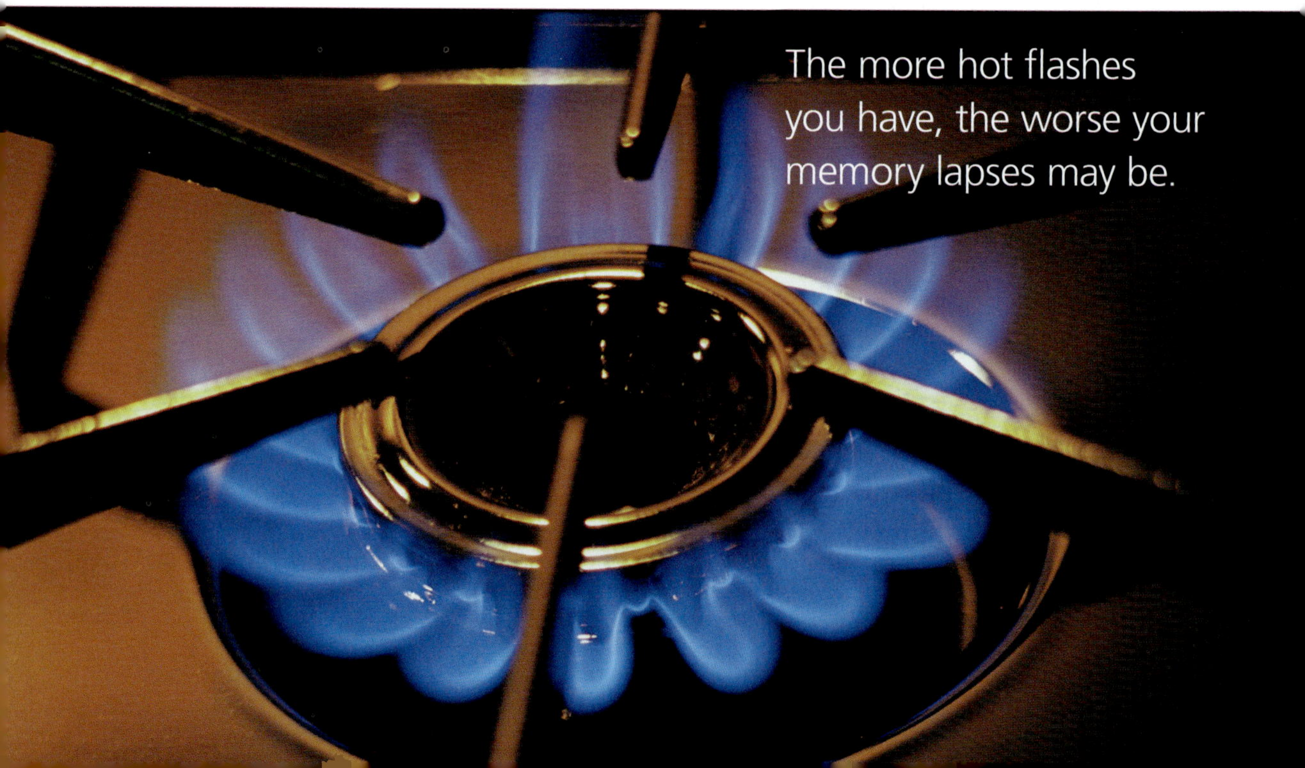

The more hot flashes you have, the worse your memory lapses may be.

You're not alone. When University of Arizona researchers interviewed 110 women who were entering menopause about their most distressing symptoms, 92 percent named forgetfulness. It was second only to sleep problems, which affected 95 percent. The more hot flashes you have, the worse your memory lapses may be. When 29 menopausal women wore skin monitors for 24 hours to detect every hot flash, researchers found that those who had the most flashes also performed the worst on memory tests. "The hot flash–memory relationship is not all in a woman's head," notes lead researcher Pauline M. Maki, PhD, of the University of Illinois.

Researchers aren't sure what causes fuzzy thinking and memory problems in women approaching menopause. Declines in estrogen are apparently not to blame, leaving stress and lack of sleep as likely culprits. Shifting hormones may disrupt a woman's slumber. You may have more trouble falling asleep or staying asleep or find yourself waking up earlier in the morning. In the University of Illinois study, researchers also found that the fewer hours a woman slept—and the more nighttime hot flashes she had—the worse her memory the next day.

What to do? Hormone therapy and most drugstore and health-food store remedies do little to help your memory. We recommend strategies that will help you get a good night's sleep, diminish hot flashes, and reduce other stresses in your life. Also refer back to Vaccine #6: Sleep, beginning on page 130, for more tips.

Cultivate a stellar sleep routine. Stick with set hours for going to bed and waking up, exercise several times a week (a Stanford University study shows it can help you fall asleep 15 minutes faster and get an hour more shut-eye each night), abolish caffeine after noon, and banish TVs and computers from the boudoir. Keep the room cool and, if night sweats are a problem, keep yourself cool, too: Sleep with a fan blowing on you and, if you tend toward p.m. hot flashes, check out pajamas made of sweat-wicking materials and marketed specifically for women with night sweats. A search online for "pajamas" and "hot flashes" will point you to several brands.

Develop a smart strategy for coping with hot flashes. If you want to try a hot flash remedy, consider the herb black cohosh. Some studies suggest it may help a little, though it could take more than 6 weeks to see results. (If you aren't seeing improvement by then, stop.) You can also ask your doctor about taking a low-dose antidepressant to help regulate your body temperature and curb hot flashes. And of course, short-term estrogen use is an option if your personal health history doesn't take it off the table (read more in Vaccine #3: Drugs, beginning on page 98). But your best bet may be a do-it-yourself mosaic of strategies: Avoid hot baths and showers, skip spicy foods, and dress in layers.

Deal with the other stresses in your life. Stress is a major brain drain—and it's typically rampant at midlife. One small study from the University of Rochester Medical Center found clues that women going through perimenopause had difficulty learning and remembering new information due largely to stress. Cut stress where possible and learn to cope with the rest by regularly practicing a stress-reduction strategy that you like. This could be daily exercise, calm breathing, progressive muscle relaxation (tense and then release one muscle group at a time) before bed, 10 minutes of morning yoga, or regular chats with a friend who makes you laugh.

CATCH HEARING LOSS EARLY

Like tufts of grass waving in a breeze, tiny hairlike cells deep within your inner ear move in time to the sounds in your life. A child's winsome "hello!" might trigger a gentle shimmy, the BANG! of fireworks could act more like gale-force winds, silencing a few of these sound-transmitting cells forever. Lose enough of them, due to aging, noise exposure, or certain illnesses, and you have hearing problems that can be socially isolating—and bad for your brain.

A little hearing loss is normal with age. Between 24 percent and 40 percent of adults over age 65 have difficulty hearing, as do up to half of people over age 75. In one University of California study of people ages 50 to 94, researchers found that hearing loss was tied with loss of memory and cognitive skills. The reason: You may spend so much mental energy trying to figure out what people are saying that your brain doesn't have a chance to focus on the information. On a practical level, hearing problems also simply mean more social isolation and less brain stimulation, both risk factors for brain drain. How can you save your ears? These three steps are a great place to start.

See your doctor if you suspect you've lost some hearing. If she suggests a hearing aid, be patient. The results are worth the effort it takes to get used to the device—and it could help you stick with activities that can foster brain health.

Sometimes, the solution is even simpler. In one large study of people with hearing problems, researchers had to excuse 1 in 10 study volunteers before the experiment even began—because their hearing problems improved significantly when doctors removed earwax!

Turn the music down. If you use headphones or earbuds, your tunes are turned up too loud if others can identify what you're listening to.

Stash earplugs everywhere. Wear them when you'll be exposed to any sound over 85 decibels, such as a lawn mower, a rock concert, a wedding with loud music, even time in a loud health club. Don't rely on cotton balls or bits of paper stuffed in your ears; they'll screen out only about 7 decibels, while foam earplugs can block up to 32 decibels. Need more protection? Buy sound-deadening earmuffs.

When Everybody's Mumbling: Is It *Your* Ears?

You may have early signs of hearing loss—and should see your doctor—if you:

- Have trouble hearing on telephone calls
- Have trouble following conversations when two or more people are talking
- Turn up the TV volume so loud that others complain
- Have trouble hearing when there's background noise
- Think everyone is mumbling

ADDRESS ADULT ADHD

At least 1 in 25 adults has Attention Deficit-Hyperactivity Disorder (ADHD), lifelong trouble with concentration, focus, planning, organizing, and remembering. While kids are often diagnosed early, adults today never had that opportunity. The result: Many struggle silently, despite the fact that there's proven help out there.

Many kids with ADHD may simply have brains that mature a little later than average, which could explain why 40 to 70 percent of kids outgrow the disorder. But researchers are also uncovering the reasons why it can persist for a lifetime. For one thing, ADHD may be an outward sign of a differently shaped brain. In one recent study from the Kennedy Krieger Institute in Baltimore, researchers found that boys with ADHD had smaller basal ganglia, a part of the brain associated with controlling physical movement. Other studies have found differences in the shape and size of the frontal cortex, the brain stem, and the cerebellum. All of this may help explain why people with ADHD have trouble focusing. There's also evidence that in ADHD, some regions of the brain produce lower-than-usual levels of the chemical dopamine, which could help explain ADHD-related thinking and memory problems.

If you've felt that staying organized, remembering things, and controlling impulsive behavior has been a problem for you since childhood, you may have ADHD. Doctors know more than ever before about how to spot this condition in adults, and how to treat it.

Ask for an evaluation. Start with your family doctor, and ask for a referral to a mental health professional who can perform an ADHD evaluation.

Consider treatment. The same medications that help kids with ADHD focus can help you, too. They work by increasing levels of the brain chemicals dopamine and norepinephrine. Drugs approved for use in adults are two stimulants, extended-release mixed amphetamine salts (Adderall) and dexmethylphenidate hydrochloride (Focalin XR), and the nonstimulant drug atomoxetine (Strattera).

Try therapy. Cognitive behavioral therapy (CBT), a practical type of therapy that helps people solve problems and adjust their thinking and their behaviors, is a good type to try. One recent study from Massachusetts General Hospital found that a combination of drug therapy and CBT was more effective at controlling ADHD than drug therapy alone. Look for a psychologist specifically trained in this type of therapy.

Seeing, and Thinking, Straight

There's a hidden connection between vision-robbers like age-related macular degeneration (AMD), glaucoma, and dementia. When researchers followed 206 people with AMD for 3 years, they discovered that nearly 15 percent showed signs of a decline in memory and other thinking skills, most likely because vision loss caused people to drop out of some of their activities. The take-home lesson? Get regular eye exams to help preserve your vision, and do all you can to keep participating in the activities you love.

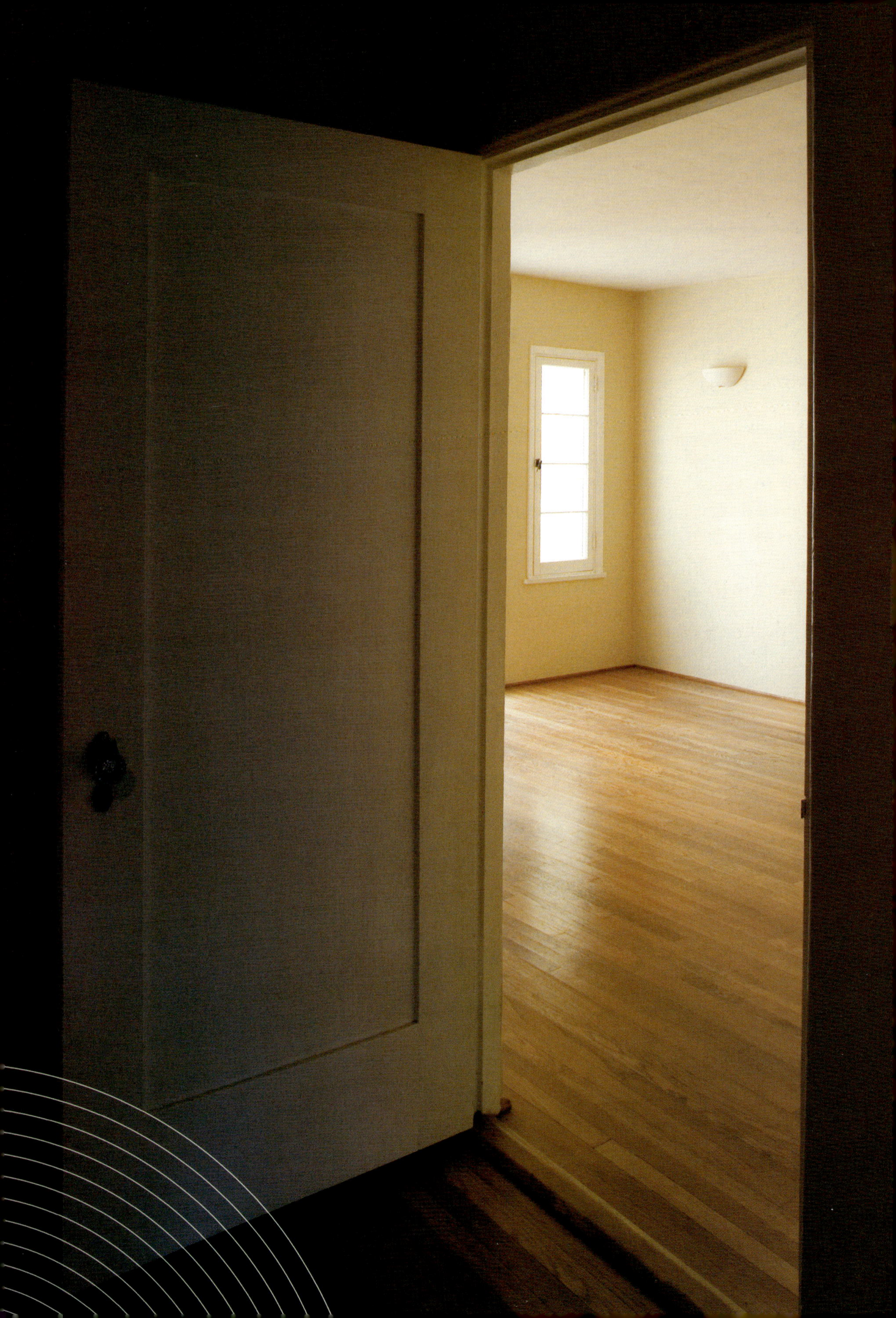

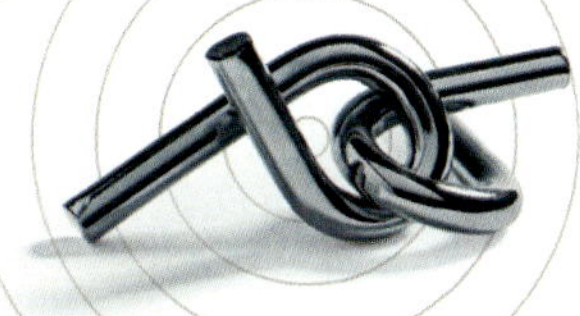

DRAIN #6

alzheimer's disease and other dementias

Many adults fear Alzheimer's disease far more than they fear heart disease (the number one killer), diabetes, or even cancer, and it's no wonder: Losing our minds equates with losing our very selves. While there isn't yet a vaccine or cure for Alzheimer's, there is tremendous new knowledge of how to prevent or put off this disease and other forms of dementia.

"There's no magic bullet, but there is plenty of evidence that most people can prevent, delay, or lessen the impact of these brain disorders," says Richard E. Powers, MD, chairman of the Alzheimer's Foundation of America's Medical Advisory Board and associate professor of neurology at the University of Alabama School of Medicine. Emphasis on most people.

"Some people will do everything right and still develop dementia, others will do practically nothing and never develop it," says Dr. Powers. But, he adds, "I think we know enough right now to advocate many ways to protect yourself."

What about those scary statistics, especially the one that says that one in two people over age 85 develop dementia? It's true, but it's only part of the story. Your odds of developing Alzheimer's rise from 5 percent at age 65 to 17 percent at age 75 to nearly 50 percent by age 85—but not if you exercise or eat well or take care of your health in other ways.

The proof: In one study that looked at how physical activity affects dementia risk, people who exercised three times a week saw their risk rise more slowly than those who exercised less often. Their risk increased to 50 percent only at age 92—and by then, infrequent exercisers had a 75 percent risk. How does exercise help? By lowering high blood pressure, protecting against diabetes, boosting blood circulation, and encouraging the growth of new brain cells.

What you eat every day also heavily influences your likelihood of developing dementia. In a Columbia University study of 1,882 older people (average age 77), those with faltering memories who followed a healthy Mediterranean-style diet were 48 percent less likely to develop full-blown Alzheimer's disease than those who didn't. Experts aren't certain why, but they do know that this style of eating pampers blood vessels and helps reduce inflammation, which may play a role in the development of brain diseases.

Keeping your brain engaged and stimulated is also important, as you've read throughout this book, as is maintaining an active social network throughout life. "The evidence is pretty convincing that the combination of social, physical, and mental activity, along with good control of medical conditions like diabetes, high blood pressure, and high cholesterol, gives you the best chance of either preventing or delaying cognitive decline," says Kristin Fargher, MD, assistant director of the University of South Florida's Eric Pfeiffer Suncoast Alzheimer's and Gerontology Center.

It's your brain. Here's how to protect it.

new thinking

Most dementia isn't Alzheimer's alone. When researchers at Rush University Medical Center performed autopsies on the brains of 50 people who had dementia during their lifetimes, they made a surprising discovery: Nearly all had been diagnosed with Alzheimer's disease, yet most actually had a mix of dementias—an important clue that points to an easy target for preventing memory and thinking problems. Just 30 percent had "pure" Alzheimer's disease: Their brain tissue was packed with plaques and tangles. More than 40 percent had Alzheimer's plus vascular dementia. And another 12 percent only had vascular dementia.

Follow Three Key Rules

Rule #1
KEEP BLOOD VESSELS HEALTHY

Many people diagnosed with Alzheimer's disease also have a condition called vascular dementia (see "New Thinking" at left). The second-most common form of dementia, it causes memory and thinking problems when blood vessels in the brain can't deliver enough oxygenated blood to brain cells. This may happen when blood vessels are narrowed by atherosclerosis, contain leaks that damage surrounding brain tissue, or have been damaged by a stroke.

Experts know more about preventing vascular dementia than they do about preventing or slowing Alzheimer's at this point. You can take steps now to keep the blood vessels in your brain healthier, such as losing weight if you need to, exercising regularly, and eating more fruits and vegetables to help keep your blood pressure low. Healthy blood vessels can help protect you even if you do develop signs of Alzheimer's. In some studies, they seem to be the reason people whose brains contain the characteristic neurofibrillary tangles (twisted bits of protein inside nerve cells) and plaques (clusters of dead and dying cells) of Alzheimer's disease show no memory loss, confusion, or behavior problems. On the flip side, in one recent Johns Hopkins University study, people with Alzheimer's disease who also had the most severe cardiovascular disease—high blood pressure, irregular heartbeats, and/or chest pain—saw their memories and thinking skills decline the most rapidly.

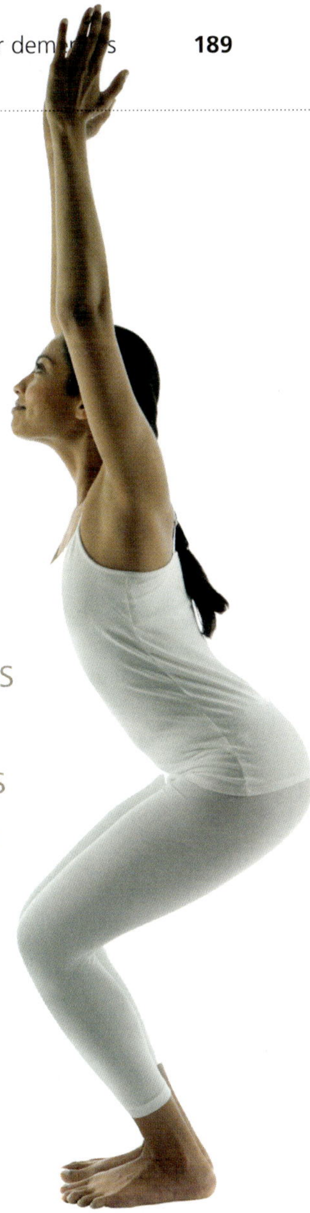

Regular exercise helps keep the blood vessels in your brain healthier.

Rule #2
MAINTAIN A COGNITIVE RESERVE

If having healthy blood vessels can help protect you from ever developing dementia, having a brain brimming with healthy nerve cells and connections between them can help protect you from cognitive problems if your brain does develop signs of Alzheimer's disease. When Rush University scientists looked at the brains of 91 supposedly dementia-free people, 37 had enough plaques and tangles to qualify as Alzheimer's patients, yet they had no noticeable problems with memory or thinking.

"When you have a lot of cognitive reserve, you can retain more cognitive abilities even in the face of Alzheimer's disease," Dr. Powers says. "You build and maintain cognitive reserve by challenging your brain, keeping blood vessels healthy, and keeping your brain healthy so it can grow new cells, as needed."

Exercise and stress reduction help brain cells regenerate, and mental challenges build new connections.

Rule #3
TAKE AN ACTIVE APPROACH TO PREVENTION

Perhaps you've been thinking, "What if Alzheimer's runs in my family?" It's true that the disease is partly genetic. But again, that's not the whole story. Genetics is a deciding factor in *early-onset* Alzheimer's, an uncommon type that develops before age 65 and affects 5 to 10 percent of all people with Alzheimer's. It generally runs in families; if a parent or grandparent developed Alzheimer's early on, your own risk is higher.

Most people with Alzheimer's develop the late-onset type that appears after age 65. Two genes have been identified that raise your risk: One is a mutation called APOE4, carried by 15 to 20 percent of us, the other a more recently discovered mutation called SORL1. "These genes are not deciding factors," Dr. Powers says. "Inheriting the APOE4 gene from one parent means that you could develop Alzheimer's 8 years earlier than someone without it. Inheriting it from both parents could mean that you could develop it 16 years sooner. But it doesn't always work that way. There are people who inherit a copy from each parent who never develop Alzheimer's, and people who don't inherit it at all who *do* develop Alzheimer's or other forms of dementia," he adds.

Why this news matters: If late-onset Alzheimer's runs in your family, consider it a wake-up call, not your destiny. The flip side is also true: If your family tree is dementia-free, you're not off the hook. The same healthy lifestyle strategies lower the risk for people in both groups.

Should You Get Your Genes Tested?

If early-onset Alzheimer's (before age 65) runs in your family, a blood test for one of the genes behind this devastating, yet fairly rare, condition could help you and your family prepare for the future. Talk with your doctor and meet with a genetic counselor first to be sure that you're ready for whatever you discover.

Tests for APOE4, the best-studied gene involved in the development of late-onset Alzheimer's, are used mostly in research studies. But for several hundred dollars and a saliva sample, companies on the internet promise to analyze your risk. Should you, or shouldn't you? "I don't recommend it," says psychiatrist Kristin Fargher, MD, assistant director of the University of South Florida's Eric Pfeiffer Suncoast Alzheimer's and Gerontology Center. "It doesn't really tell you what your real risk is. Some people with the gene never develop the disease, and people without the gene do develop it."

Top Anti-Alzheimer's Strategies

If you follow these ten tips, you'll be doing everything you can to avoid dementia later in life.

Don't smoke. Smoking doubles Alzheimer's risk and increases your risk for all types of dementia and cognitive declines by 40 to 80 percent, say Australian researchers who analyzed 19 studies involving more than 26,000 smokers, former smokers, and nonsmokers. If you smoke now, will quitting provide some protection? In this study, it did: Compared to current smokers, former smokers were 70 percent less likely to develop Alzheimer's disease and cognitive decline, and slightly less likely to develop vascular dementia, presumably because their blood vessels were healthier.

Abstain from heavy drinking. While moderate alcohol consumption (up to one drink a day for women, two for men) may protect against dementia (one study found that it reduced risk for vascular dementia by 71 percent), overdoing has the opposite effect. In fact, some experts suspect that one in ten cases of dementia is the result of brain-battering heavy drinking. Binge-drinking in middle age—downing a bottle of wine or five bottles a beer at least once a month—tripled the risk for dementia 25 years later, according to one Finnish study of 554 women and men.

Maintain healthy blood pressure. High blood pressure increases the risk for all types of dementia by 50 percent, studies show. It damages the brain by making small blood vessels leak, by triggering silent strokes, and by causing major strokes. If you don't have high blood pressure, the strategies here and in Drain #5: Medical Causes, beginning on page 174, will help you prevent it.

If you already have it, do whatever it takes to bring it down to healthy levels (optimal is below 120/80 mmHg) and keep it there. Studies show that using blood pressure drugs to control hypertension can reduce the risk for Alzheimer's disease by up to 40 percent and lower the risk for other forms of dementia almost to those of someone with naturally healthy blood pressure.

Keep a lid on blood sugar. Diabetes significantly increases a person's likelihood of developing vascular dementia and Alzheimer's disease. But even if you don't officially have diabetes, high blood sugar

Drive-Thru Dementia

The next time you pull into the drive-thru for a quick meal or snack, do your brain a favor: Order unsweetened iced tea and a salad with grilled—not fried—chicken and a splash of olive-oil vinaigrette. You'll avoid two big dementia threats that dominate fast-food menu boards.

Saturated fat. In lab studies, Canadian researchers found that diets rich in the saturated fat found in hamburgers, cheese, creamy salad dressings, and milkshakes boosted levels of Alzheimer's-related brain proteins up to eight times higher than the diets rich in the "good" fats found in fish and nuts.

Sugar. Sweet drinks lowered memory scores and doubled the number of amyloid plaque deposits—a hallmark of Alzheimer's disease—in a lab study from the University of Alabama. A great reason to say "no thanks" to soda, sweet tea, and fast-food desserts like cookies and pie.

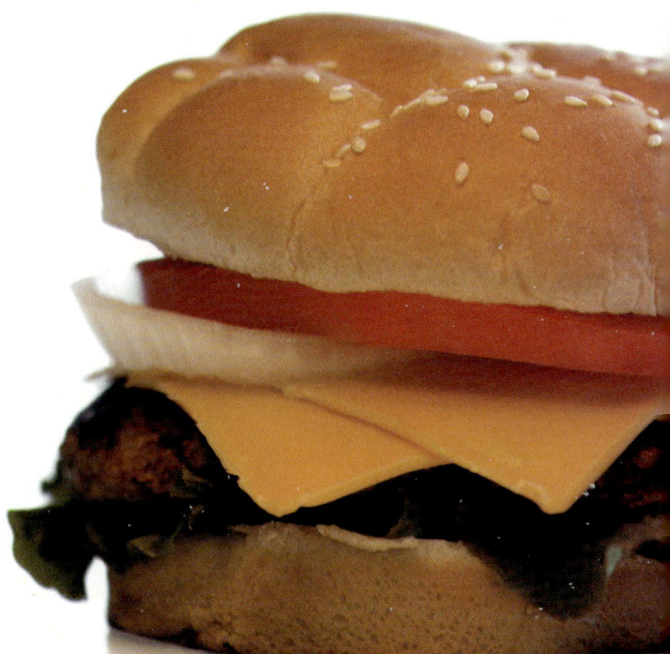

levels spell trouble. In one Swedish study, "borderline" diabetes, a reading of 100 to 125 mg/dL on a fasting blood sugar test, increased dementia risk by 67 percent and Alzheimer's disease risk by 77 percent.

Prevent it by maintaining a healthy body weight, exercising regularly, and eating smart. Keep calories in check and ease off simple carbohydrates such as white rice and white bread, along with all sugary foods and drinks. If you're at risk for diabetes, work with your doctor to be sure your blood sugar levels are checked often enough to spot problems early. If you do have diabetes, make tight blood sugar control a priority. Research shows it really does protect the brain.

Exercise at least twice a week. Walking, swimming, gardening, washing the car...whatever you do, make sure you do it at least twice a week (the minimum exercise frequency found to lower dementia risk in studies). "Light" exercise (gardening or strolling) was associated with a 35 percent lower risk for Alzheimer's disease and dementia in one recent Swedish study of 3,334 sets of twins. Regular, moderate exercise lowered risk by 50 percent.

Exercise protects against dementia even if you're older, inactive, or carry the gene for late-onset Alzheimer's disease. In one study of 2,263 men ages 71 and older, inactive volunteers who started an exercise program cut their risk of dementia in half compared to those who did not. In another study, people who exercised just twice a week were half as likely to have dementia 21 years later as those who were inactive, even if they had inherited the APOE4 gene for late-life Alzheimer's.

Exercise helps the brain use blood sugar more efficiently, avoiding gluts and shortages that may harm some brain regions. It also boosts blood circulation, protects brain cells from injury, and helps fuel new cell growth in areas we use for complex thought.

Eat like you're sitting beside the Mediterranean. The combination of foods plentiful in the traditional Mediterranean-style diet—fruits, vegetables, whole grains, fish, nuts, and olive oil—lowered the risk for Alzheimer's disease by 40 percent in one Columbia University Medical Center study. The effects of this diet even protected the brains of people who were beginning to show signs of mild cognitive impairment. In a 2009 study that followed 1,842 people for 4 1/2 years, the same team of researchers found that those with early signs of memory and thinking trouble lowered their odds for progressing to Alzheimer's disease by 45 to 48 percent if they ate "Mediterranean."

The closer you stick with this eating style—by eating the foods mentioned above and passing up fatty meats, full-fat dairy products, white bread, and sweets—the bigger the brain benefits. Among people with no known memory or thinking problems at the start of the study, those who followed the diet faithfully reduced their risk for developing early cognitive problems by 28 percent; those who followed it some of the time lowered their risk by 17 percent.

Watch your waistline. When researchers at the Kaiser Permanente Division of Research in Oakland, California, tracked more than 6,000 women and men for 30 years, they found that those who had the biggest waists in middle age were 65 percent more likely to develop dementia 30 years later compared to those with the trimmest waists. Keeping your waistline well below 35 inches for women and 40 inches for men will help.

Challenge your brain every day. "The brain is a use-it-or-lose-it organ," Dr. Powers notes. "When you challenge your brain, you're building and maintaining connections, so you have more cognitive reserves—you maintain thinking and memory ability longer, even if other connections are weakened."

When researchers from Albert Einstein College of Medicine followed 450 older people for 21 years, they found that those who were the most mentally active—they played chess and board games, kept up their skills on musical instruments, or attended lectures and visited museums—were 75 percent less likely to develop Alzheimer's and other forms of dementia than those who were least active.

There's no need to buy pricey brain-building software to get this benefit. "Attempting something that's new and different is all that matters," Dr. Powers says. "In other words, if you're an accountant, try learning a new language instead of reading another accounting book. If you tend to play Scrabble and do crossword puzzles, try a math puzzle."

Wear a helmet if you bike or ski. Experts are divided over whether mild head injuries (like the time you slipped on the ice and banged your noggin hard) increase dementia risk. But they're certain that moderate and severe head injuries do. So wear protection whether you're bungee-jumping, biking around the block, or skiing the slopes.

Stay in touch with friends and family. Maintaining regular contact with three, four, or more friends—in person, on the phone, or even via e-mail—is one key to protecting your brain and your memories. Staying social reduced dementia risk by 26 percent in one Kaiser Permanente study of 2,200 women, and the same amount in men in a study from Johns

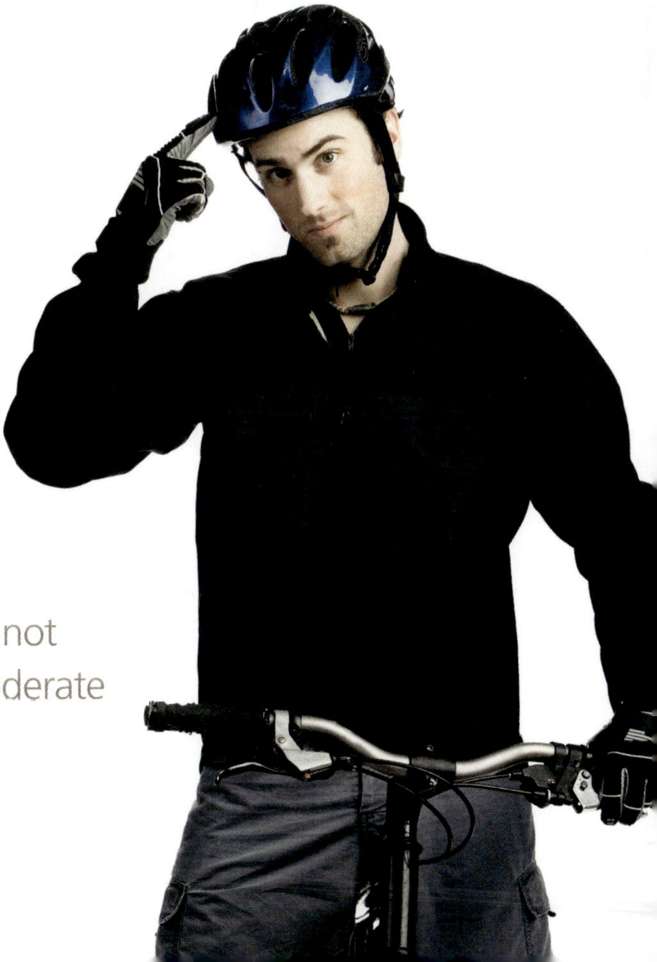

Mild head injuries may or may not increase dementia risk, but moderate and severe ones certainly do.

Hopkins Bloomberg School of Public Health. Socializing at home with your spouse may not be enough; the Kaiser researchers found that women with large social networks who made daily contact with friends had the lowest risk for dementia, but being married didn't make a difference.

Medicating Alzheimer's Disease

Until we know exactly what causes Alzheimer's, we probably won't be able to develop drugs to cure it. In the meantime, a handful of drugs have been approved by the FDA to help stall the progress of the disease. Each is believed to be most helpful when taken beginning in the early stages of Alzheimer's, though most are approved only for moderate to severe cases—all the more reason to check with your doctor if you suspect you have memory loss.

CHOLINESTERASE INHIBITORS

In your brain, chemicals called neurotransmitters are crucial to carrying messages from one brain cell to the next. People with Alzheimer's disease are often low on one of them, called acetylcholine, because cells that produce it are damaged or destroyed. The following drugs help preserve acetylcholine by inhibiting an enzyme called acetylcholinesterase, which breaks it down. (These drugs are also known as cholinesterase inhibitors.) They don't cure Alzheimer's (only 30 to 50 percent of people on these drugs show any improvement) but, in some people, they can help slow the course of the disease.

Tacrine (Cognex). Tacrine was the first drug approved by the FDA for treatment of Alzheimer's. It is rarely prescribed now because it can be dangerous to the liver.

Donepezil (Aricept). The second drug approved by the FDA, donepezil is the most widely prescribed in its class. While it's often prescribed to help slow the progression of diagnosed Alzheimer's, several international studies have found that it may also help protect higher function of patients with mild cognitive impairment as well as vascular dementia.

Rivastigmine (Exelon). In a large double-blind, placebo-controlled clinical trial in Italy, this drug was shown to improve cognition and performance of everyday activities in people with mild to moderate Alzheimer's disease.

Galantamine (Razadyne, Reminyl). The newest drug in this class, galantamine boosts acetylcholine and also helps the brain use it more effectively.

NMDA ANTAGONISTS

There is such a thing as too much of a good thing. In normal quantities, the neurotransmitter glutamate activates neurons. But too much glutamate can be toxic to the brain and may cause some of the neuron degeneration that occurs with Alzheimer's disease. These drugs work by blocking the receptors on cells that normally receive glutamate, thereby reducing the "static" between cells and allowing them to "talk" better to each other. They have been used in Germany from the 1980s on, for any kind of dementia, and also for depression.

Memantine (Akatinol, Namenda). Approved in 2004, memantine is currently the only FDA-approved drug of this type. While it's typically prescribed only for moderate to severe Alzheimer's, several studies are investigating it as an option for early Alzheimer's.

COMBINATION THERAPIES

Sometimes two drugs are better than one. One recent study, funded by the National Institute on Aging, found that a combination of a cholinesterase inhibitor and an NMDA antagonist showed the most promise. Researchers followed 382 patients for 2 1/2 years. Some received no drugs, some received a cholinesterase inhibitor, and some received a combination of a cholinesterase inhibitor and memantine. The researchers found that patients who'd been on both drugs showed the least cognitive decline. These effects increased over time, and researchers projected that the benefits would continue building the longer the patients were on the drugs.

Some doctors believe the combination is better because the methods of action complement each other. One drug works by allowing signals to be clearer, and the other works by allowing the substance that transmits the signals to be more plentiful.

If you are managing the care of a loved one with Alzheimer's, even mild dementia, talk to the doctor about trying combination therapy.

OTHER DRUGS IN THE PIPELINE

These drugs are a few years away from completed testing, but show some promise. Of course, the drug company that eventually happens upon the most successful Alzheimer's drug will be handsomely rewarded, so expect to see many other drugs undergoing trials in the future.

Selegiline (Eldepryl). Currently used in the United States as a treatment for Parkinson's disease, this drug raises the levels of certain brain chemicals by inhibiting an enzyme known as monoamine oxidase. It may also slow cognitive decline in Alzheimer's disease by protecting nerve cells.

B-secretase inhibitors. Researchers have shown that amyloid proteins, which accumulate in the brains of people with Alzheimer's disease, trigger inflammation in the brain and destroy brain cells. These drugs may stop the formation of amyloid plaque and halt the progression of dementia. They seem to work on the plaque, though they aren't specifically developed for targeting plaque in the brain.

Intravenous immune globulin (IVIG). Administered by IV, this "drug" contains antibodies from the blood of more than a thousand blood donors. This treatment has been used for other conditions, such as leukemia and immune system disorders, for more than 30 years. Now researchers have begun to study it in patients with Alzheimer's disease. IVIG contains antibodies that bind to amyloid proteins, which form the brain plaques characteristic of Alzheimer's disease. Initial results are promising. The problem? The cost is prohibitive—over $100,000 a year.

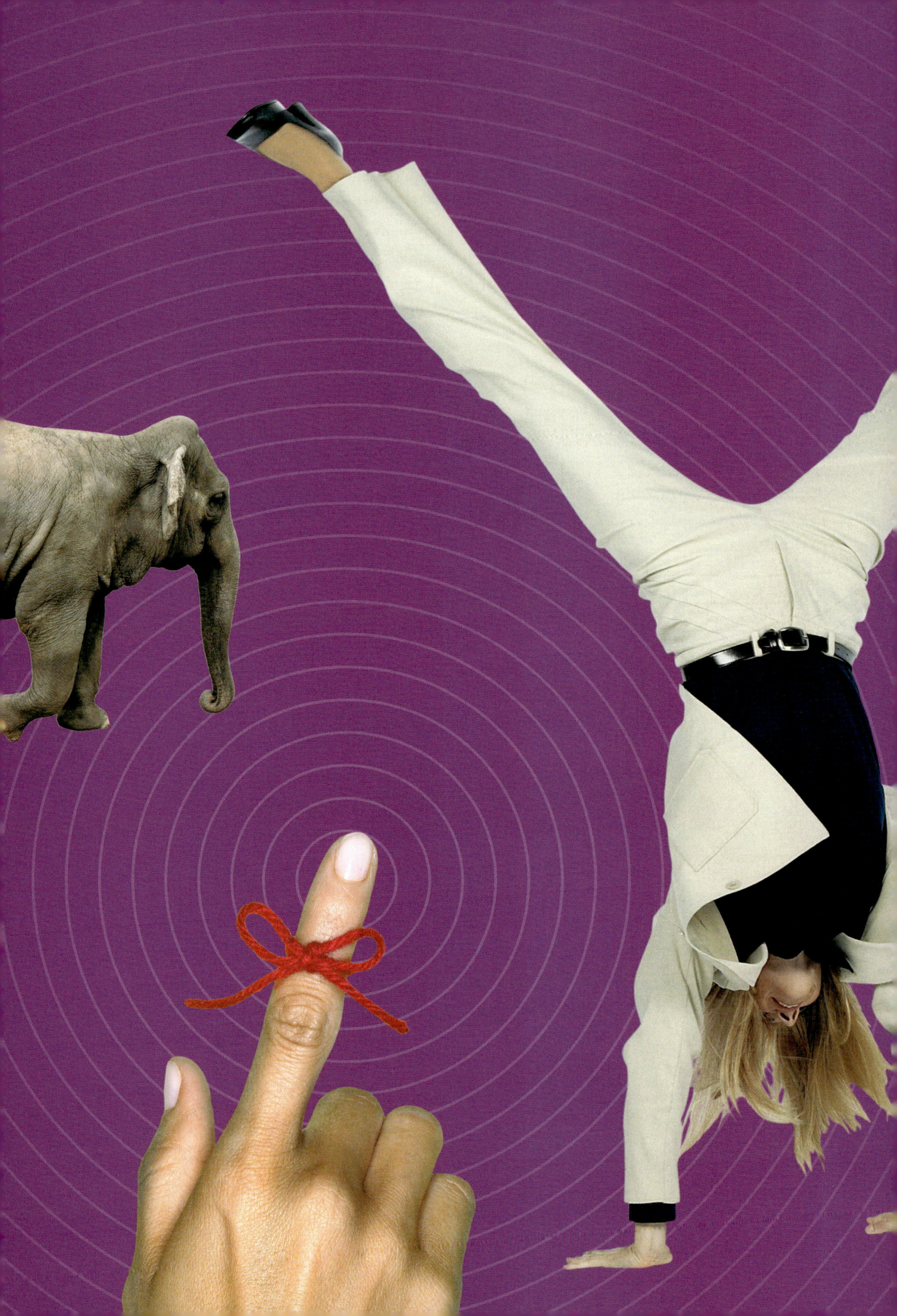

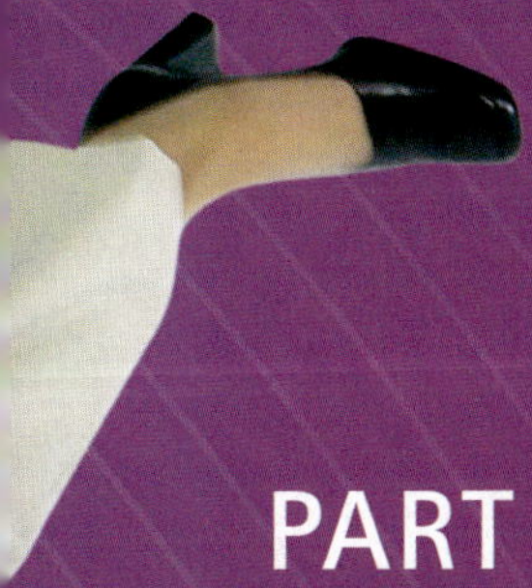

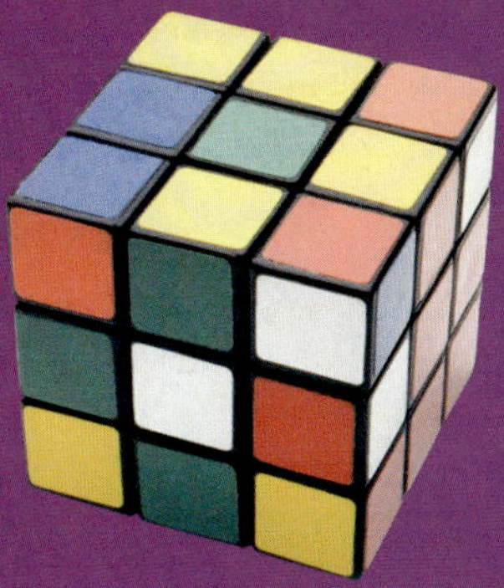

PART FOUR

your brain fitness program

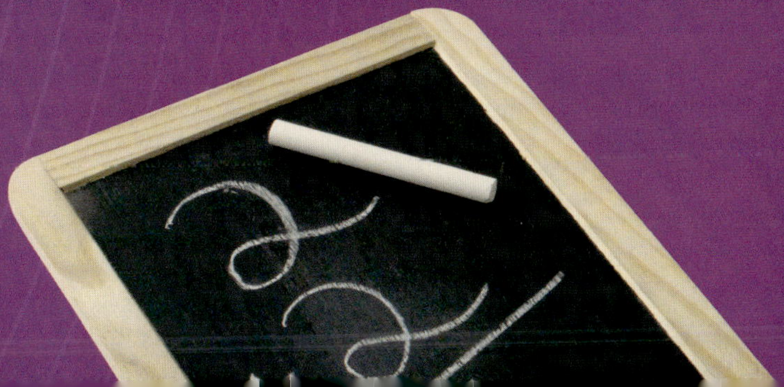

INCREASE YOUR Brain power IN MINUTES A DAY

The big brain breakthrough of the past decade is proof of plasticity—confirmation that the brain is in a constant state of change and adaptation. By challenging the brain, we can actually encourage it to grow new brain cells and form new connections between those cells for faster, more-efficient, more-effective thinking.

In retrospect, it seems odd that the medical community would be so surprised by this discovery. Every other part of the body changes, including the bones, which seem rock solid but are constantly breaking themselves down and building themselves back up. The more we tax our bones with weight-bearing exercise, the stronger they are forced to grow. Likewise, the more we challenge our brains, the stronger they will become.

That's why we created this brain fitness program. The exercises are designed to improve your skill in six main areas of cognitive function: attention and focus, memory, processing speed, verbal skills, number skills, and reasoning. If you apply yourself to these and similar exercises for at least 20 minutes a day, you should start to see improvements in your memory almost immediately. The growth of new neurons will take a few weeks, but you should feel more alert and "with it" almost instantly once you give your brain a jolt of stimulation.

THE PROOF

You know that scientists are pretty darned sure that staying mentally active can help boost brain power when the prestigious *New England Journal of Medicine* prints an article with the title "Use It or Lose It." That article appeared in 2003 after a 5-year study by researchers at Albert Einstein College of Medicine of Yeshiva University in the Bronx showed that leisure activities—including reading, playing board games, playing a musical instrument, and dancing—could reduce the risk of developing dementia by more than half.

That's an amazing benefit of doing such fun activities. Of course, it makes sense; if the brain is always looking for challenges and reasons to grow, then everything we do short of staring off into space should have some positive effect. The next big question was whether specific brain training would also reduce dementia. The answer turned out to be "yes."

In 2006, the *Journal of the American Medical Association* published results of the study known as ACTIVE—Advanced

Cognitive Training for Independent and Vital Elderly. People over age 65 received lessons in ways to improve memory, reasoning, and processing speed, and then were evaluated immediately and 5 years later. The researchers found that after 10 short sessions, people who received the training did better in those areas than those who were not trained. Astoundingly, trainees maintained their superior skills when they were retested 5 years later. Imagine taking a shower every day for 10 days and still being clean a year later!

What all this research tells us is that, yes, we absolutely can reduce brain drain and combat some of the less-welcome biological realties that occur with age, such as slower processing of new information and a slightly smaller capacity for storing short-term memory. Spend some time in this "brain gym" and you just might remember the name of the next acquaintance you meet, and maybe their phone number and birthday, too! And, with a few helpful tricks you'll discover here, you'll find yourself losing your car keys, struggling for words on the tip of your tongue, and forgetting appointments less often.

BEFORE YOU BEGIN

Do you remember the quiz you took at the beginning of the book? (We certainly hope so!) It tapped into six main facets of cognitive ability. Your scores in these six areas can point you in the direction of your greatest areas of cognitive weakness. Go back and look at your quiz answers, then see "Where Am I Weakest?" below to learn which of the six areas you should focus on the most.

It is important to remember that these exercises should be the beginning of your brain training, not the end. This is your cognitive kindergarten. Your advanced studies need to take place out in the world. Opportunities to use and expand your brain power are all around you; you just need to reach out and take them.

Where Am I Weakest?

In the quiz you took on pages 8–10, the questions addressed six areas of cognitive function. The more True answers you had in a particular category, the more help you need in that area. Pay special attention to the pages indicated.

COGNITIVE FUNCTION	QUIZ QUESTIONS	PAGE NUMBERS
Attention and Focus	4, 11, 15, 16	200-215
Memory	1, 5, 6, 8, 13, 14, 26, 28, 29, plus the 3 words you were asked to remember	216-233
Processing Speed	7, 17	234-241
Verbal Skills	2, 3, 30	242-247
Number Skills	9, 10, 18, 27	248-255
Reasoning Skills	19, 31, 32, 33, 34	256-263
Lifestyle/Health Issues	12, 20, 21, 22, 23, 24, 25	Stress: 142 ; Drugs: 98; Medical Causes: 174; Exercise: 86; Diet: 64

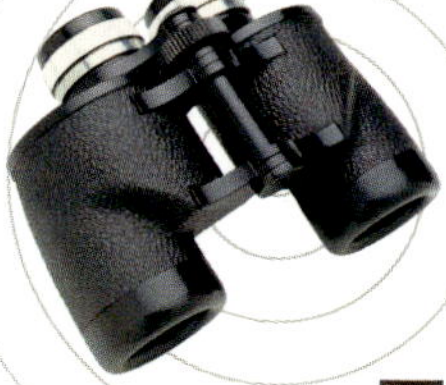

Improve your attention and focus

When was the last time you really lost yourself in a good book or became so enthralled with a project that hours flew by like minutes? It happens all the time in childhood, but as you get older, your ability to focus intensely goes the way of your ability to turn cartwheels. No one knows exactly why this happens, but one of the most popular theories is that younger people have a system of inhibition that keeps irrelevant and extraneous information from interfering with attention.

Think of this system as mulch in a garden to keep down the weeds. A kid in high school has "mulch" so thick that he can do math homework with music blaring and occasionally stop to answer a text message. With age, though, the "mulch" thins, allowing more and more distractions to creep in. When too many get through, they can affect how well we learn and remember, as well as how we perform certain tasks. Let's say you're driving along and spot a bit of garbage on the side of the road, which makes you think about whether you remembered to take the trash bag out of the kitchen, which reminds you that you need to pick up onions for dinner, which leads to thoughts of crying and eyes and the fact that you have an appointment with the optometrist next week. All of a sudden, your focus switches back to the road and you see that you've driven miles without realizing it, and maybe even missed your exit.

ATTENTION, PLEASE!

No one can pay attention to everything. Information blasts into your senses constantly. Every color, object, sound, taste, odor, or physical sensation is taken into the brain and processed. Most of these inputs are ignored, as they should be—it would be exhausting to be hypervigilant to every piece of information at every moment, and there's no real need to remember whether the bird that just flew by the window was brown, red, or blue. Instead, you choose which bits of information to pay attention to, like the e-mail you were reading when the bird flew by. It's that information that you hold in your short-term memory.

Unfortunately, as you get older, you have less working memory (also called short-term memory); unless you pay close attention, the information just doesn't stick as well as it used to. That's one reason an older person may have trouble moving back and forth between one task and another. Let's say you're trying to read alternately from two chapters in a book. When you switch chapters, you may lose your place in the previous chapter and struggle to get reoriented, while a younger person with greater working memory would have less difficulty.

A kissing cousin to attention is focus. If you think of attention as turning on a light in a dark room, focus is turning a laser beam on a specific object in the room. Focus is that intense level of attention you bring when you feel as though you are burning memories into your brain. You lose some of that ability as you age, too. The small details simply vanish. If you read a passage in a book, you might remember the gist of it, but a younger person will be more likely to be able to recall exact sentences. You don't lose your ability to focus entirely; it's just that it takes more energy and interest. What you gain is the ability to absorb a broader, bigger-picture view of the world—a sum of the parts. Younger people tend to see the parts, but might miss how the parts fit into the big picture.

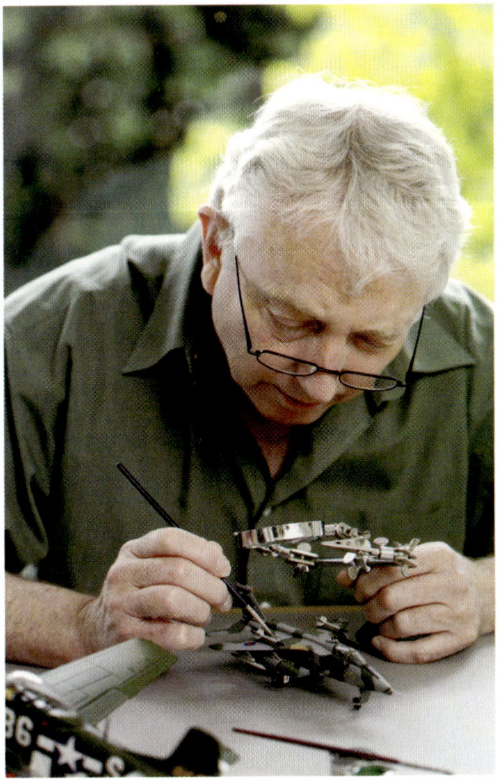

The tips and exercises in this chapter are designed to help you improve both your attention and focus, so you can make it through *War and Peace* if you choose to, or at least a newspaper feature article. Who knows, maybe you'll even be able to sit down and figure out how to program your VCR once you're done here!

Smart Everyday Strategies

All of us get distracted and lose our focus now and then. If it happens to you a lot, get in the habit of using these strategies to help compensate.

Take notes. Writing forces you to pay attention and also helps move the information from short-term memory into long-term memory. And, of course, it provides a solid record if you need it later on.

Carry a pocket-size recorder. For years, patient advocates have been advising people to take a small cassette or digital recorder when they see a doctor. When people are nervous or under stress, they may not accurately or fully remember what was said in an office visit. The same strategy can help in everyday life. If you carry a recorder, you can use a voice-activation feature to capture important conversations or even personal memos to yourself. You can then review the recording anytime you want.

Invest in a pair of noise-reducing headphones. Unlike earplugs, these gadgets reduce or eliminate ambient sound while slightly muffling distinct sounds. For example, if you wear them in the office, you'll eliminate the hum of machinery and background chatter, while allowing you to hear someone speaking to you or the sound of a telephone ringing.

Control sensory distractions. Take charge of the controllable distractions around you by turning off the music, television, and radio. If you are cold, put on a sweater. If you are hungry, eat. If the air feels stagnant, open a window. The more comfortable you are, the better you'll be able to focus.

Find a quiet corner. If you don't have total noise control, take yourself to another location. Libraries are often quiet, or at least quieter than a busy home.

Boost concentration with caffeine. Researchers from the University of Arizona in Tucson discovered that people over age 65 who felt that their attention was highest in the morning (as opposed to "night owls" who concentrate best late at night) could improve their focus by drinking 12 ounces of regular coffee. Decaffeinated coffee didn't work. And this trick only works if you are already a coffee-drinker. If not, the side effects of caffeine—that jittery buzz—will only disrupt your attention.

exercises

These exercises challenge your attention and focus, training your brain to really pay attention. Regardless of how well you do or how quickly you complete each exercise, you win! Your prize is no more brain drain.

DETAILS, DETAILS

For this exercise, you'll need a pen or pencil.

Below, you'll find a series of short essays. Read them carefully, trying to remember as much detail as possible. Then, without looking back at the essay, answer the questions on the next page. You'll probably notice that it's easier to retain details when reading about topics with which you're already somewhat familiar. The same is true in real life.

Details, Details #1

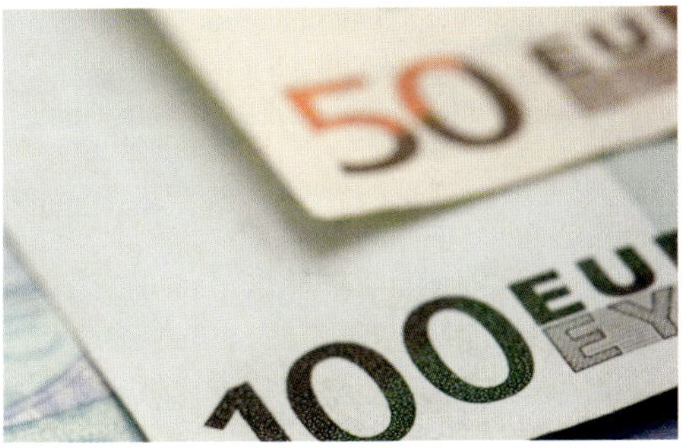

The Euro is the official currency of most of the member nations of the European Union. The nations that use the Euro exclusively form what's known as the Eurozone. Euro coins and banknotes entered circulation on January 1, 2002, as the national currency of 11 countries: Austria, Belgium, Finland, France, Germany, Ireland, Italy, Luxembourg, the Netherlands, Portugal, and Spain. The Euro is managed and administered by the Frankfurt-based European Central Bank. The inspiration for the distinctive € symbol was the Greek letter Epsilon, a reference to the cradle of European civilization.

The Euro is divided into 100 cents. Euro coins come in eight different denominations, ranging from 1 cent to 2 Euros, although by Finnish law, cash transactions are rounded to the nearest 5 cents, so that 1-cent and 2-cent coins aren't needed. There are seven Euro banknote denominations, from 5 through 500 (€5, €10, €20, €50, €100, €200, and €500). Each denomination has its own size and color, in part to assist visually impaired people in recognizing them.

Questions

1. What is term for the group of European nations that uses the Euro? ______________________

2. In what year did the Euro enter circulation? ______________________

3. What was the first nation not on the European mainland to adopt the Euro? ______________________

4. How many different Euro banknote denominations are there? ______________________

5. What nation doesn't use the two smallest Euro coin denominations? ______________________

Check your answers by rereading the essay.

Details, Details #2

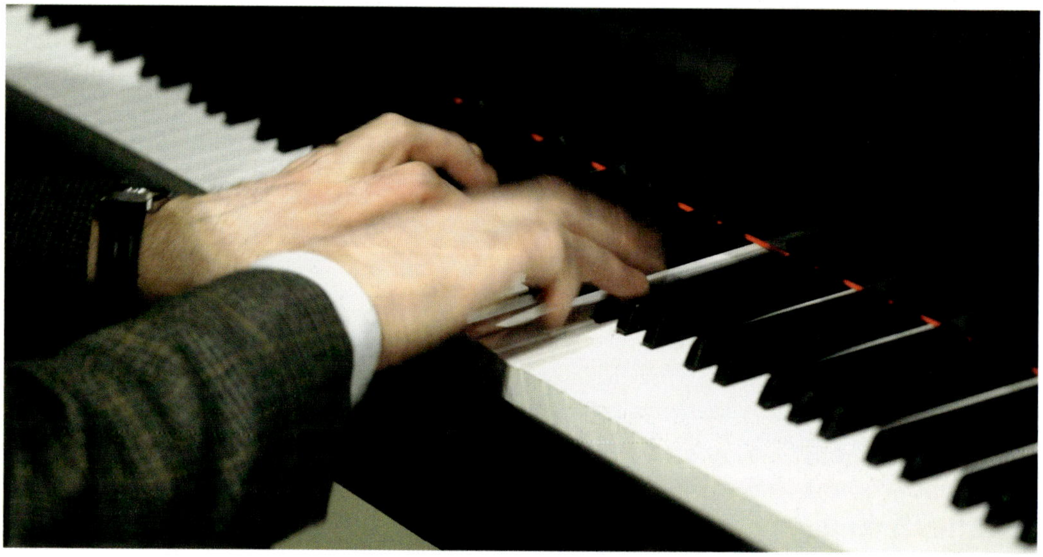

Many people who enjoy solving crosswords have wondered how crosswords are made. Those who have tried making a puzzle of their own, perhaps for a friend's birthday, were probably surprised at how difficult it was. They likely discovered that solving crosswords and making them are two very different talents, each requiring its own set of skills. Sure, there's some overlap. You'll need a good vocabulary and a wide-ranging base of general knowledge to do both successfully. But the skill intersection pretty much ends there.

Consider this analogy from the world of music. Playing the piano is very different from composing a symphony. There are, of course, people noted for excelling at both composition and performance—Leonard Bernstein, George Gershwin, and Franz Liszt come to mind.

It's safe to say that solving crosswords is much easier than making them. About 50 million Americans do crosswords regularly, but fewer than 1,000 Americans are known to create crosswords for a living or as a professional hobby. And just in case you've ever wondered whether puzzle-writers create the clues or the word diagram first, here's a hint: Try to make your own 3-by-3 crossword by writing the clues first, and you'll quickly see the answer for yourself.

Questions

1. Who is the non-American composer mentioned? ____________________

2. About how many million Americans do crosswords regularly: 30 million, 40 million, or 50 million? ____________________

3. The two skills required both to solve and make crosswords are a wide-ranging base of general knowledge and what else?

____

4. What celebratory occasion is mentioned in the passage? ____________________

5. As implied by the passage, do crossword-writers create the clues or the word diagram first? ____________________

Check your answers by rereading the essay.

Details, Details #3

Do soufflés get a bum rap? They've been the butt of jokes for ages, especially in cartoons and kids' programs, where only a tiny poke or a loud noise will make them collapse.

Well, those shows stretch the truth, but only a little. *Soufflé* actually means "to blow up" in French—in the "inflate" sense, not the "explode" sense. Whether prepared as a savory main dish or a sweet dessert, every soufflé is made from two basic components: a base made from custard or flavored cream sauce and egg whites that are beaten into a soft meringue. The base provides the flavor, while the egg whites provide the lift. Soufflés are traditionally served in flat-bottomed, round porcelain containers called ramekins.

If prepared correctly, your soufflé will be puffed up and fluffy when you take it out of the oven. But be sure to serve it quickly—they generally fall within 5 to 10 minutes.

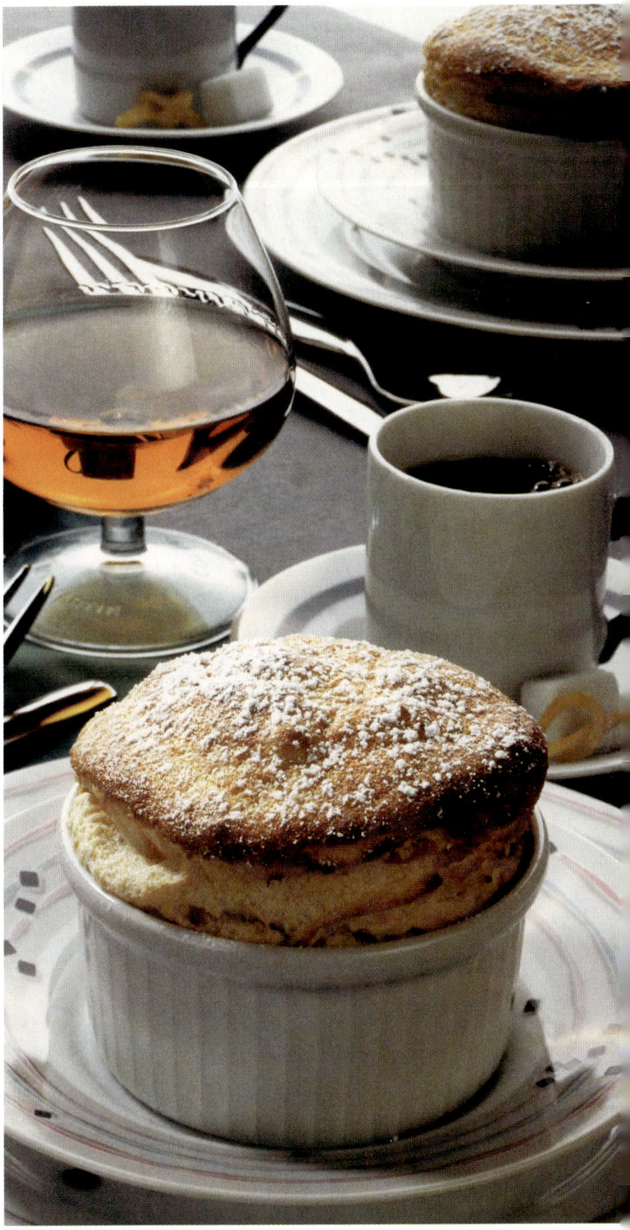

Questions

1. What does "soufflé" mean in French?

____

2. What ingredient provides the lift in a soufflé? ______________________

3. What are soufflé containers called?

____

4. What form do the egg whites take when beaten? ______________________

5. How soon after being taken out of the oven will soufflés generally fall?

____

Check your answers by rereading the essay.

STACK TRACKING

For this exercise you'll need:

- **A pen or pencil**
- **A watch or clock with a second hand**

Below you'll see a grid containing geometric shapes with the names of the shapes underneath. Your goal is to assure that the shapes and names match, so that each shape has a correct name in the corresponding position on the grid. If you run across a mistake, circle the incorrect word and continue on.

For example:

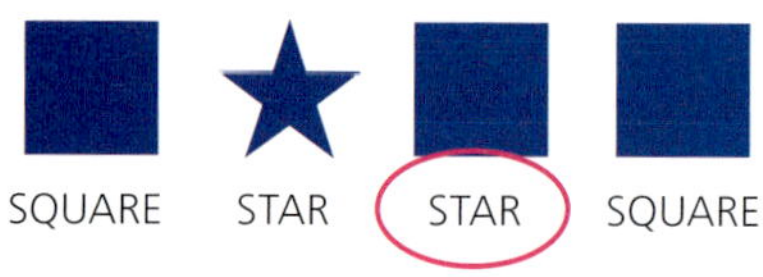

Third word ("star") should be circled.

These exercises will be scored for accuracy. But time is also important, so work as quickly as possible. When you have completed each page, write down the amount of time you needed to finish in the space provided at the bottom. Score the exercise before moving on to the next one. When you are ready, set the timer and begin!

Stack Tracking #1

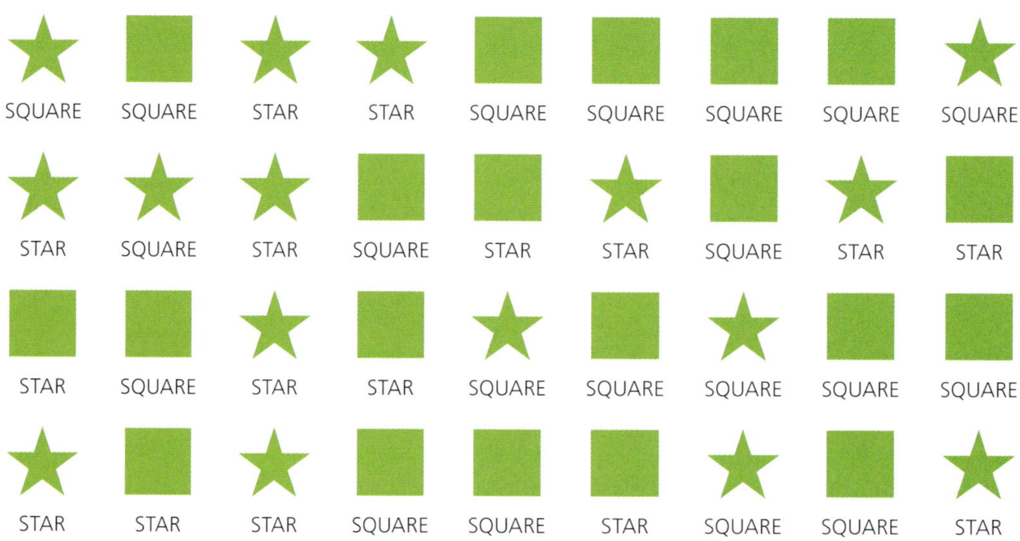

TIME ____________ ITEMS CIRCLED INCORRECTLY __________ MISSED MISTAKES __________

Answer on page 264

Stack Tracking #2

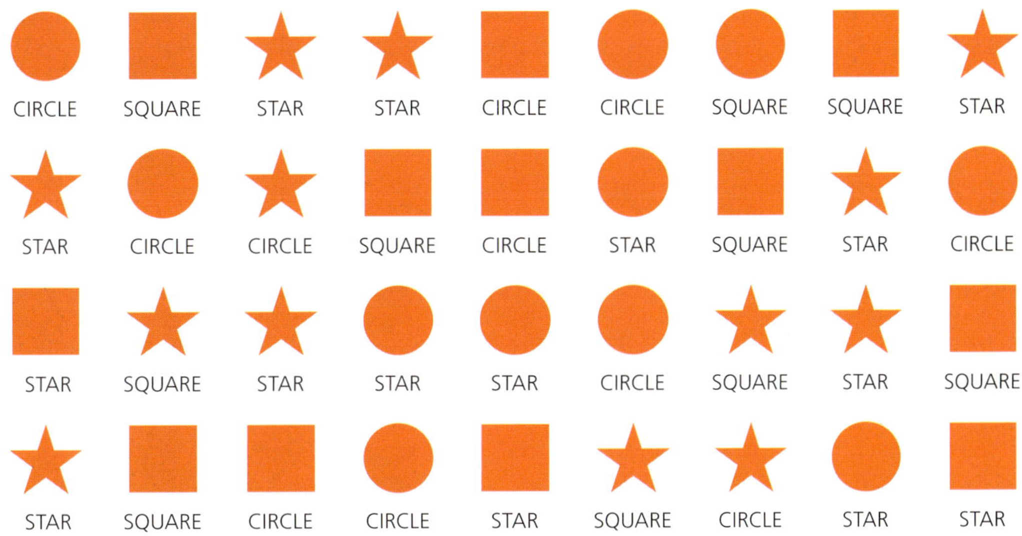

TIME ____________ ITEMS CIRCLED INCORRECTLY ____________ MISSED MISTAKES ____________

Stack Tracking #3

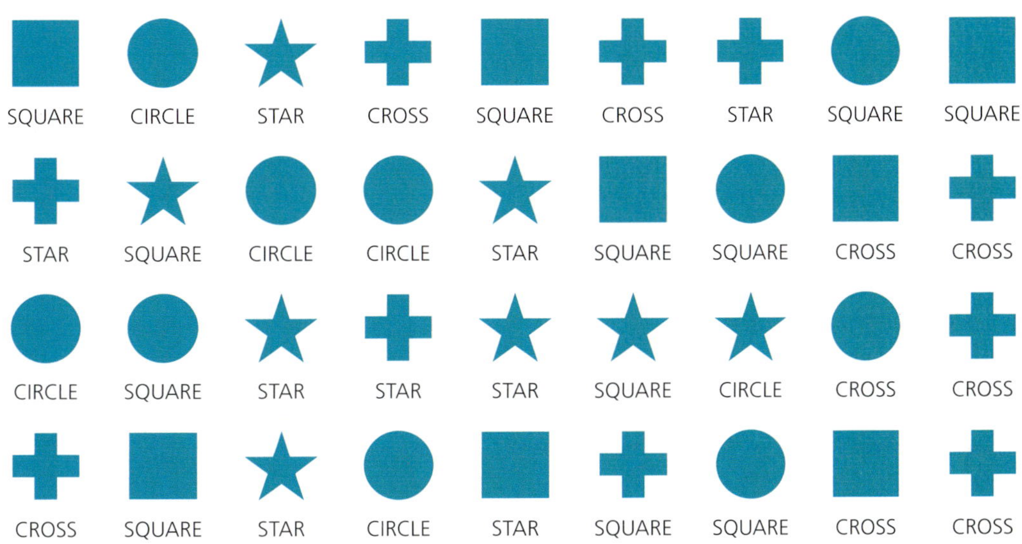

TIME ____________ ITEMS CIRCLED INCORRECTLY ____________ MISSED MISTAKES ____________

Answers on page 264

Stack Tracking #4

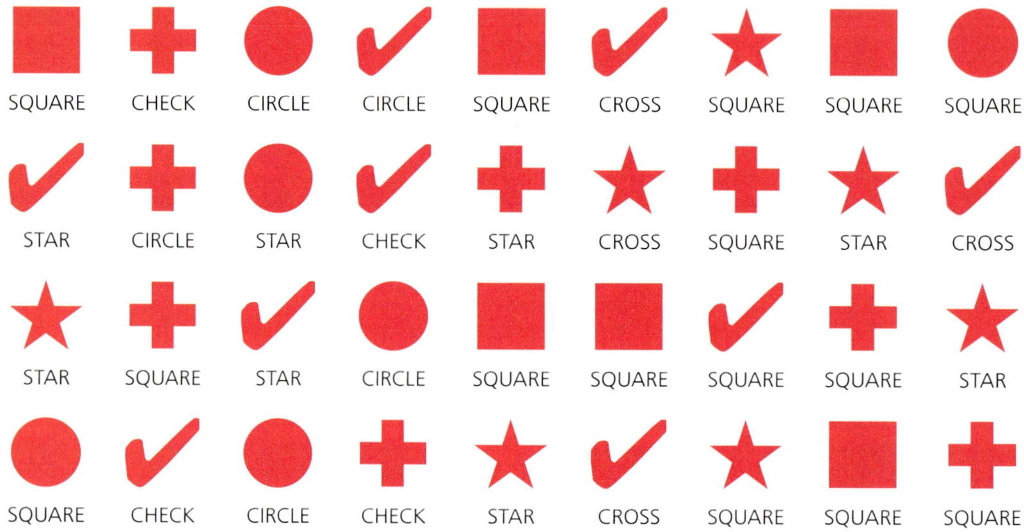

TIME ____________ ITEMS CIRCLED INCORRECTLY __________ MISSED MISTAKES __________

Stack Tracking #5

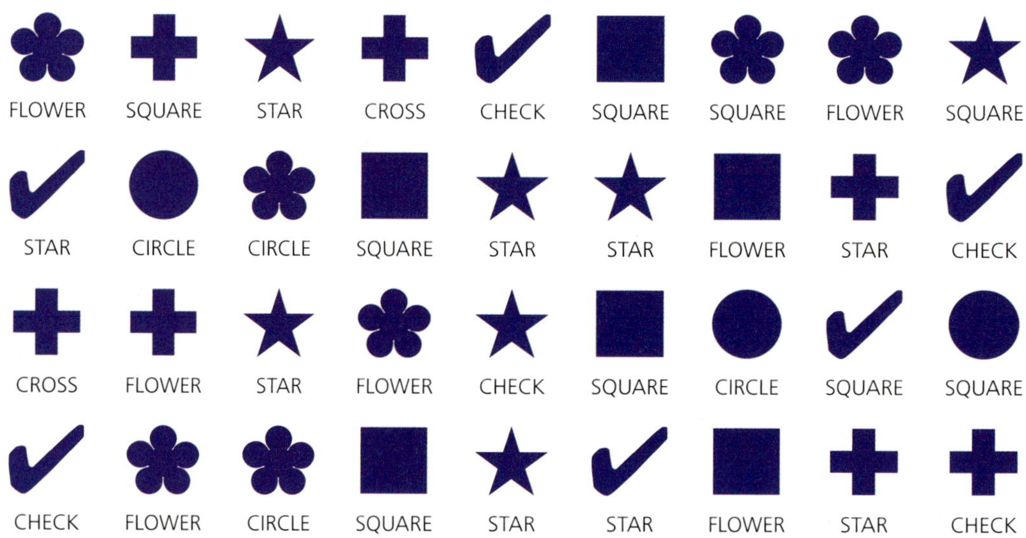

TIME ____________ ITEMS CIRCLED INCORRECTLY __________ MISSED MISTAKES __________

Answers on page 264

ONE AMONG MANY

For this exercise, you'll need a pen or pencil.

Below, you'll see what looks like several identical items. Only one item in the bunch is different from the others. Find and circle that item. This is not a timed exercise.

One Among Many #1

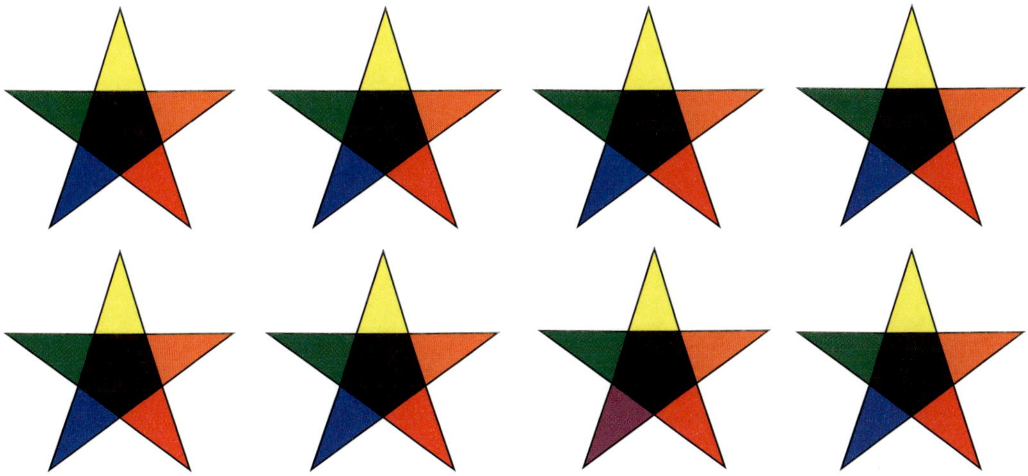

One Among Many #2

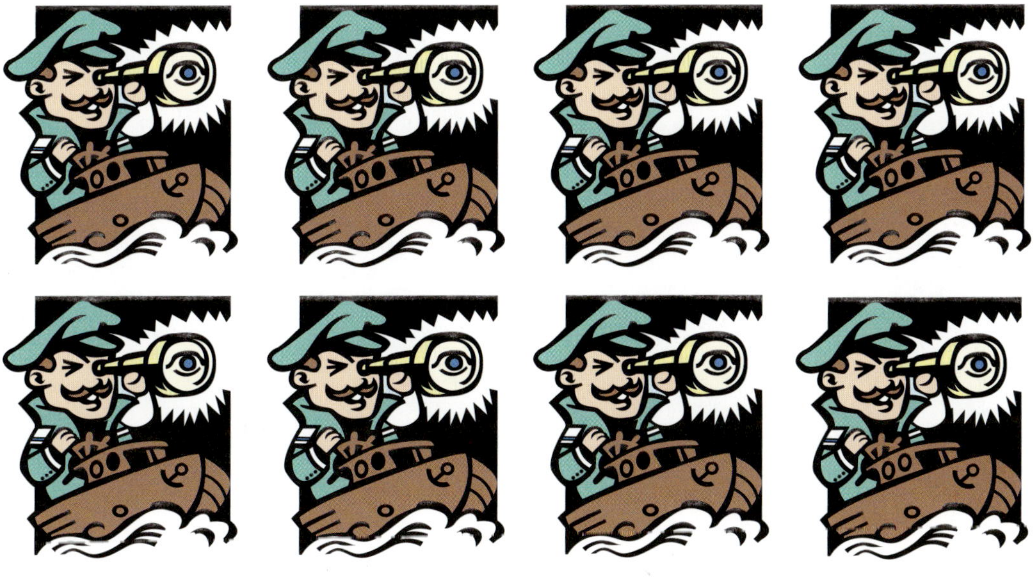

Answers on page 264

One Among Many #3

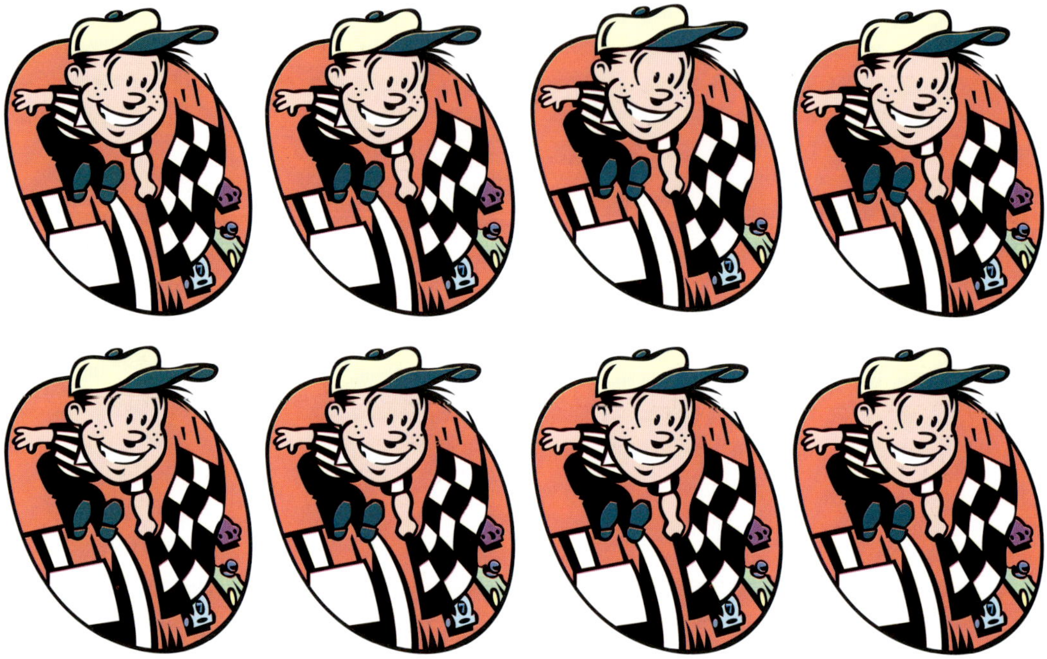

One Among Many #4

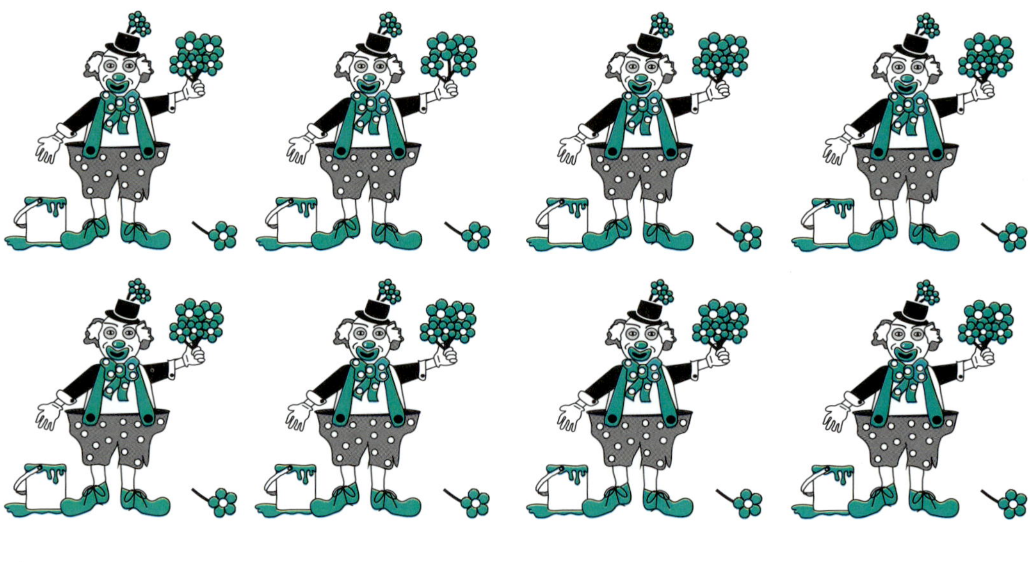

Answers on page 264

One Among Many #5

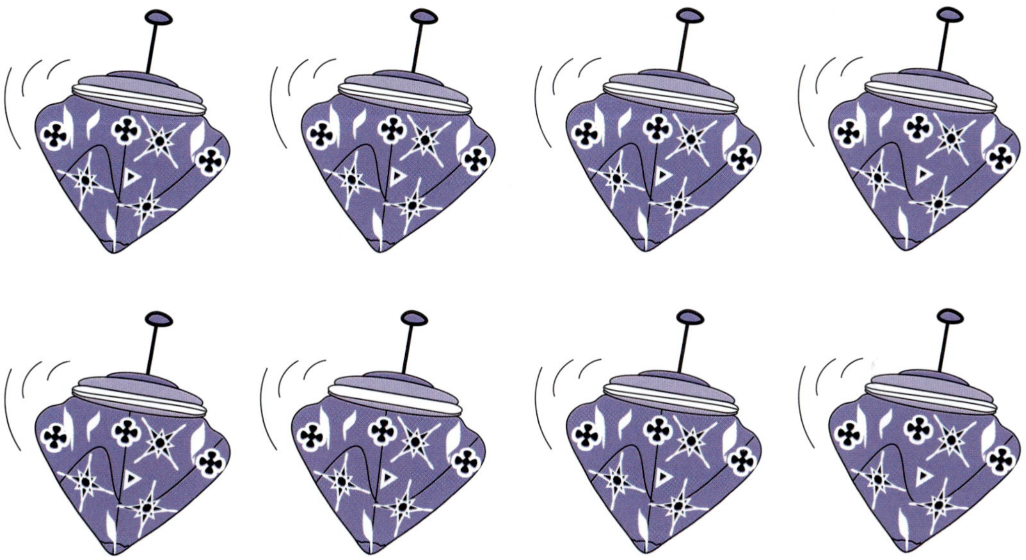

One Among Many #6

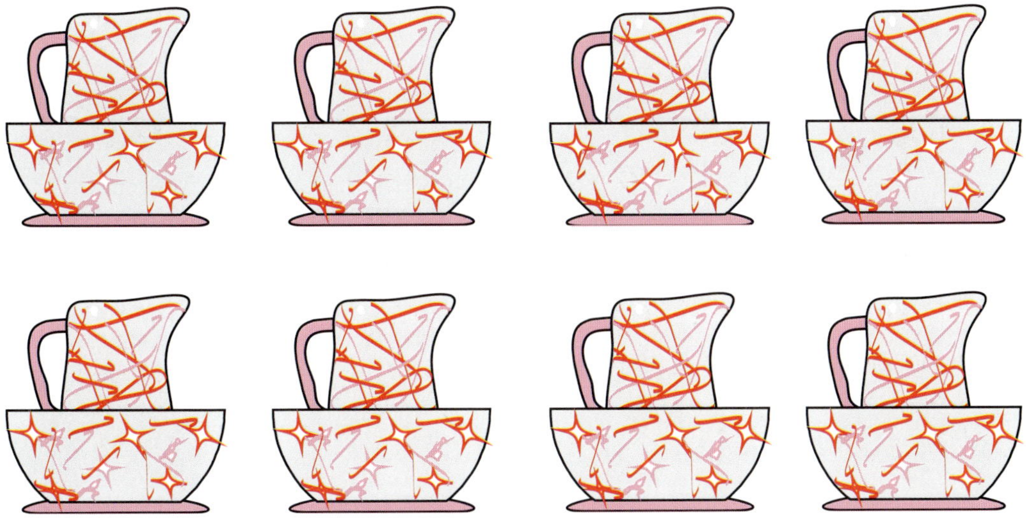

Answers on page 265

PICTURE IMPERFECT

For this exercise, you'll need a pen or pencil.

The images below are nearly identical, but not quite. Find the noted number of differences and circle them. This is not a timed exercise.

Picture Imperfect #1

Can you spot the three differences?

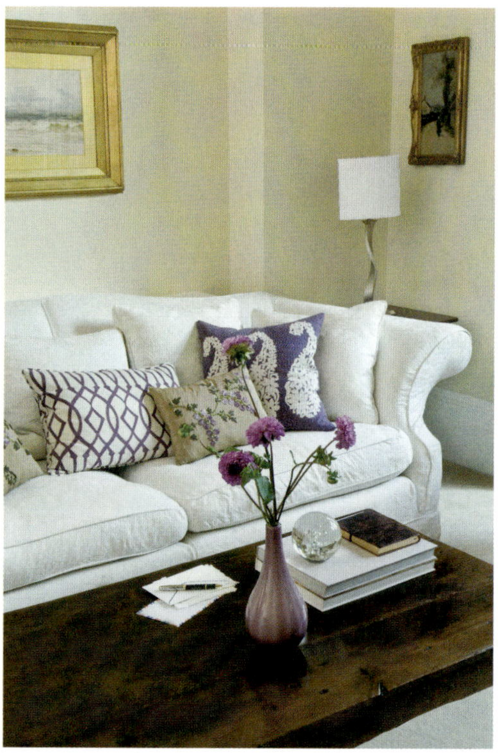

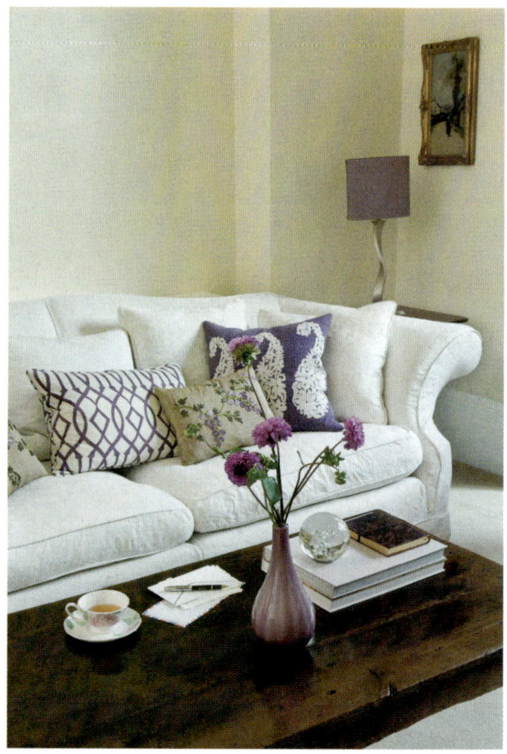

Answers on page 265

Picture Imperfect #2

Can you spot the four differences?

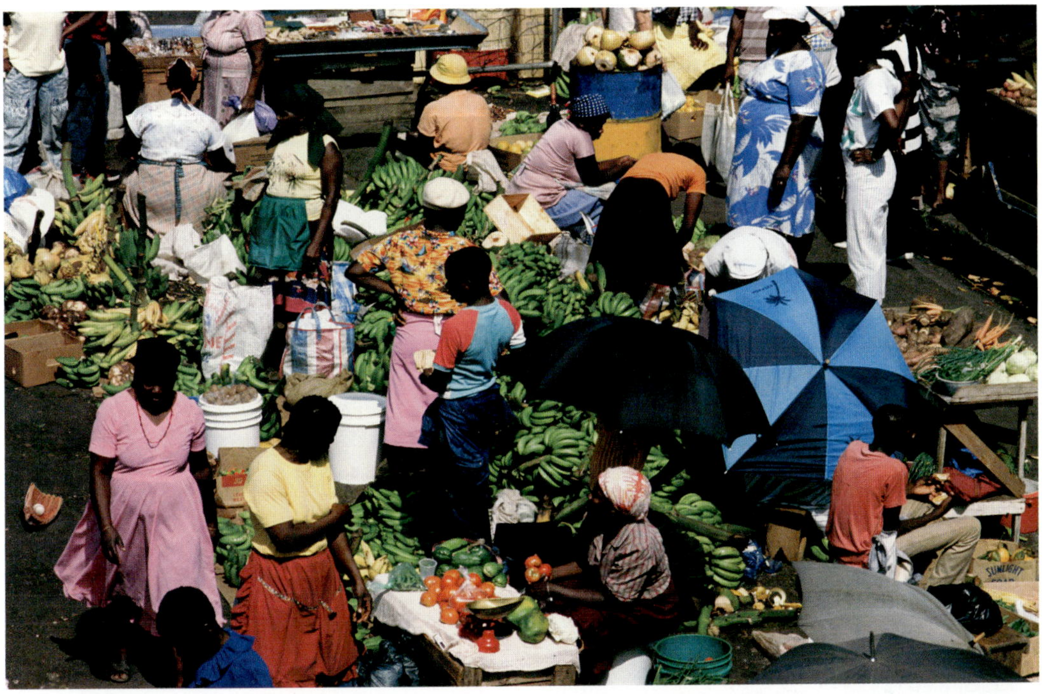

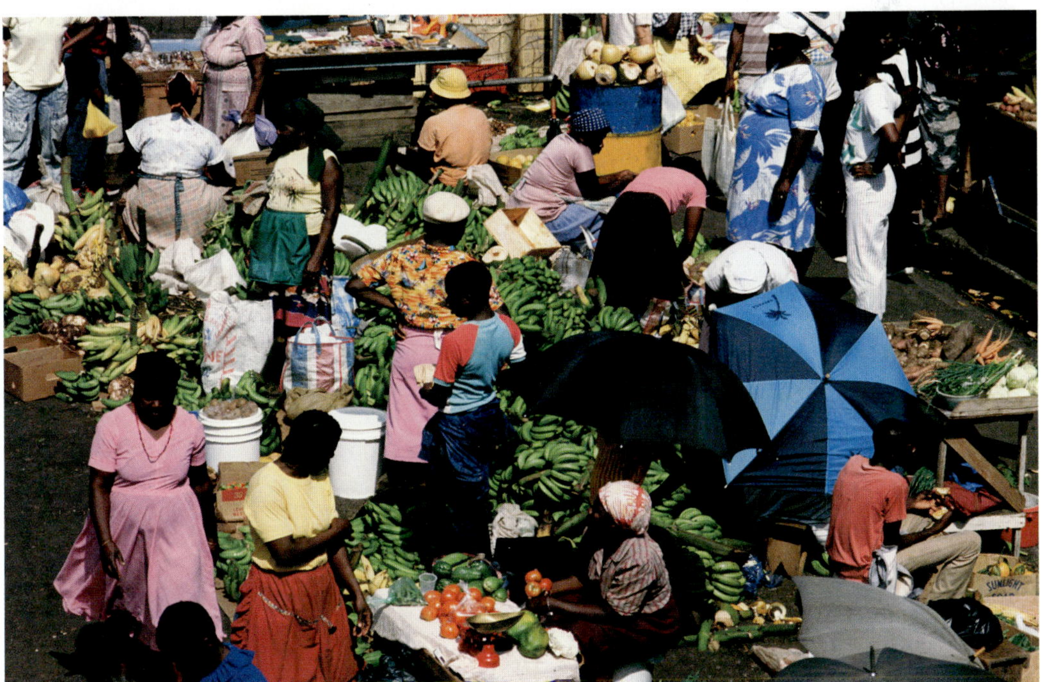

Answers on page 265

Picture Imperfect #3

Can you spot the five differences?

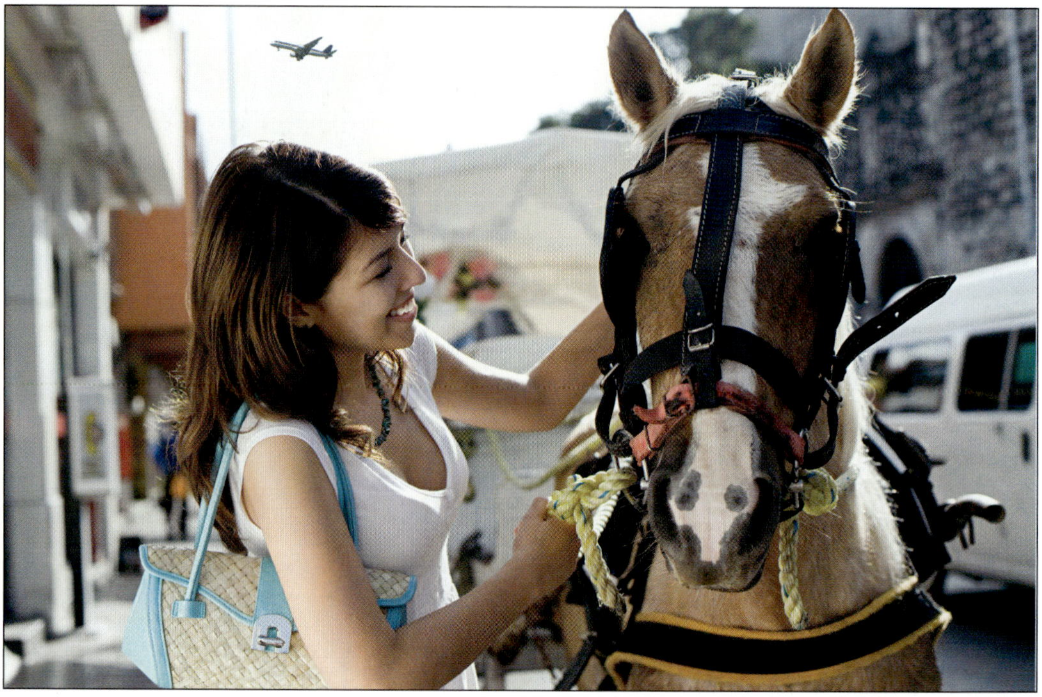

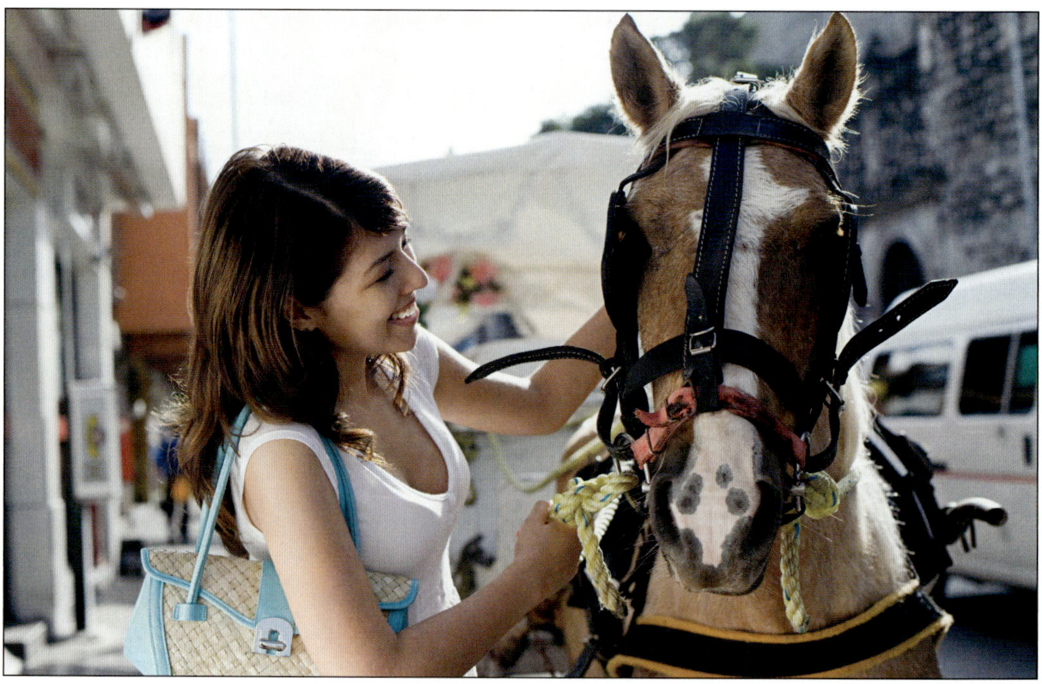

Answers on page 265

Picture Imperfect #4

Can you spot the six differences?

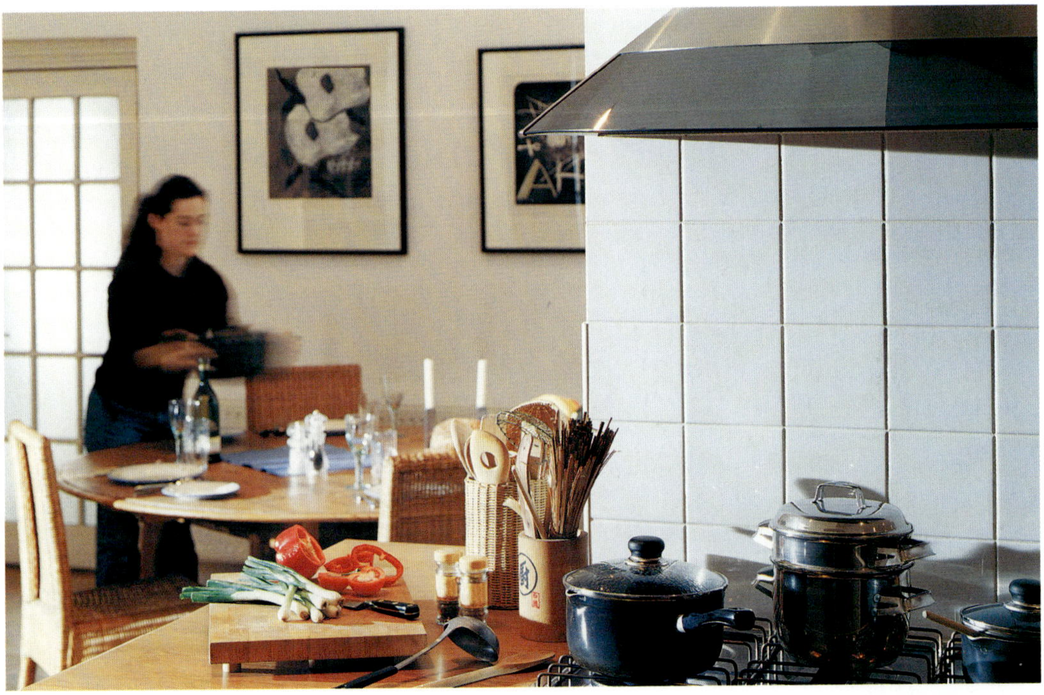

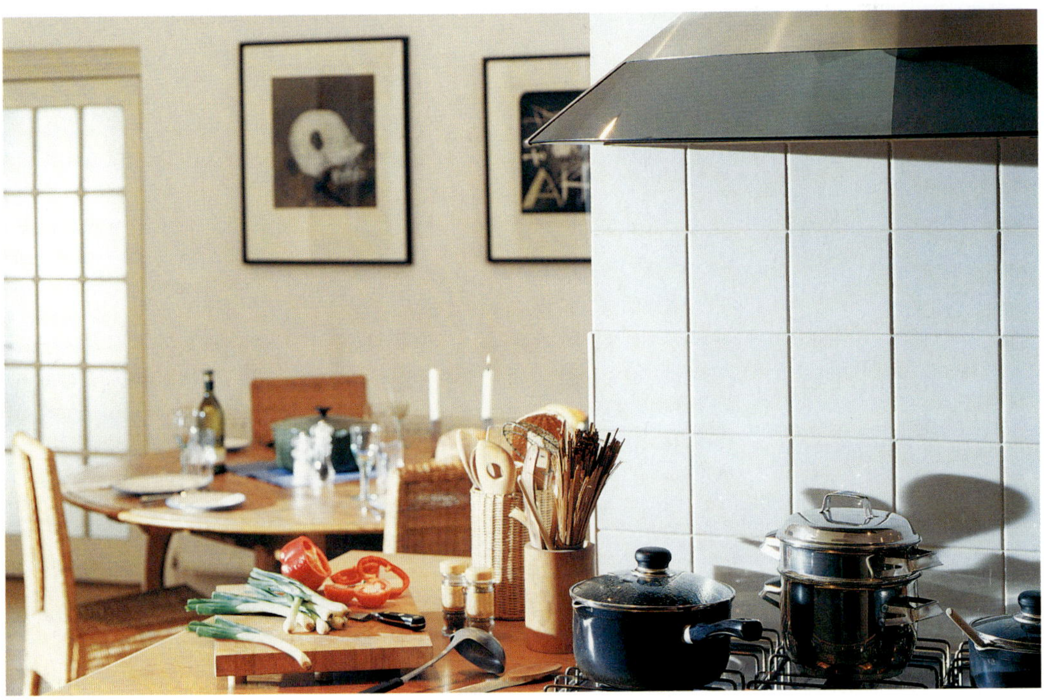

Answers on page 265

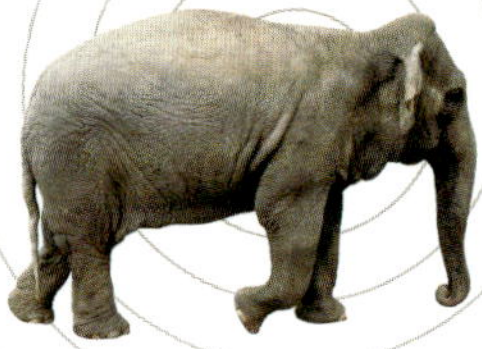

Improve your memory

When people talk about their memories getting bad, they usually mean those aspects of memory that allow them to function in the world—remembering appointments, the location of car keys, items on a to-do list, work deadlines, even basic facts. We can run into real trouble when our memory lets us down, especially when it comes to "remembering" future events. One woman who forgot to send in the payment for her health insurance was dropped from the plan. That slip cost her thousands of dollars in uncovered medical bills. Fortunately, most memory slips are more benign.

KEEPING TRACK

Keys, sunglasses, cell phone, car in a parking lot—if you haven't "lost" one of these items in the past month, then you're doing great in the memory department. Misplacing objects is normal at any age, especially when you're under stress. You lose track of items because the brain is so darned efficient. When you perform routine tasks, it lets the body go on automatic pilot. Let's say that every day, you come home and throw the keys in the same general location. But if something interrupts you—perhaps the phone is ringing as you open the door—then your brain is preoccupied with the new task. Your automatic pilot disengages, you drop the keys somewhere new, and you later have to search to find them.

RECALLING THE PAST

The ability to pull up memories of past events declines with age. Recognition remains strong, but recall weakens. This is a fine but important distinction. Recall is the ability to pull up a memory simply by thinking about it. Recognition is the ability to remember once prompted with a cue. For example, if you were asked to name all the places to which you have ever traveled, your list would probably be incomplete. But if you were asked if you had ever been to Egypt, you could definitively answer yes or no.

If you want to remember on your own, you need to provide your own cues. That's one reason people purchase souvenirs—to remind them of the details of a trip. For everyday purposes, we can use our imaginations instead.

"REMEMBERING" THE FUTURE

The most bothersome of all memory problems involves *prospective memory*—remembering something that is yet to happen, such as an appointment or an anniversary. When this type of memory fails, we may forget to take medication, stop at the store for milk, or return a DVD on time. Mark McDaniel, PhD, of Washington University in St. Louis, a leading expert on prospective memory, calls this remembering to remember.

As far as the brain is concerned, this is much more difficult to pull off than other types of remembering. Thank the gap in time between intending to do something and actually doing it. And you can't look at a postcard to "remind" you of something that hasn't happened yet. You can, however, write yourself a Post-It note!

Though everyone has prospective memory failures, some research has shown that these types of slips tend to become more common as we get older. But age isn't the only determining factor. Stress, lack of sleep, and side effects from medication all have been shown to influence the forgetfulness factor.

Smart Everyday Strategies

Let's face it: No one's memory is perfect. And yours doesn't have to be, either. It's easy enough never to lose the car keys again or forget another appointment simply by using some commonsense strategies. Save your brain power for other things!

Establish routines. This plan may not appeal to the spontaneous bohemian in you, but admit it: It's easier to find things if you always put them in the same place. Stick a magnetic hook on the fridge for the car keys and create a special drawer or folder for unpaid bills, for instance. As a last resort, put a catchall bin in the rooms you use the most, and use them as a multipurpose home base for those things you tend to misplace.

Say it out loud. If you must put an item in an unfamiliar place, say what you are doing out loud, as in, "I am putting my sunglasses on the table by the door." All sensory channels create their own neural links to the information. By letting your ears register the information, you increase your chances of remembering it later.

Take advantage of Post-It notes. Those sticky notes have saved careers and kept families from doing all-out battle.

Keep a pad of them in every room and stick a reminder where you are likely to see it. Afraid of forgetting a book on your way to work? Stick the note to your car window or inside your front door. Worried that you will forget to call a friend? Put one note on the phone and another in a spot that you are likely to notice during the day, such as on the television or on your computer keyboard.

Let technology remember for you. Cell phones, Blackberries and other PDAs, and other devices have calendars you can program to remind you of what you need to do during the day. Some computer softwares have a "notes" function that lets you create a note on one computer and send it to your cell phone or other device. Once you learn how to use these systems, you'll wonder how you ever got along without them. And yes, you can learn to use them. Researchers have taught people with significant memory problems—those with brain injuries and mild to moderate Alzheimer's disease—to use these devices successfully. Just make sure you keep a back-up, such as a wall calendar, day planner, or external hard drive.

Use checklists. People make lists for a reason: They work. Check off each to-do as you complete it. Bonus: If your list has several items, you're likely to refer to the it again and again, each time reinforcing your memory of the tasks there.

Plant a visual reminder. If you need to remember to bring your umbrella, hang it on the door handle. Some people have found success with old-fashioned reminders, such as a piece of string tied around a finger or moving a ring from one hand to the other. Just seeing those items can remind you that you have something to remember, and that may be enough.

Visual reminders can even help you accomplish your goals. For example, if you decide you want to begin a healthy diet tomorrow, put the oatmeal on the counter the night before.

Use imaginary cues. There are times when planting a visual clue is impossible. If you go to a museum and have to check your umbrella, how can you remember to get it again before you leave? By using your imagination. Dr. McDaniel suggests this tip: When you first realize that you will need to use prospective memory, look for physical landmarks to trigger your memory. Doors are a great example, but it may also be a statue or other permanent fixture. Then, imagine your item and the landmark together. In the museum example, you can imagine an open umbrella blocking the doorway. In studies, these imaginary cues proved to be as effective as external cues. Note, however, that imaginary cues work best when you are in an unfamiliar location or situation and therefore less likely to go on autopilot.

Do it now, not later. Although this won't work in all situations, the best way to remember to do something is to do it while you're thinking about it. Instead of telling yourself to remember to make a phone call or pay a bill, why not do it immediately? Too often it's procrastination that makes us forget.

exercises

These exercises challenge your recall of old memories as well as your retention of new information.

YOU MUST REMEMBER THIS

For this exercise, you'll need a timer.

Set the timer for 5 minutes. Read one of the questions, then close your eyes and remember all the details you can. Try to think on all sensory fronts: sight, sound, smell, taste, and touch. Don't rush the process; take the full 5 minutes. After the timer goes off, open your eyes. Did you remember more than you thought you would?

1. How did you celebrate your 13th birthday?
2. How did you get to school in the 5th grade?
3. What do you remember about your best friend's wedding?
4. What do you remember about your most recent vacation?
5. Where and with whom was your first kiss?
6. What was the best birthday present you ever got?
7. What do you remember most about your grandparents?
8. How did you spend summers as a child?
9. Which dance steps or music groups were popular when you were in high school?
10. What do you remember about the first job you ever held?
11. What books did you read in the past year?
12. What movies did you see in the past year?
13. How did you and your friends spend your time after school when you were 10?
14. What was your first pet?
15. What was your most intimidating moment?
16. When did you get your first bicycle?
17. What was your favorite book as a kid?
18. Who was your favorite grade-school teacher?
19. What did the first house you lived in look like?
20. Who was your first crush?

PICTURE PERFECT

For this exercise, you'll need:

- **A pen or pencil**
- **A timer**

Set the timer for 2 minutes and study the picture below. After 2 minutes, turn the page. There you'll find a picture that is identical to this one except for a few details.

Picture Perfect #1 (Part A)

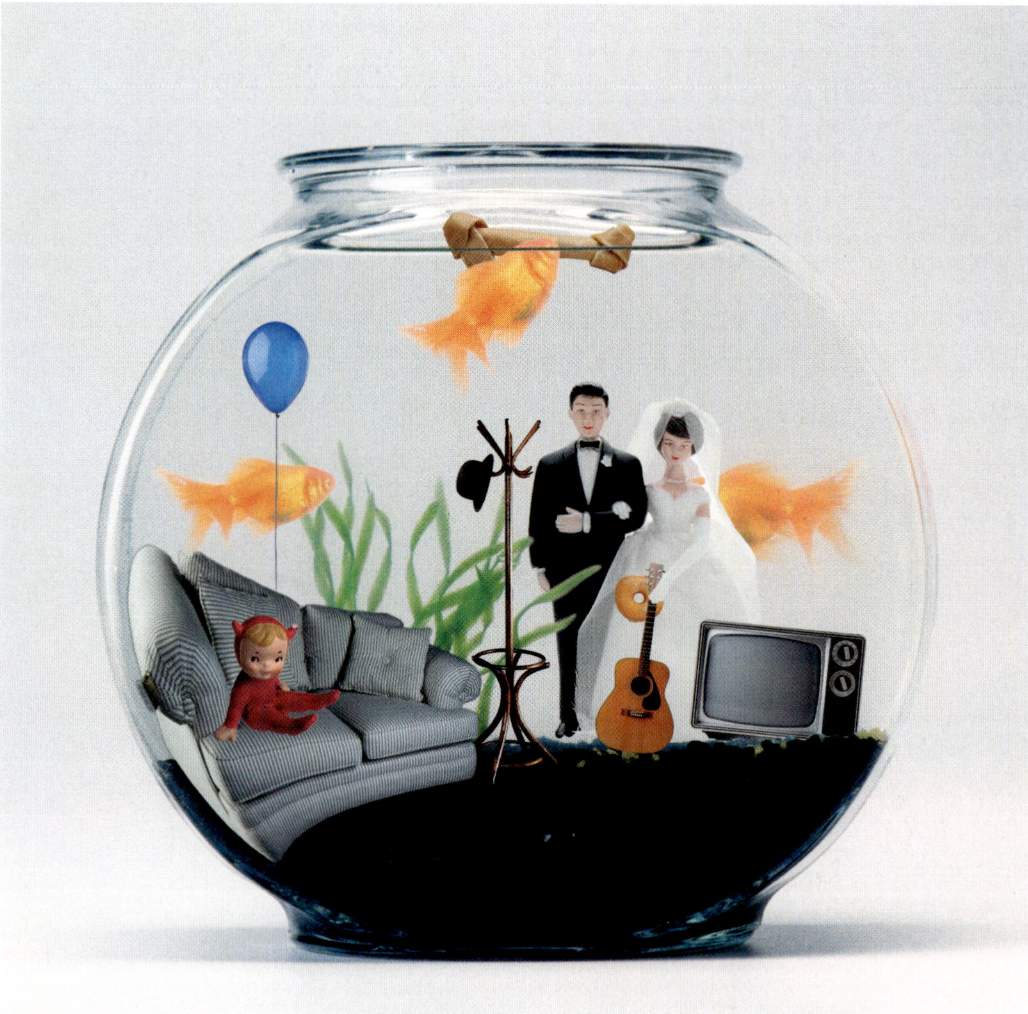

Picture Perfect #2 (Part A)

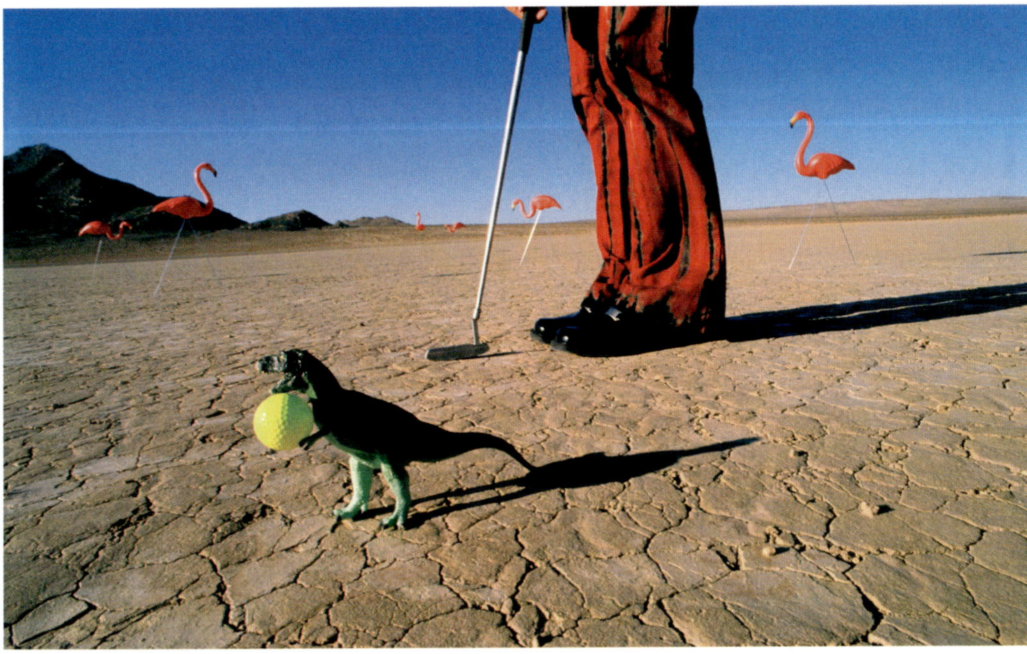

Picture Perfect #3 (Part A)

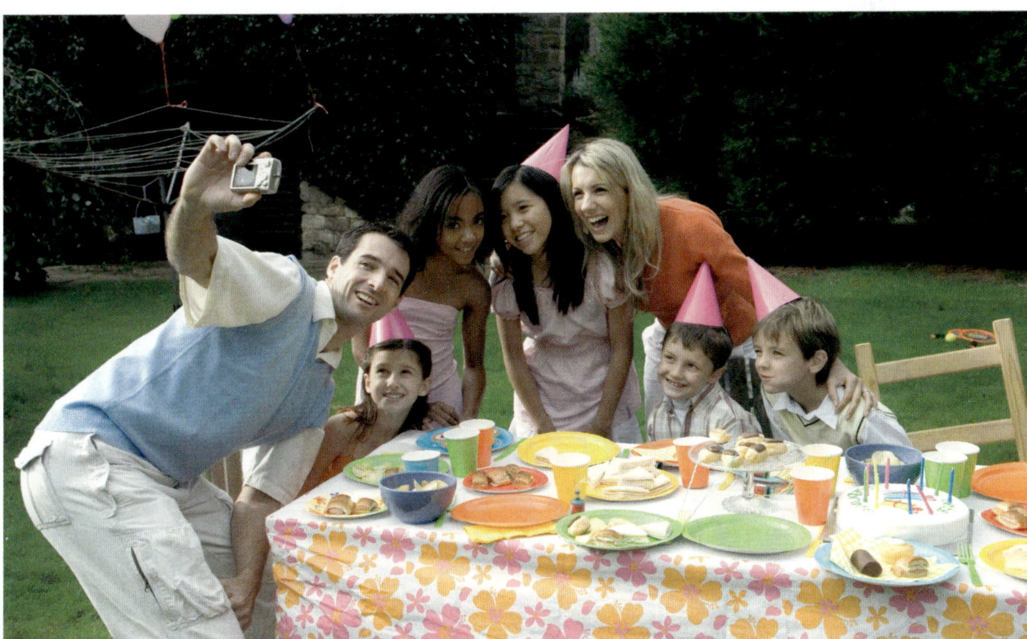

Picture Perfect #1 (Part B)

Without looking back, circle the details that have changed. How many can you identify?

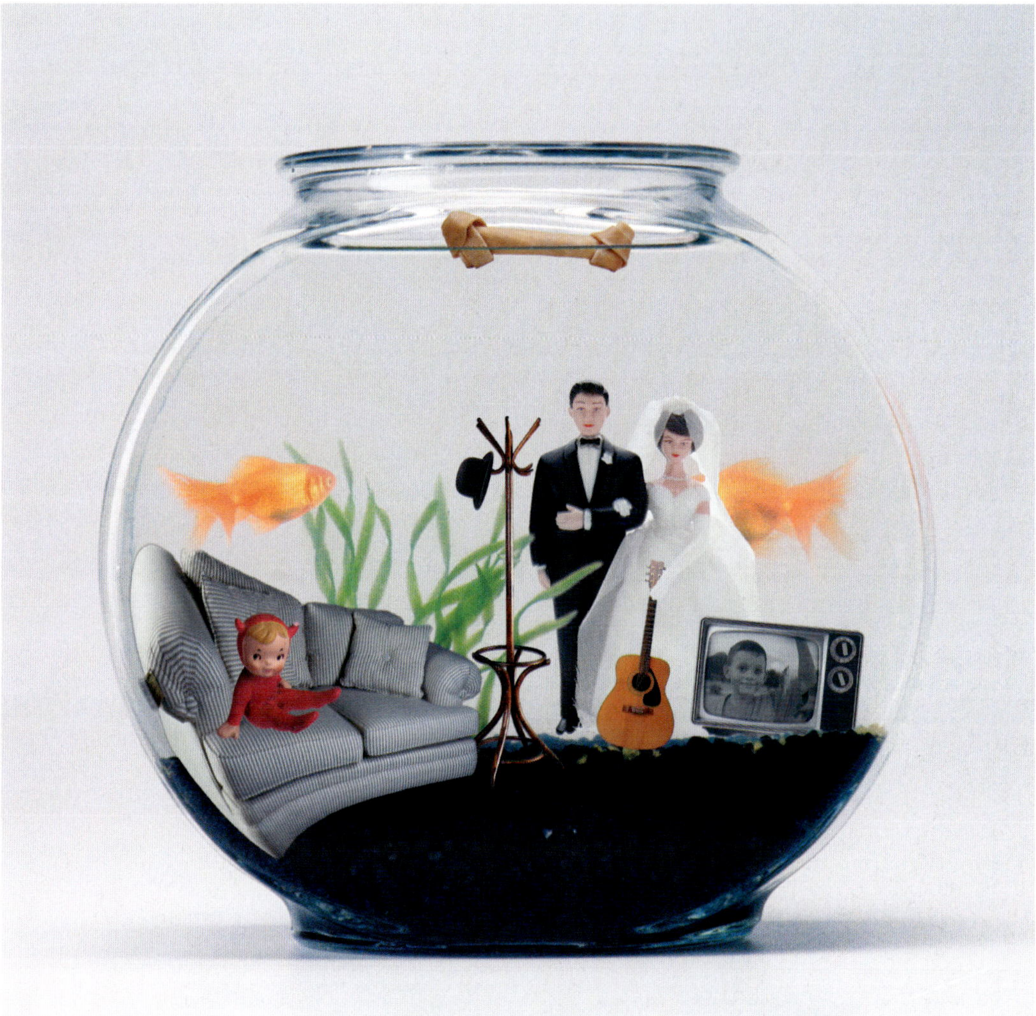

Answers on page 266

Picture Perfect #2 (Part B)

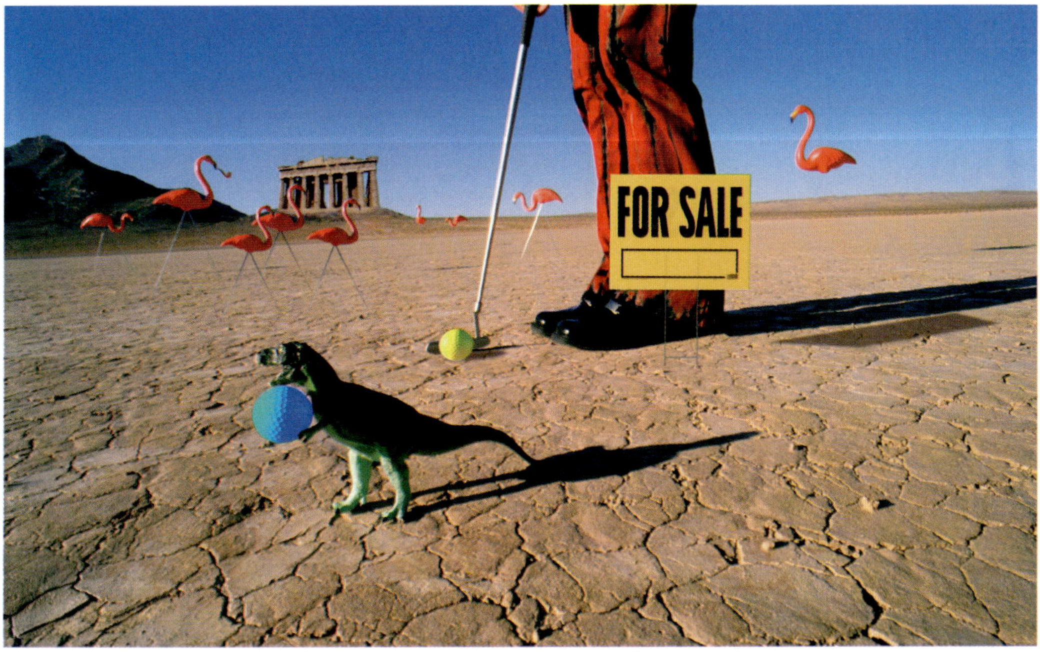

Picture Perfect #3 (Part B)

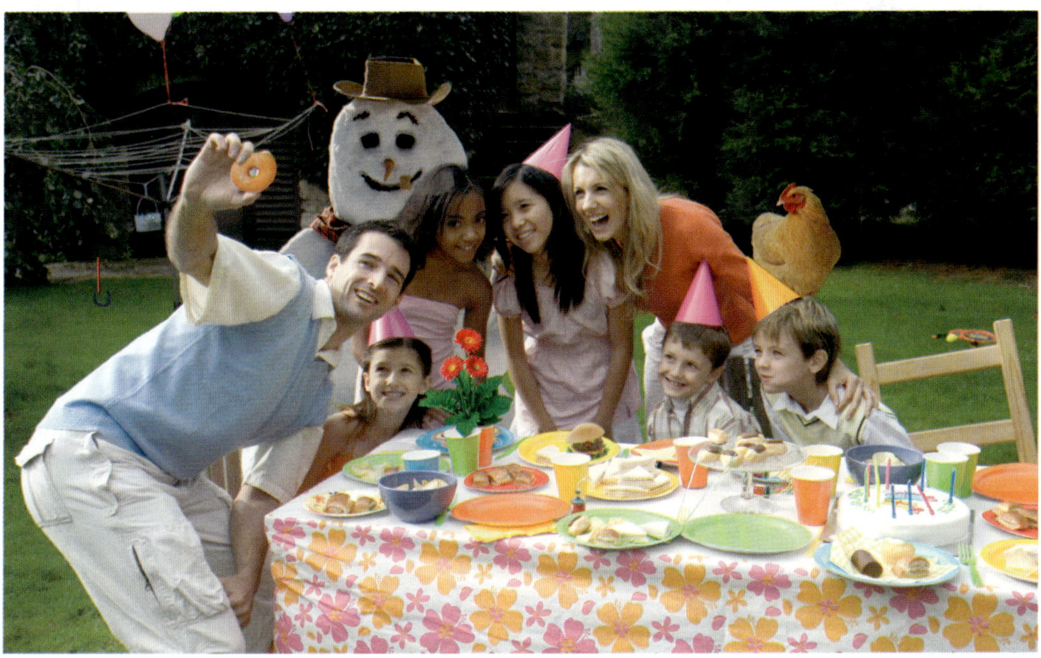

Answers on page 266

CONCENTRATION

For this exercise, you'll need:

- **A pen or pencil**
- **A timer**

Set the timer for 1 minute and study the grid below. After a minute, turn the page. There you'll find a blank grid and a column of objects. Match the objects to their proper locations on the grid.

Concentration #1 (Part A)

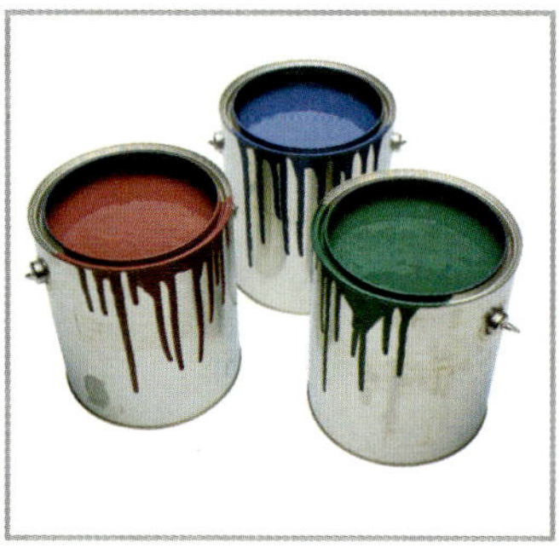
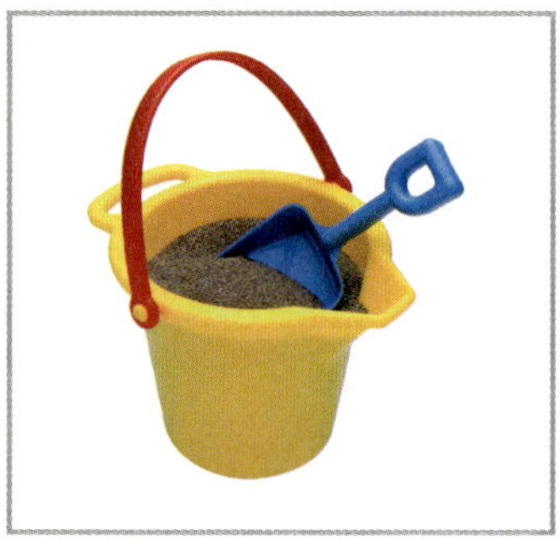
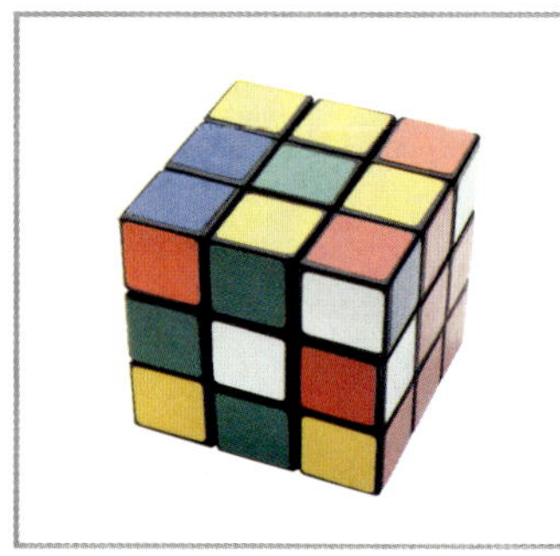
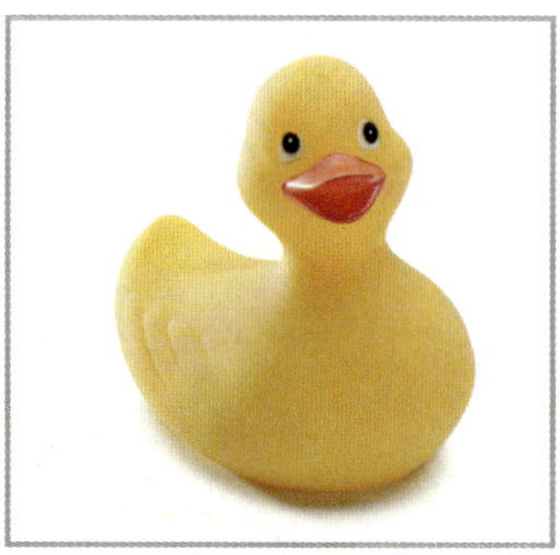
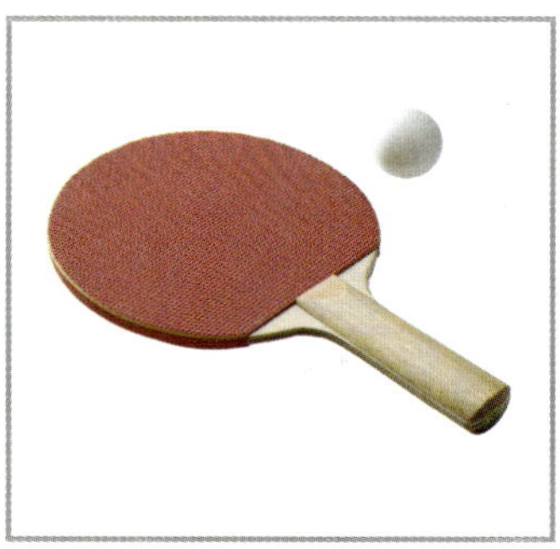
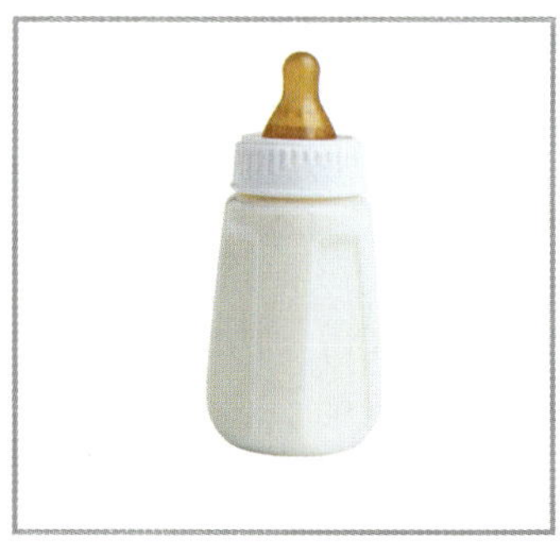
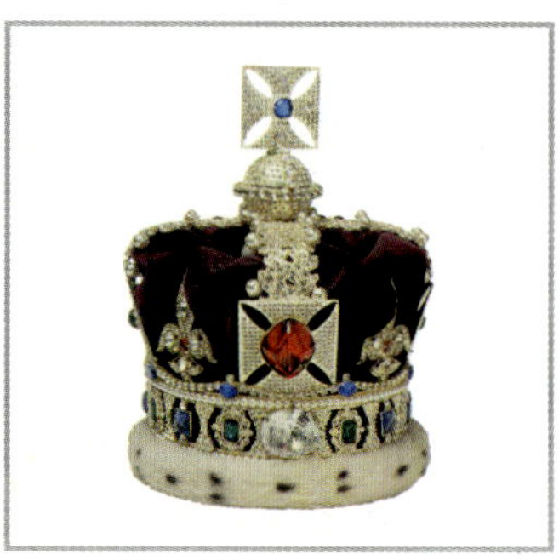
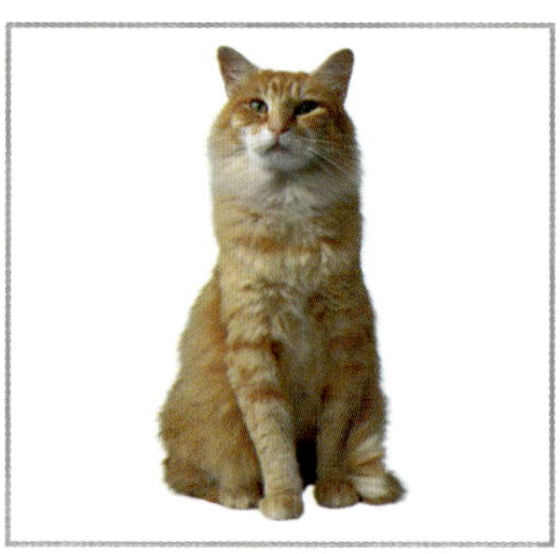
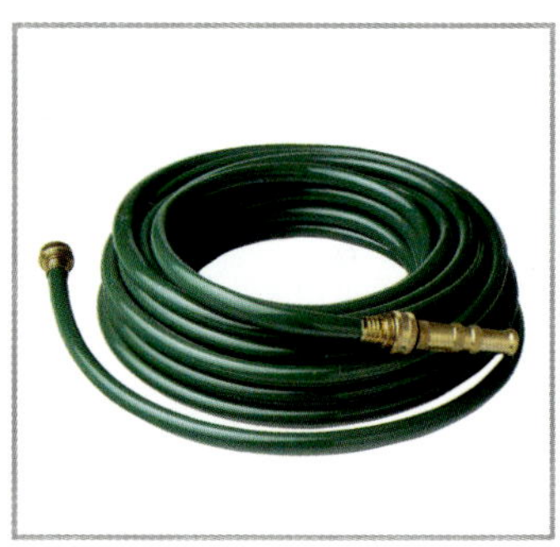

Concentration #2 (Part A)

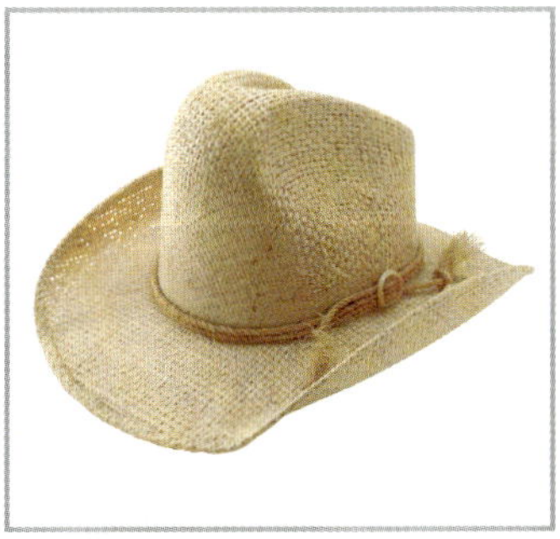
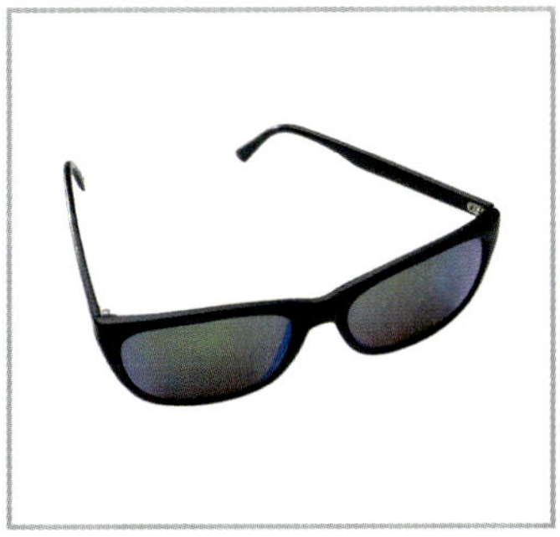
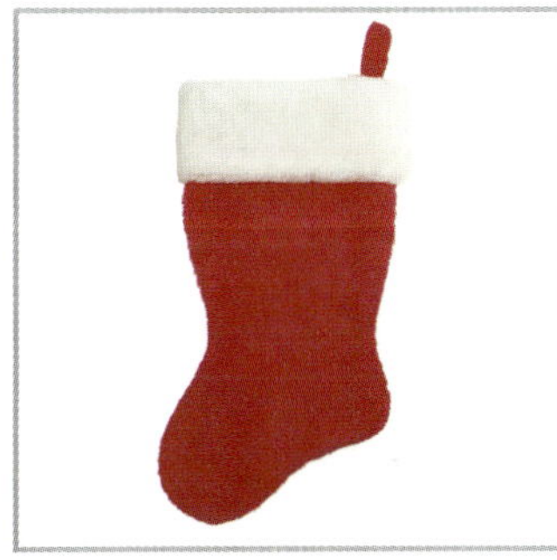
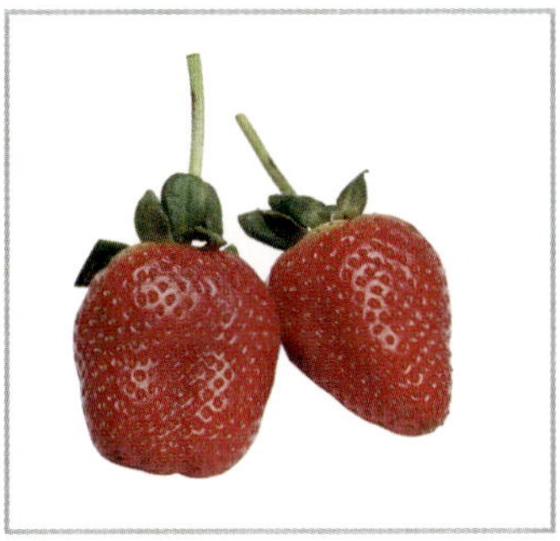
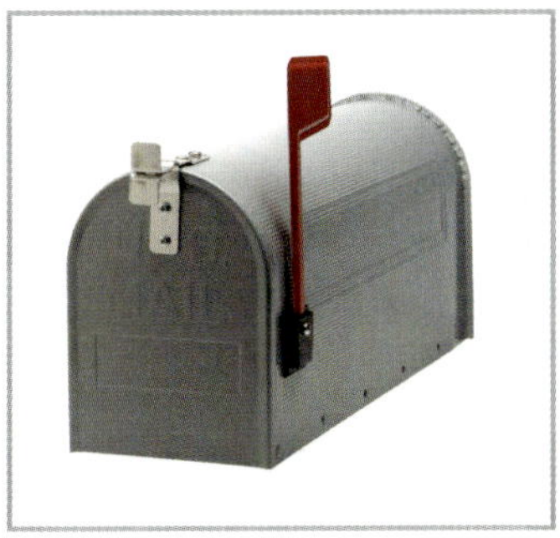
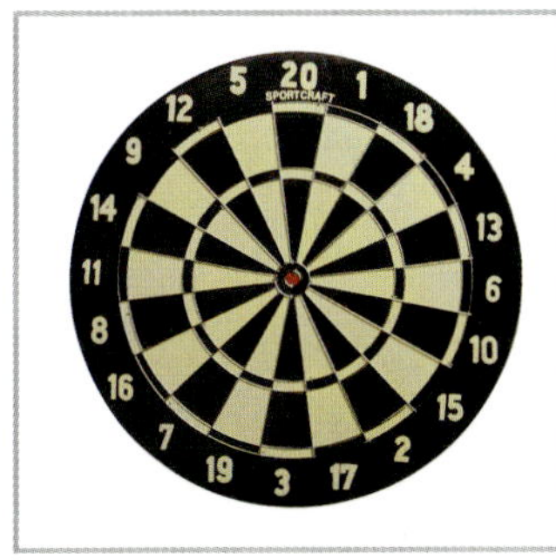

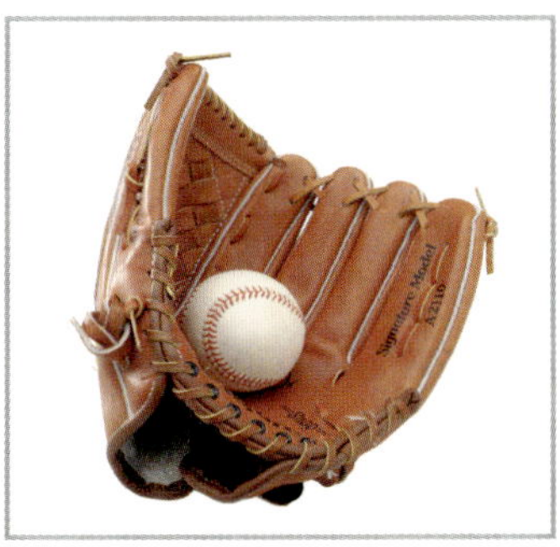
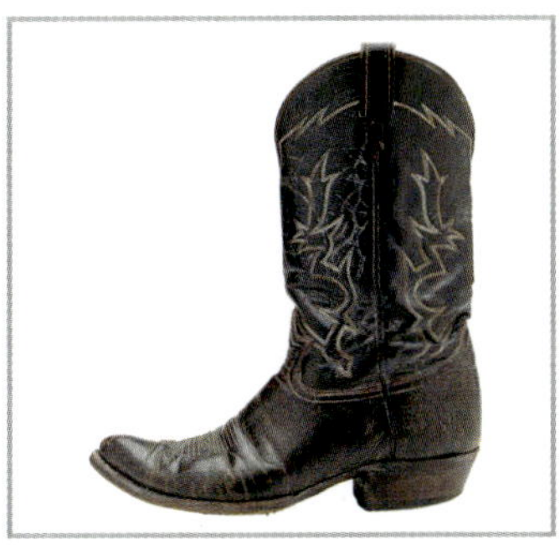
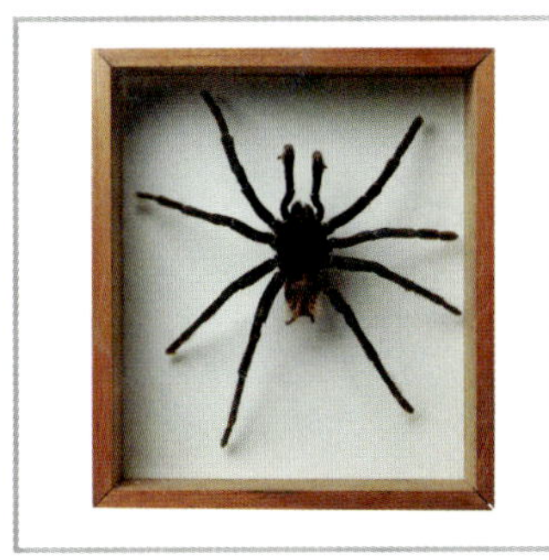

Concentration #1 (Part B)

Each picture is labeled with a letter. Try to recall where each picture was located on the grid, then write the letter associated with the picture in the proper place on the grid.

A

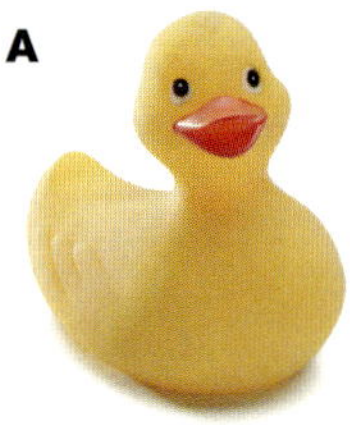

B

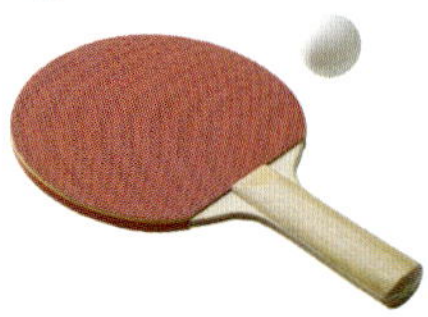

C

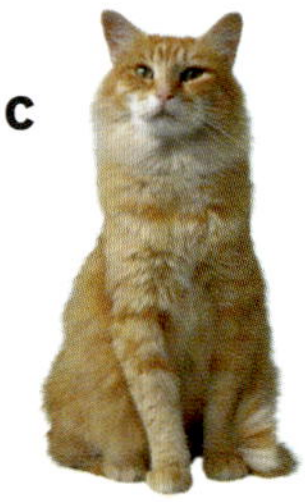

D

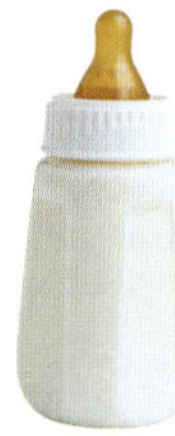

E

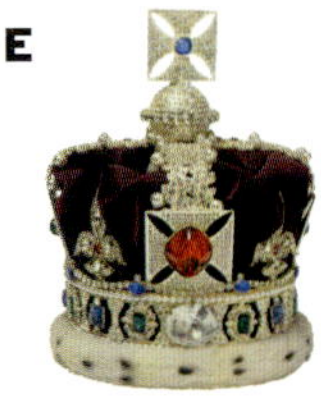

F

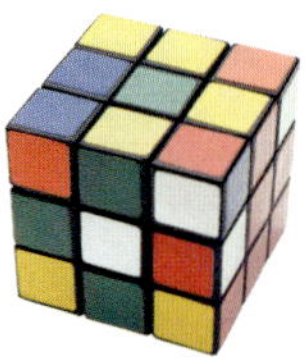

G

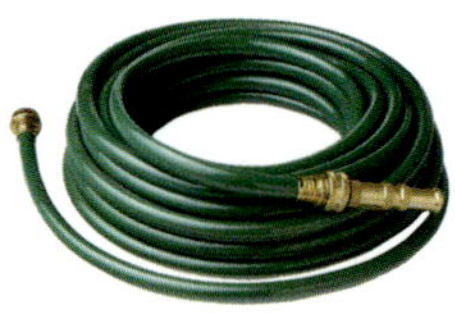

H

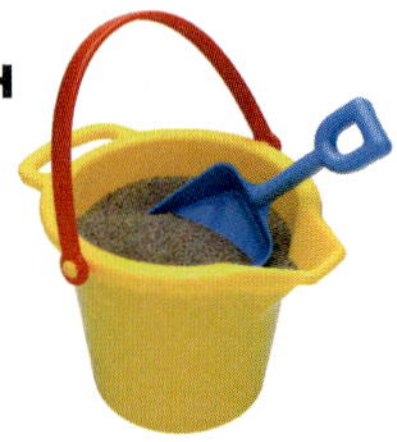

I

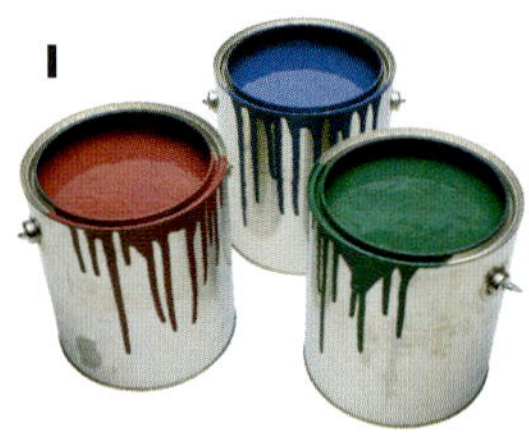

To check your answers, turn back to page 224

Concentration #2 (Part B)

A
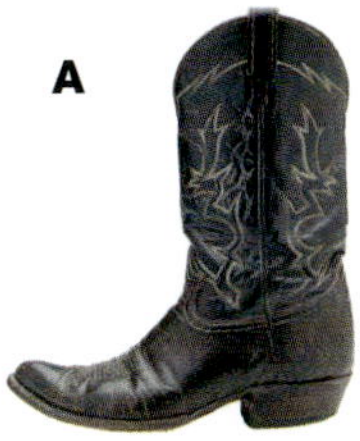

B
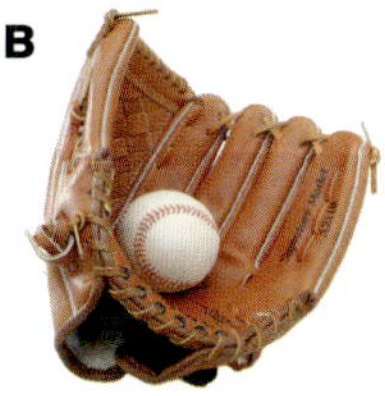

C
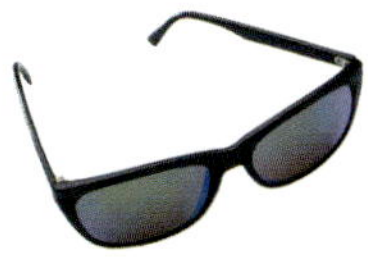

D
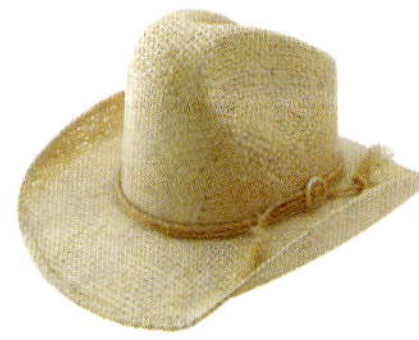

E
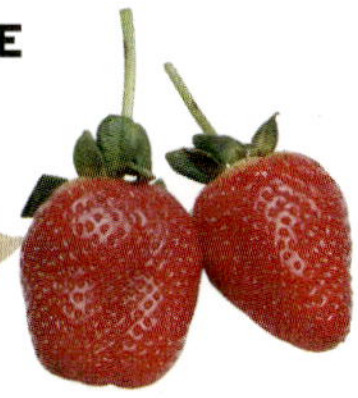

F
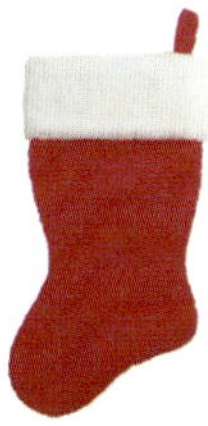

G
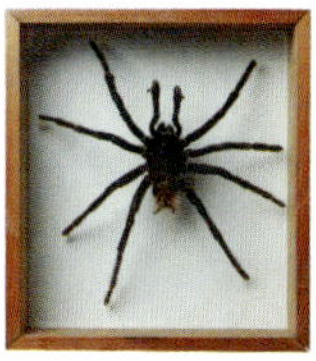

H
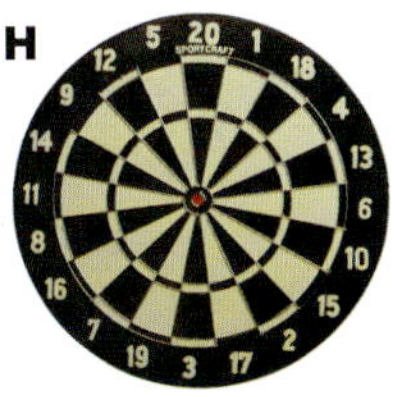

I
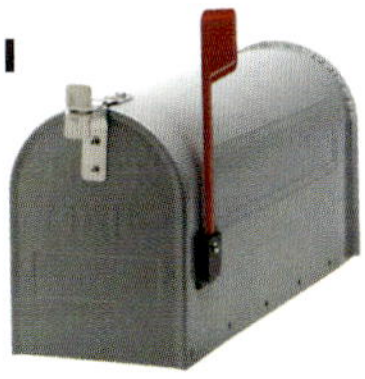

To check your answers, turn back to page 225

Concentration #3 (Part A)

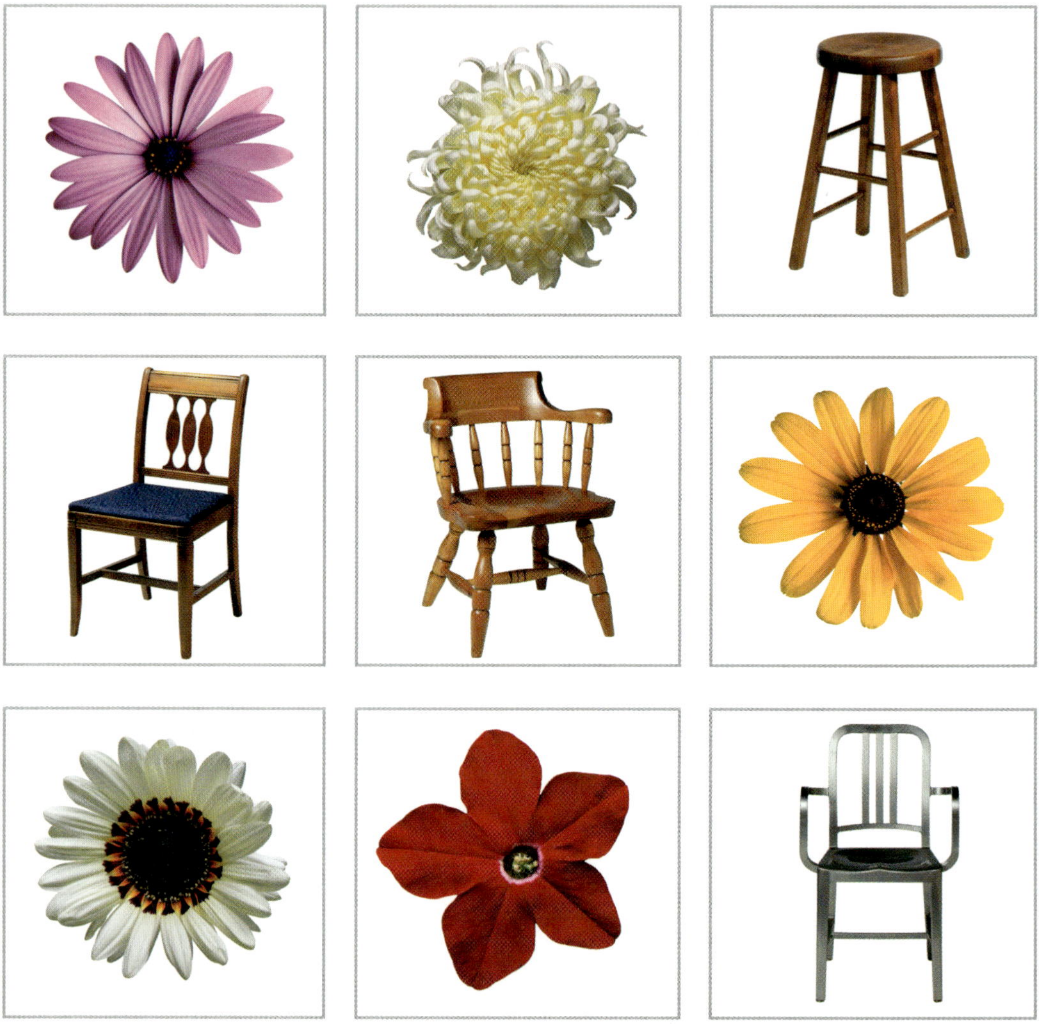

Concentration #4 (Part A)

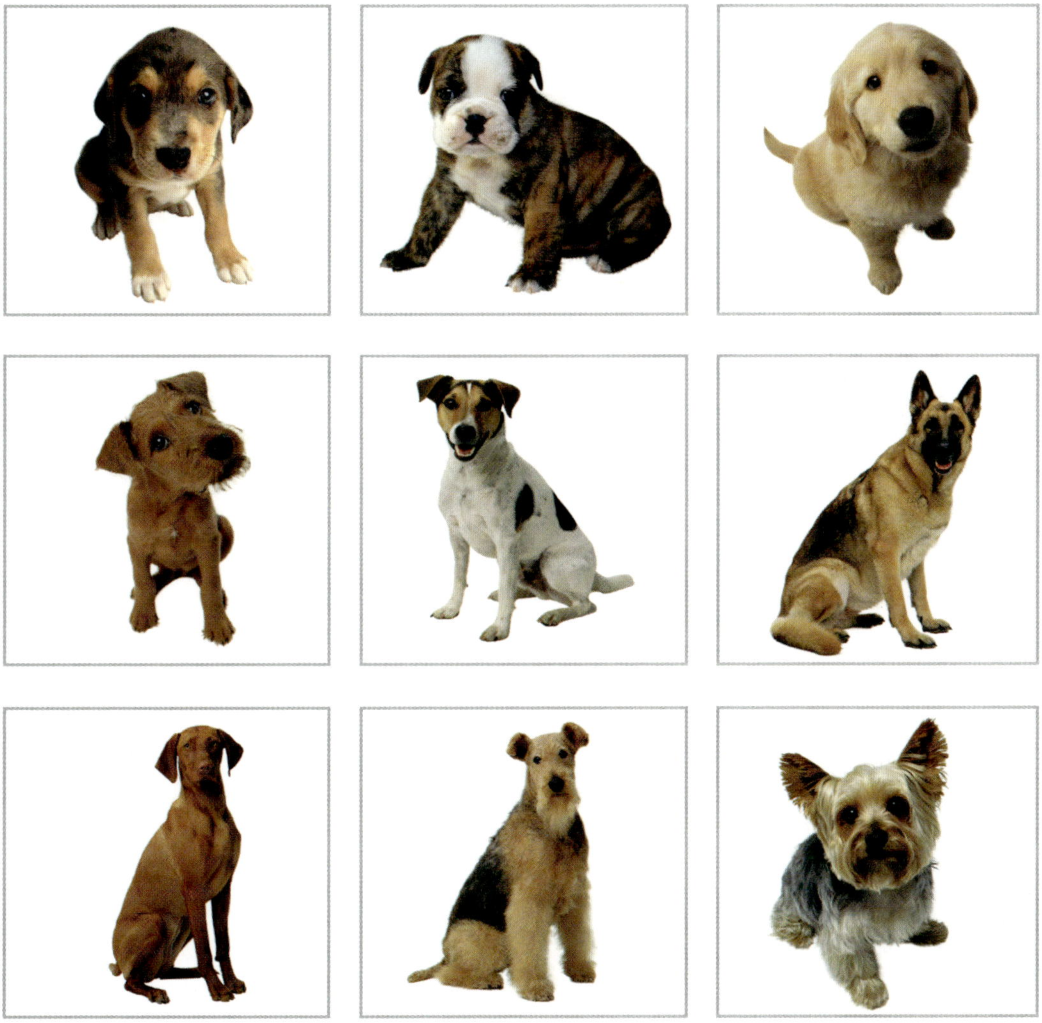

Concentration #3 (Part B)

A

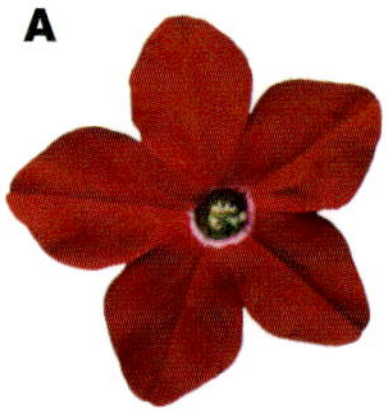

B

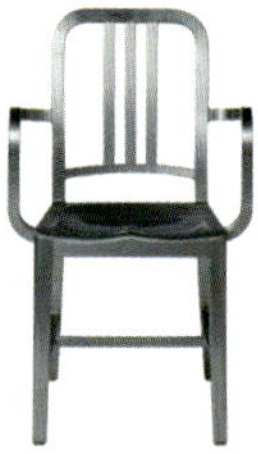

C

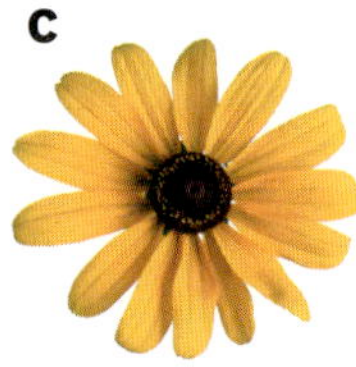

D

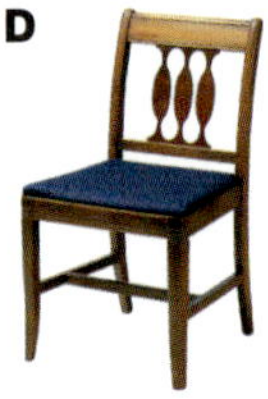

E

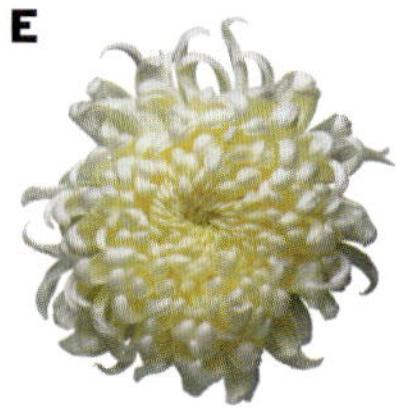

F

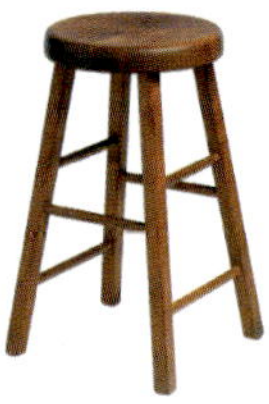

G

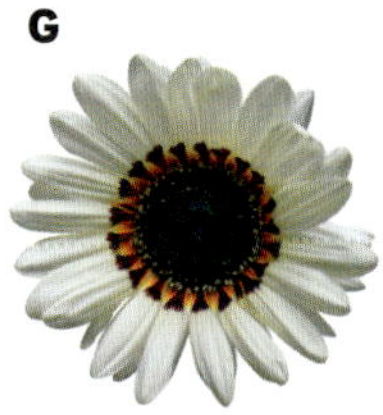

H

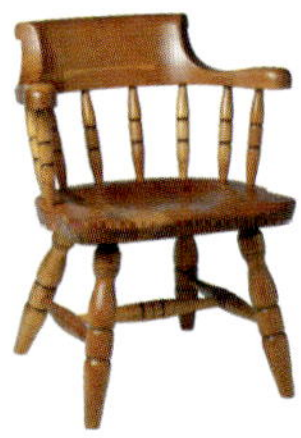

I

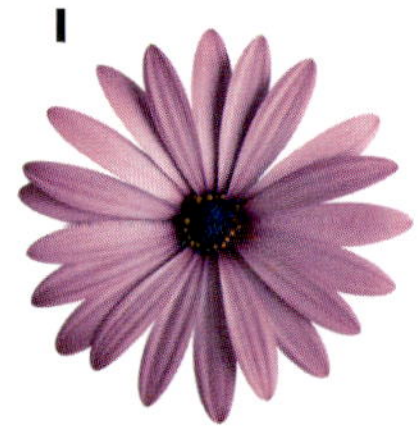

To check your answers, turn back to page 228

Concentration #4 (Part B)

A 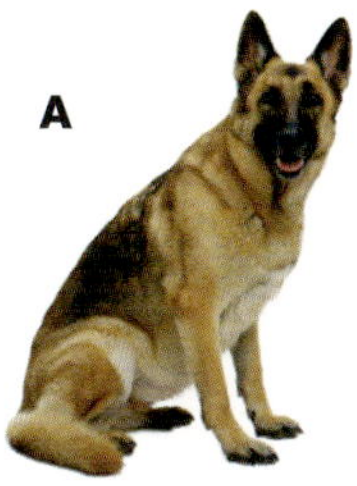

B 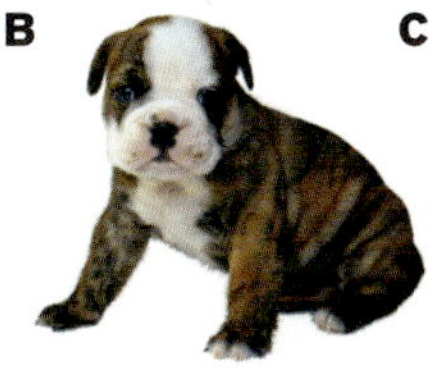

C 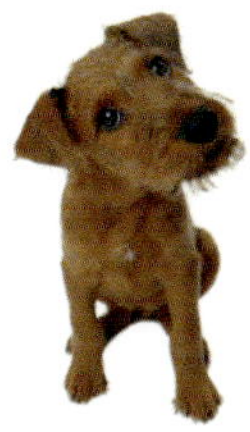

D 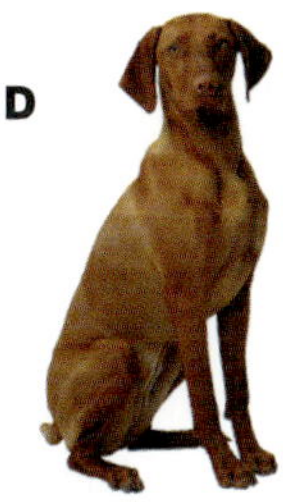

E 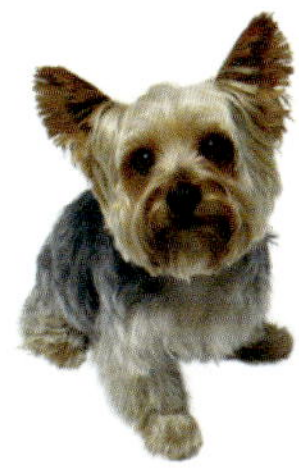

F 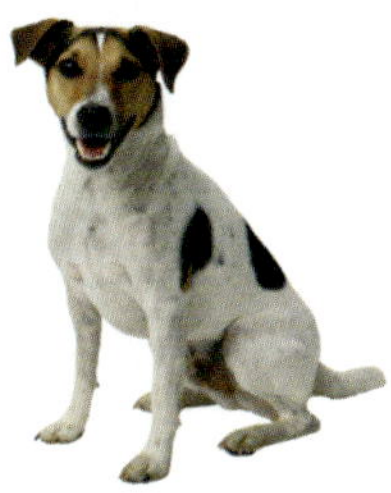

G 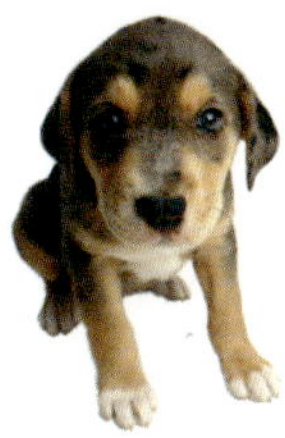

H 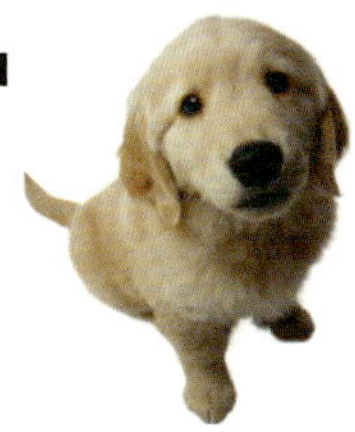

I 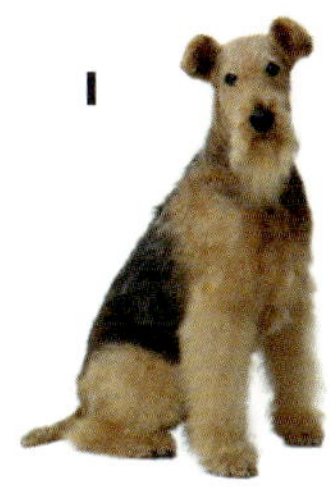

To check your answers, turn back to page 229

SCENTS AND SENSIBILITY

For this exercise, you'll need:
- **A pen or pencil**
- **A timer**

Certain scents have the amazing ability to bring you right back to a particular time, place, or moment in your life. The olfactory bulb, the area of the brain that perceives smells, is part of the brain's limbic system, which plays a major role in long-term memory, especially emotional memories.

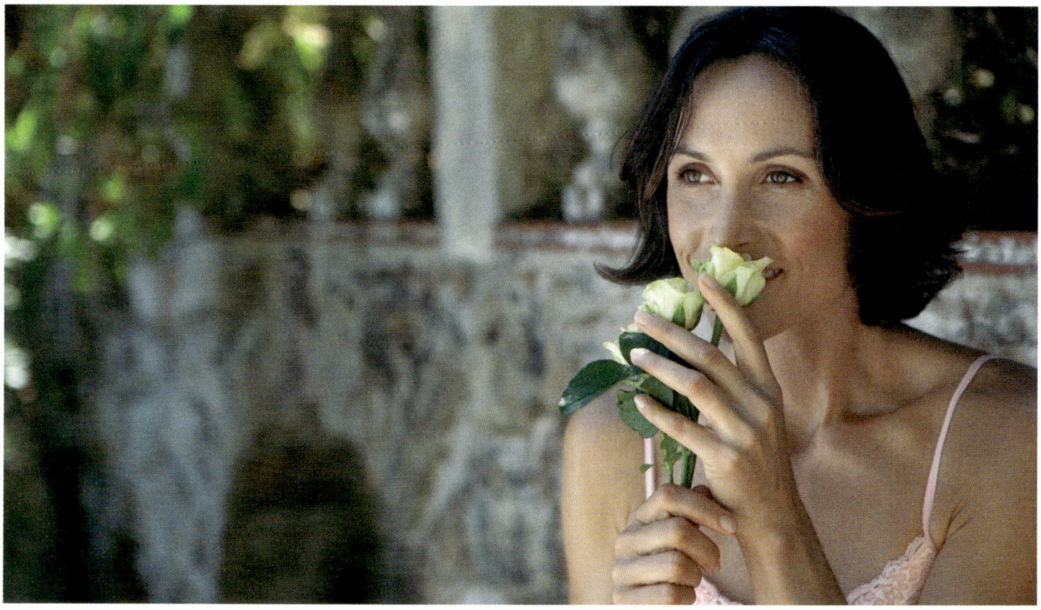

Scents and Sensibility #1

Set the timer for 5 minutes. Look at the list below and choose one of the scents. If you happen to have access to the scent, take a good whiff. Then, sit down without any distractions and imagine the smell as best you can. Let your mind recall every detail of the memories it evokes. Don't rush the process; take the full 5 minutes. Later, come back and do this exercise with other scents from the list.

Cinnamon
Warm apple pie
Warm chocolate chip cookies
Freshly sharpened lead pencil
Fresh pine (or a pine-scented candle)
Roses
Musk
Skunk
Floral perfume

Baby powder
Cut grass
Worms after a rainstorm
Manure
Homemade chicken soup
Mulled wine
Musty books
Wood smoke
Hay
Tobacco

Rubbing alcohol
Aftershave
Nutmeg
Shoe polish
Baking bread
Burning leaves
Stinky cheese
Strawberry lip gloss
Lake water
Chlorine

Scents and Sensibility #2

Think of a scent that has special meaning for you. Maybe it's the perfume your mother wore to church on Sundays, an old lover's after-shave, chicken fat from your grandmother's kitchen, a sycamore tree from your childhood backyard, a leather chair from your father's study, machine oil or melting solder or sawdust from your uncle's workshop, or burnt marshmallows from summer camp. The possibilities are endless. For each scent you think of, write down the memory you associate with it.

Scent: ______________________________

Memory: ______________________________

____

____

____

Scent: ______________________________

Memory: ______________________________

____

____

____

Scent: ______________________________

Memory: ______________________________

____

____

____

Scent: ______________________________

Memory: ______________________________

____

____

____

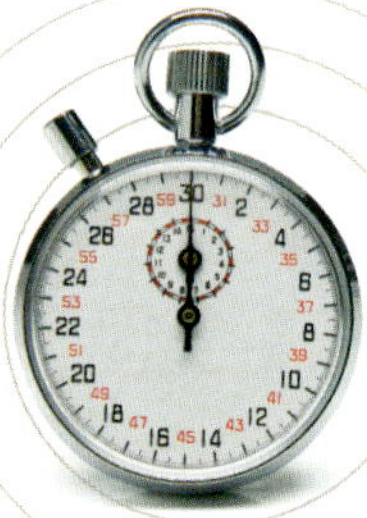

Improve your processing speed

Have you watched a young child in action lately? They don't walk; they run. They don't sit; they fidget. As we get older, our bodies slow down. The same goes for our brains. We can learn and remember almost as well as we used to, but it might take our brains a bit longer.

That's because we naturally produce fewer neurotransmitters, the all-important brain chemicals that carry information across the gaps between brain cells. We also lose some of our white matter, the fatty goop that insulates the brain's high-speed information "cables" (bundles of nerve fibers, really) that enable faster transmission of electrical signals from one part of the brain to another.

Lagging speed can affect our ability to understand a fast-moving scene in a movie, count change at the store checkout, balance a checkbook, or react to a car swerving in front of us on the highway. It can even affect how "fast" the brain hears. Sounds that enter the ear take an extra moment or two to be registered and translated in the brain. Many older people are sent for hearing tests by family members who are later confused when the tests show normal hearing. The delay between hearing and responding is often interpreted as a hearing problem, when it actually is just a natural, if frustrating, slowdown in the brain.

That slowdown is also the reason we can't burn in new memories as quickly or

Can Playing Computer Games Make You Smarter?

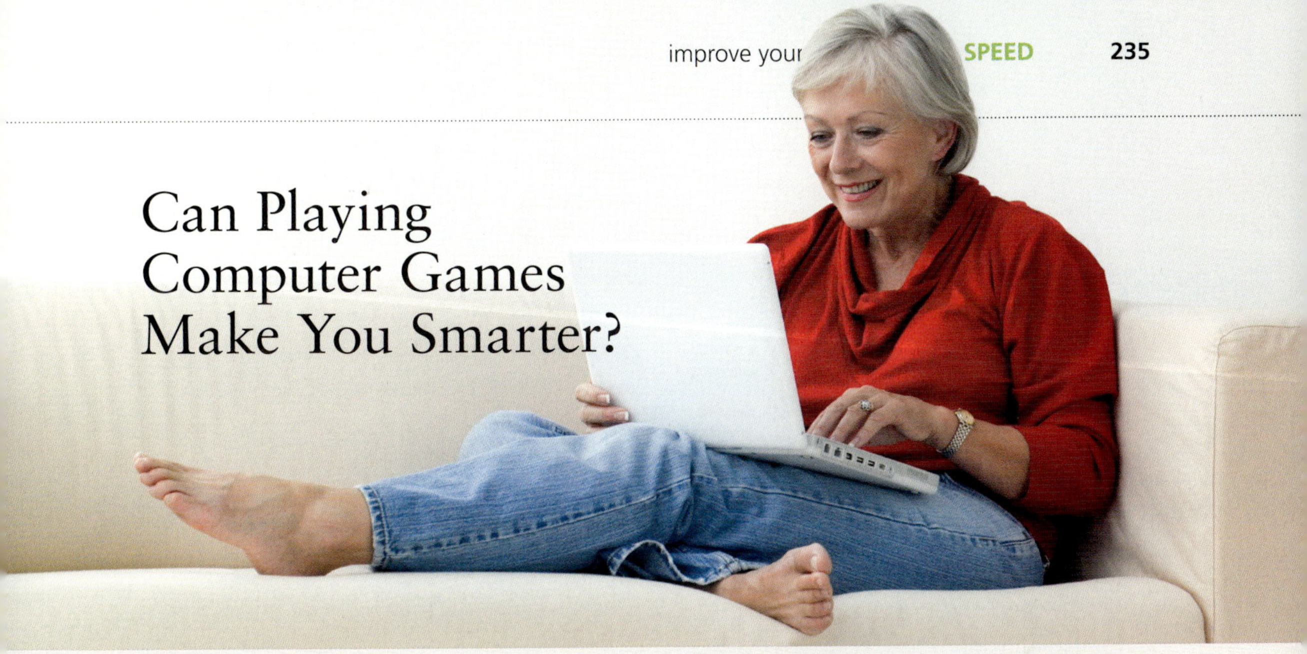

With so many baby boomers living in fear of brain drain, it's no wonder that computer games designed to improve brain fitness have sprouted like so many gray hairs on an aging head. There's Nintendo's Brain Age, Posit Science's Brain Fitness, and CogniFit's MindFit, to name a few, plus Web-based programs such as www.lumosity.com and www.happy-neuron.com. But do they work? The answer is a definitive yes...and no. It comes down to a question of what your goals are, how hard you are willing to work (or, in this case, play), and which software you use.

Imagine a teenager who wants to improve his overall athletic ability. What should he do? He could start running on a track to improve his speed and endurance, but that won't help him on the basketball court. He could spend weeks perfecting his dribbling technique, but that won't help his ability to land a jump shot. And none of that training will help his golf game.

That's how it is with brain training, too. Cognitive abilities come in many distinct types. The best programs—usually those designed with the help of neuropsychologists—work on several types, including processing speed, visual acuity, listening, concentration and focus, reasoning, spatial orientation, and memory. These encourage general brain improvement, as opposed to what might be called the Sudoku effect—if you work Sudoku puzzles day and night, you might get really quick at filling squares with numbers, but you won't be any better at counting change at the grocery store.

Detractors say that there is no proof that any of the games really help improve mental function, and that the business is overwhelming the science. But the science in support of several of these products is growing. For instance, Posit Science tested its 8-week program on older adults (ages 60 to 97) and found that memory improved significantly, even months later. Larger studies are underway at most of the serious brain fitness companies that will eventually show whether these games can prevent or delay age-related memory problems or even Alzheimer's disease.

Bottom line: The games can't hurt anything but your wallet. Many people enjoy them, and experts agree that keeping your mind active helps delay or even prevent dementia associated with aging. "Everything you do helps in one way or another" says Alan Castel, Ph.D., assistant professor of psychology at the University of California, Los Angeles, and an expert in memory and cognitive aging. Dr. Castel believes that these programs are not a cure for memory loss, but that they can play an important part in keeping our thought processes agile.

Just don't neglect the rest of the world; there are lots of noncomputer ways to challenge your mind.

as completely as we once did. The good news: Although we can't expect to keep the pedal to the metal, there is no need for the mental equivalent of shuffling. Like Lance Armstrong training for a bike race, we can train our brains to go faster.

Smart Everyday Strategies

While you're using the exercises in this book to help increase your processing speed, also consider these strategies.

Be deliberate and calm. As with all mental processes, speed suffers when you are stressed. If you find yourself feeling pressured by your own or others' expectations, take a deep breath, relax, and remind yourself that you deserve to take as much time as you need.

Practice. Everything you do, you can do faster with practice. The general reaction to doing poorly at tasks is to give up trying, but if speed is your problem, avoidance of the task will only make it worse. Work at small projects by practicing them again and again, the way you would practice if you were learning to play a musical instrument, and soon your brain will find the "notes" in no time.

Check out computer games. The same computer games your kids and grandkids play can help improve your ability to see, process, and react to fast-moving objects. You can also train your brain using video games designed specifically to improve cognitive abilities, including processing speed (see "Can Playing Computer Games make You Smarter?" on page 235). These can be played on a home computer or video game system.

exercises

If our reaction time slows, the world can pass us by. We become frustrated, and it's not difficult to feel that others are annoyed with us, as well. These exercises were designed to improve the brain's processing speed. Do them every day, at least once a day.

SORT FOR SPEED

Repeat three times every day, if possible.

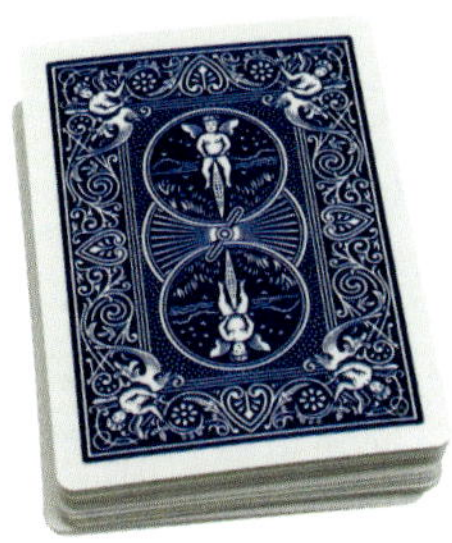

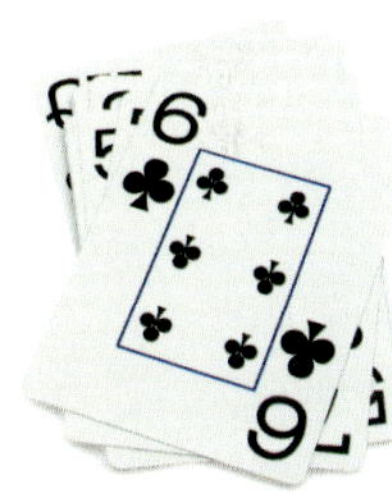

For this exercise, you'll need:

- **A pen or pencil**
- **Paper**
- **A watch or clock with a second hand**
- **A deck of playing cards**

Sort for Speed #1

a. Prepare

Shuffle the deck well and place it facedown in front of you.

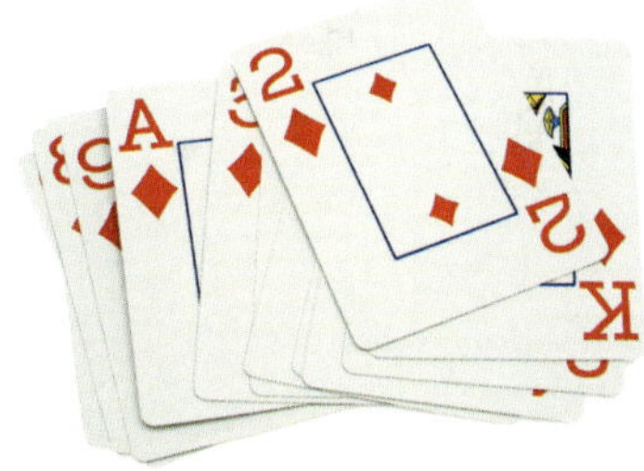

b. Begin

Note the time when you begin. Pick up the deck and sort the cards into four piles by suit. Do this as quickly as you can. When you finish sorting, look at the clock and note the time.

c. Finish

Write down how long it took you to complete the exercise—and try to beat your time next time. Then, for your own information, look through the piles to see how accurate you were.

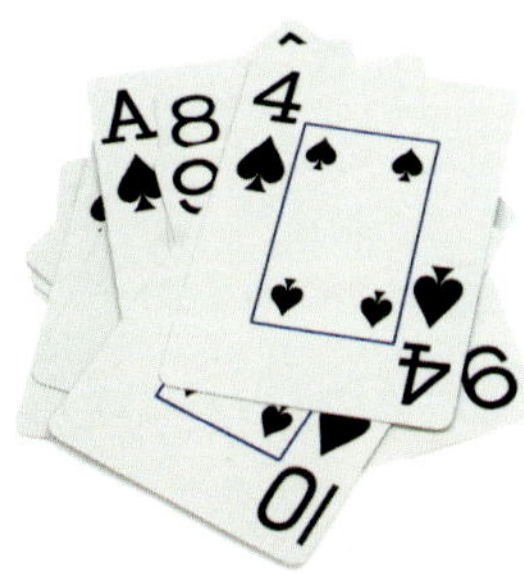

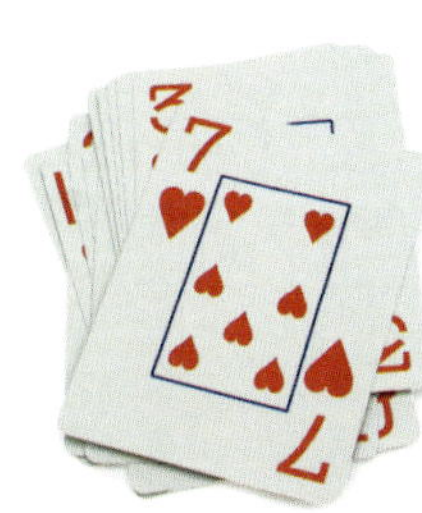

TIME ________________

NUMBER OF MISTAKES ________________

Sort for Speed #2

One Step Harder

Note the time you begin. Quickly separate the deck into piles by suit, then take each pile and order the cards by number, with aces low and face cards in this order: jacks, queens, kings. Do not record your time until both phases of the exercise are complete.

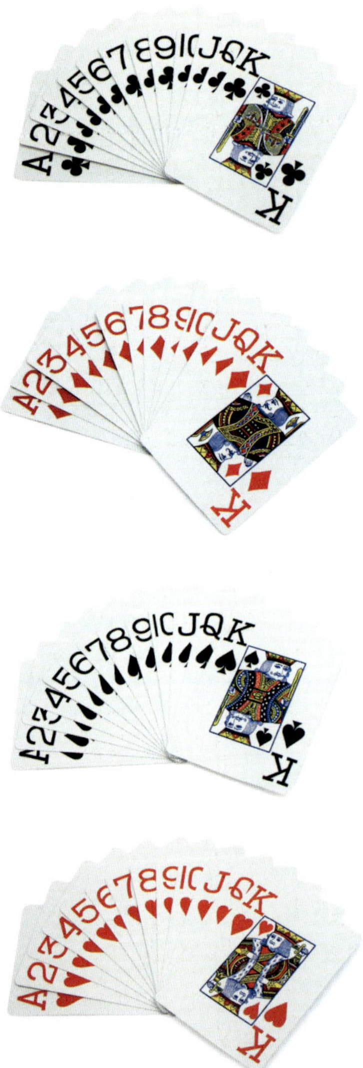

TIME ________________

NUMBER OF MISTAKES ________________

Sort for Speed #3

Two Steps Harder

Note the time you begin. Separate the deck into six piles—aces in one pile, face cards in a second pile, and four piles of numbered cards by suit. Do not record your time until all phases of the exercise are complete.

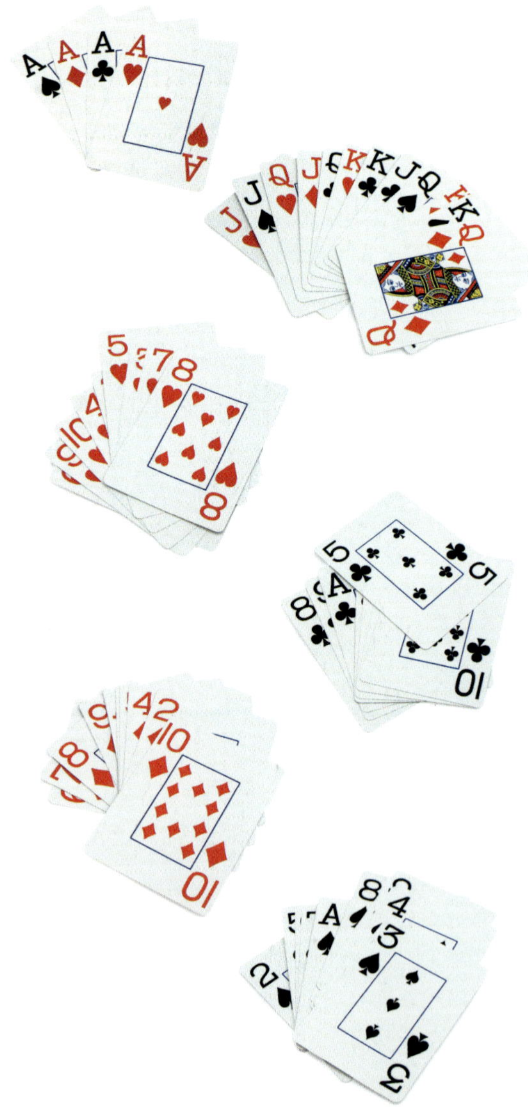

TIME ________________

NUMBER OF MISTAKES ________________

LETTER SEARCH

For this exercise, you'll need:

- **A pen or pencil**
- **A stopwatch or watch or clock with a second hand**

Letter Search #1

In the grid below, find all appearances of the letter *R*, both capital and lower-case, any color. When you are ready, set the stopwatch or note the time. Circle every letter *R*. Then go back and count how many appear in capital and how many in lower-case. Finally, count how many *R*s appear in **red**. Note how long it took you, and see if you can beat your time in subsequent exercises.

K	a	N	M	r	r	N	c	N	m	n	k	A	r	X	c	X	m	x	r	N	a
k	R	n	n	r	k	r	X	B	k	k	M	z	N	r	n	k	r	X	N	Z	N
a	x	m	Z	r	R	r	K	Z	N	X	k	R	X	n	k	k	n	R	a	k	X
x	r	x	n	Z	k	m	X	R	r	Z	c	m	x	Z	r	Z	m	X	Z	r	R
m	Z	c	Z	N	a	Z	n	Z	R	m	N	r	R	M	z	A	Z	m	c	k	R
R	m	z	n	X	r	Z	m	N	K	z	x	N	a	z	R	z	M	r	z	X	r
X	z	N	k	m	M	c	z	Z	r	c	X	R	N	n	z	K	R	a	K	k	n
c	m	z	R	z	k	c	M	N	Z	x	m	z	B	a	x	X	M	R	X	m	m
x	X	N	z	m	r	R	x	A	X	n	z	m	Z	X	N	z	M	n	X	a	X
n	X	A	k	r	n	m	x	R	a	X	R	R	r	m	c	R	n	B	a	k	z
k	x	z	M	Z	k	N	z	m	R	N	X	a	k	r	R	x	r	k	X	r	X
B	Z	r	X	r	K	a	Z	B	z	R	z	N	A	k	M	x	X	c	R	n	A
r	X	n	x	a	R	M	k	k	Z	x	r	X	k	a	c	K	x	R	n	R	z
c	x	z	N	R	x	c	M	m	R	n	z	B	M	x	R	z	n	R	z	x	M
N	R	r	R	z	r	R	n	Z	R	n	m	R	A	a	X	X	r	m	R	n	Z
R	z	R	z	N	z	B	x	R	R	r	Z	x	R	n	X	a	z	m	R	x	n

TIME ______________ NUMBER OF CAPITAL *R*s ____________

NUMBER OF LOWERCASE *R*s ____________ NUMBER OF RED *R*s ____________

Answers on page 266

Letter Search #2

In the grid below, find all appearances of the letter *N*, both capital and lower-case, any color. When you are ready, set the stopwatch or note the time. Circle every letter *N*. Then go back and count how many appear in capital and how many in lower-case. Finally, count how many *N*s appear in **blue**. Note how long it took you.

K	a	N	M	r	r	N	c	N	m	n	k	A	r	X	c	X	m	x	r	N	a
k	R	n	n	r	k	r	X	B	k	k	M	z	N	r	n	k	r	X	N	Z	N
a	x	m	Z	r	R	r	K	Z	N	X	k	R	X	n	k	k	n	R	a	k	X
x	r	x	n	Z	k	m	X	R	r	Z	c	m	x	Z	r	Z	m	X	Z	r	R
m	Z	c	Z	N	a	Z	n	Z	R	m	N	r	R	M	z	A	Z	m	c	k	R
R	m	z	n	X	r	Z	m	N	K	z	x	N	a	z	R	z	M	r	z	X	r
X	z	N	k	m	M	c	z	Z	r	c	X	R	N	n	z	K	R	a	K	k	n
c	m	z	R	z	k	c	M	N	Z	x	m	z	B	a	x	X	M	R	X	m	m
x	X	N	z	m	r	R	x	A	X	n	z	m	Z	X	N	z	M	n	X	a	X
n	X	A	k	r	n	m	x	R	a	X	R	R	r	m	c	R	n	B	a	k	z
k	x	z	M	Z	k	N	z	m	R	N	X	a	k	r	R	x	r	k	X	r	X
B	Z	r	X	r	K	a	Z	B	z	R	z	N	A	k	M	x	X	c	R	n	A
r	X	n	x	a	R	M	k	k	Z	x	r	X	k	a	c	K	x	R	n	R	z
c	x	z	N	R	x	c	M	m	R	n	z	B	M	x	R	z	n	R	z	x	M
N	R	r	R	z	r	R	n	Z	R	n	m	R	A	a	X	X	r	m	R	n	Z
R	z	R	z	N	z	B	x	R	R	r	Z	x	R	n	X	a	z	m	R	x	n
c	x	z	N	R	x	c	M	m	R	n	z	B	M	x	R	z	n	R	z	x	M
n	x	z	M	Z	k	N	z	m	R	N	X	a	k	r	R	x	r	k	X	r	X
R	m	z	n	X	r	Z	m	N	K	z	x	N	a	z	R	z	M	r	z	X	r

TIME ____________ NUMBER OF CAPITAL *N*s____________

NUMBER OF LOWERCASE *N*s____________ NUMBER OF BLUE *N*s____________

Answers on page 266

Letter Search #3

In the grid below, find all appearances of the letter *K*, both capital and lower-case, any color. When you are ready, set the stopwatch or note the time. Circle every letter *K*. Then go back and count how many appear in capital and how many in lower-case. Finally, count how many *K*s appear in **green**. Note how long it took you.

K	a	N	M	r	r	N	c	N	m	n	k	A	r	X	c	X	m	x	r	N	a
k	R	n	n	r	k	r	X	B	k	k	M	z	N	r	n	k	r	X	N	Z	N
a	x	m	Z	r	R	r	K	Z	N	X	k	R	X	n	k	k	n	R	a	k	X
x	r	x	n	Z	k	m	X	R	r	Z	c	m	x	Z	r	Z	m	X	Z	r	R
m	Z	c	Z	N	a	Z	n	Z	R	m	N	r	R	M	z	A	Z	m	c	k	R
R	m	z	n	X	r	Z	m	N	K	z	x	N	a	z	R	z	M	r	z	X	r
X	z	N	k	m	M	c	z	Z	r	c	X	R	N	n	z	K	R	a	K	k	n
c	m	z	R	z	k	c	M	N	Z	x	m	z	B	a	x	X	M	R	X	m	m
x	X	N	z	m	r	R	x	A	X	n	z	m	Z	X	N	z	M	n	X	a	X
n	X	A	k	r	n	m	x	R	a	X	R	R	r	m	c	R	n	B	a	k	z
k	x	z	M	Z	k	N	z	m	R	N	X	a	k	r	R	x	r	k	X	r	X
B	Z	r	X	r	K	a	Z	B	z	R	z	N	A	k	M	x	X	c	R	n	A
r	X	n	x	a	R	M	k	k	Z	x	r	X	k	a	c	K	x	R	n	R	z
c	x	z	N	R	x	c	M	m	R	n	z	B	M	x	R	z	n	R	z	x	M
N	R	r	R	z	r	R	n	Z	R	n	m	R	A	a	X	X	r	m	R	n	Z
R	z	R	z	N	z	B	x	R	R	r	Z	x	R	n	X	a	z	m	R	x	n
k	R	n	n	r	k	r	X	B	k	k	M	z	N	r	n	k	r	X	N	Z	N
B	Z	r	X	k	K	a	Z	B	z	K	z	N	A	k	M	x	X	c	R	n	A
q	X	N	z	m	r	R	x	A	X	n	z	w	Z	X	K	z	p	n	X	a	Z

TIME ________________ NUMBER OF CAPITAL *K*s____________

NUMBER OF LOWERCASE *K*s____________ NUMBER OF GREEN *K*s____________

Answers on page 266

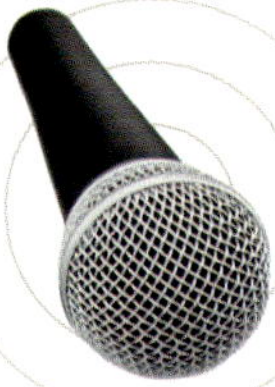

Improve your verbal skills

The ability to communicate with others is perhaps the single most valuable skill a person can have because it gives voice to the self. In prisons, solitary confinement—separating an individual from nearly all human contact—has been known to unloose men from their psychological moorings and drive them crazy. Most of us will never experience solitary confinement, of course, but even small reductions in our ability to communicate and express ourselves can be distressing. When we are speaking and suddenly forget a word or a name, for instance, we feel as if our brains are betraying us.

The tip-of-the-tongue phenomenon, in which the word or fact we want feels close by but just out of reach, is universal. The information is right there, encoded in nerve cell pathways in our brains; we just can't always access it when we want to, especially as we get older.

You don't have to feel backed into a verbal corner. The research clearly shows that people who practice mental tricks to help them remember—known as mnemonic strategies—have an easier time recalling words, names, and facts than people who wing it and hope for the best. You can improve your word recall in minutes simply by applying one of the techniques below. Psychologists used to think that there was a single best mnemonic, but new theories suggest that using *any* mnemonic technique is helpful. Read through them and try the one that fits your personal thinking style, or use more than one to meet different needs.

Smart Everyday Strategies

While you're working on your word skills with the exercises in this chapter, also learn and practice the following strategies, which will help ensure that you can access the words you need, when you need them.

Make up a story. For lists of words you want to remember short-term, such as a grocery list or a to-do list, experts recommend making up a story that links the words. The story should be as visual as possible (otherwise you're just creating words to remember other words) and as silly or ridiculous as you can imagine. For example, let's say you have three words to remember—lamp, strawberries, car. You could imagine turning on a lamp outdoors and finding strawberries growing inside the car and overflowing out the windows. The more imaginative or elaborate your mental pictures, the better your chances for remembering the items.

Group words together. For long lists of words that don't have to be memorized in order, group similar words together. You decide which categories to use. If you have a grocery list, you can "chunk" the items by location in the store, by food group, by size, by price, or by where you will store the items when you get home.

Listen for the name. When you meet someone for the first time and want to remember his name, the first step is to listen! Most people are so focused on making a good impression that they forget to pay attention to the person they are meeting. Focus on hearing the person's name. Immediately repeat the name ("Nice to meet you, Frank"), and use it again when addressing the person in conversation.

Let a name tell a story. When you hear the name, think about how the name sounds and what images it evokes. For example, if you meet Marina Taylor, you can easily visualize a marina full of boats, and a tailor sitting on the dock mending sails. You can take the exercise a step further to help you recall this person, and their name, in the future. If Marina is a red head, let every boat in the marina be painted red. It will be almost impossible to forget her name after such an elaborate visual image.

Not all names will be so easily translated into images. In those cases, use whatever associations come to mind. For example, if you meet Ted Sutton, who is balding, you might think that you have a cousin named Ted who is also balding. And that your cousin was married to a woman who used to live in New York City, which reminds you of Sutton Place. So you can imagine your cousin Ted sitting in the middle of a New York street.

Sound out difficult names. The first time you meet Wojciech Cieszko, you'll probably have a tough time coming up with a story that fits his name. In such a case, ask him to repeat his name slowly. As he does, sound it out in your head and imagine writing the phonetic spelling out on a slip of paper. Now, mentally staple the paper to a mental snapshot of the person.

exercises

Of all the memory problems people struggle with, weakened verbal skills may annoy us most because we use those skills every day. The exercises below make it possible to regain much of what was lost—and help prevent any further erosion.

IRREGULAR WORDS

For this exercise, you'll need a pen or pencil.

Below are groups of words. Within each group, one of the words does not fit in the same category as the others. Circle the irregular word.

1. Broccoli, Carrots, Spinach, Peas
2. Wristwatch, Bubble, Baseball, Globe
3. Eagle, Sparrow, Ostrich, Swan
4. Tennis, Ping-Pong, Polo, Volleyball
5. Antagonize, Anger, Inspire, Infuriate
6. Braille, Morse Code, Dominoes, Zebras
7. Duck, Badger, Camel, Hog
8. Tree, Ball, Watch, Mitt
9. Plant, Car, Money, Cash
10. Television, Magazine, Baseball Game, Movie
11. Tea Kettle, Whistle, Bathtub, Bird
12. Plant, Pipe, Brain, Toenail
13. Ice Skates, Roller Skates, Knife, Razor
14. Boat, Kickboard, Sunglasses, Wine Cork

Answers on page 266

LINKUP

Below is a series of analogies. It's up to you to fill in the blanks. We've helped by providing the correct number of spaces needed.

DOWNPOUR is to RAIN as BLIZZARD is to: ___ ___ ___ ___

2. DOLLAR is to CENT as CENTURY is to: ___ ___ ___ ___

3. RECIPES is to COOKBOOK as MAPS is to: ___ ___ ___ ___ ___

4. BASEBALL is to BAT as TENNIS is to: ___ ___ ___ ___ ___ ___

5. BLUE is to SAPPHIRE as RED is to: ___ ___ ___ ___

6. COUGAR is to LEAP as WHALE is to: ___ ___ ___ ___ ___ ___

7. HEN is to ROOSTER as FILLY is to: ___ ___ ___ ___

8. MOON is to CRATER as PAVEMENT is to: ___ ___ ___ ___ ___ ___ ___

9. SPIDER is to CRAWL as SNAKE is to: ___ ___ ___ ___ ___ ___ ___

10. CANDY is to SUGAR as TIRE is to: ___ ___ ___ ___ ___ ___

11. AIRPLANE is to PILOT as LIMOUSINE is to: ___ ___ ___ ___ ___ ___ ___ ___ ___

12. HERD is to BUFFALO as GAGGLE is to: ___ ___ ___ ___ ___

13. SOLAR SYSTEM is to SUN as ATOM is to ___ ___ ___ ___ ___ ___ ___

14. ACROPHOBIA is to HEIGHTS as PYROPHOBIA is to: ___ ___ ___ ___

15. DOUGHNUT is to HOLE as IRIS is to: ___ ___ ___ ___ ___

16. EQUINE is to HORSE as AQUILINE is to: ___ ___ ___ ___ ___

17. TETHER is to BALL as CORD is to ___ ___ ___ ___ ___

Answers on page 266

CIRCLE-GRAMS

Try to find the word formed by the letters. Hint: The trick is figuring out where to start.

1.

U Q Y T I L A

2.

L A E R E Z I

3.

R V E D E S E

4.

T S I N A I P

5.

H C S E S E E

6.

A T E R T H E

7.

U F E P O H L

8.

M O S U O N I

9.

O D B A N E M

Answers on page 266

OPPOSITES ATTRACT

Match each word with its antonym by writing a number next to each letter.

Opposites Attract #1

1. Elated	____a. Ally
2. Inspired	____b. Support
3. Lazy	____c. Beneficial
4. Obscure	____d. Acknowledge
5. Adversary	____e. Dejected
6. Pernicious	____f. Industrious
7. Oppose	____g. Ornery
8. Deny	____h. Ignore
9. Address	____i. Evident
10. Affable	____j. Unmotivated

Opposites Attract #2

1. Futile	____a. Yield
2. Penitent	____b. Disparaging
3. Boldness	____c. Unseemly
4. Agreeable	____d. Contrary
5. Defy	____e. Remorseless
6. Incessant	____f. Loquacious
7. Taciturn	____g. Useful
8. Careless	____h. Cowardice
9. Elegant	____i. Thoughtful
10. Fawning	____j. Intermittent

KISSING COUSINS

Match each word with its synonym by writing a number next to each letter.

Kissing Cousins #1

1. Settle	____a. Resist
2. Entreat	____b. Compromise
3. Acquiesce	____c. Grave
4. Dismiss	____d. Coarse
5. Peevish	____e. Wander
6. Vulgar	____f. Enlarge
7. Rome	____g. Petulant
8. Oppose	____h. Implore
9. Amplify	____i. Ignore
10. Solemn	____j. Comply

Kissing Cousins #2

1. Egotism	____a. Evasiveness
2. Grateful	____b. Rugged
3. Approach	____c. Fixed
4. Rough	____d. Overstate
5. Immobile	____e. Unwavering
6. Imitate	____f. Vainglory
7. Secrecy	____g. Vanquished
8. Exaggerate	____h. Advance
9. Persistent	____i. Mirror
10. Conquered	____j. Appreciative

Answers on page 267

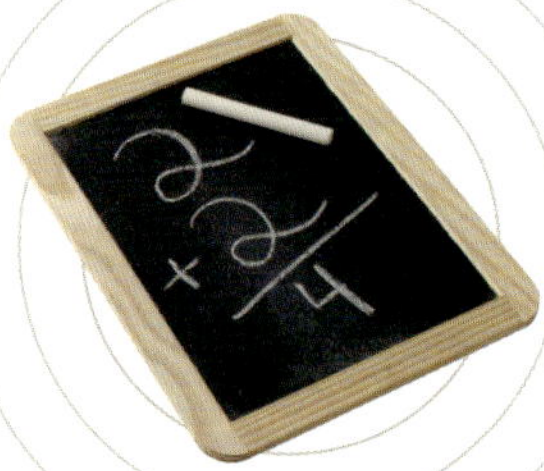

Improve your number skills

In 2006, a Japanese man set a new world record by reciting the pi, that never-ending mathematical number (taught in school as 3.14159), to 100,000 decimal places—from memory. It took him 16 hours. So why do many of us have so much trouble recalling a simple phone number?

We know that people can hold about seven digits in their working, or short-term, memory. That's why phone numbers have seven digits. Most of the time, we commit frequently used phone numbers to long-term memory simply by dialing them over and over again. But remembering other numbers from one day to the next requires a strategy. The best strategies involve finding a way to relate to the numbers, understand them, and partner them with other pieces of information so they become meaningful (and therefore memorable), instead of random.

Research shows that using number strategies can improve memory skills tremendously, and scientists have worked hard to find the best technique. Researchers from the Karolinska Institute in Stockholm, Sweden, discovered the secret: There is no single best memory strategy. As long as you use some strategy, your memory for numbers will improve significantly.

Smart Everyday Strategies

There are several classic ways to remember numbers beyond the two listed here, but we find them awfully complicated. One involves substituting words for numbers, which takes a great deal of practice. You can use the two strategies here right away.

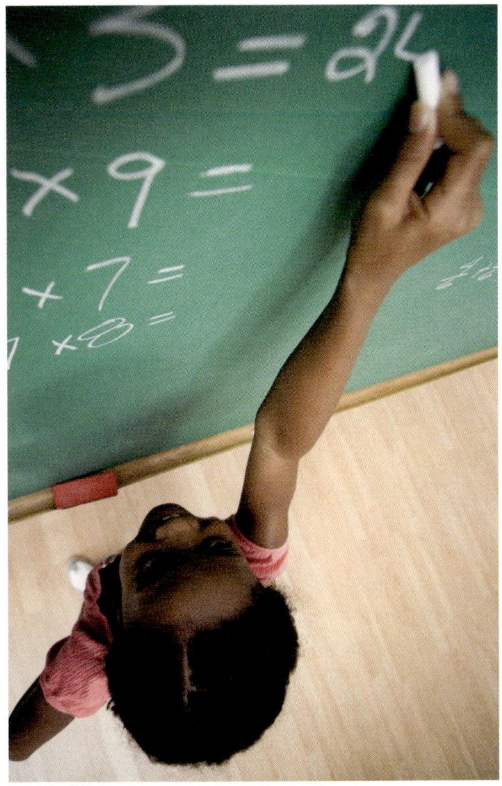

Give them meaning. Many math junkies are particularly good at remembering numbers because they manage to find meaning in them. For instance, show a math wizard the number 4824 and he might immediately think, four-digit number with the first two digits doubling the second two. If you don't happen to be gifted in this manner, find a different way to relate to the number. For example, a history buff may relate all numbers to significant dates, a librarian may place numbers in the context of the Dewey Decimal System, and a football fan may associate them with a favorite player's numbers or game scores. You can also relate them to the ages and birthdates of family members, or any other numbers you know that pop quickly to mind.

"Chunk" them. Chunking larger numbers into small groups makes them easier to remember. Think of a phone number. In the United States, we break the number down into three chunks: an area code followed by three digits followed by four digits (555-231-1002). We read them aloud in the same chunks, and we expect people to say them in the same chunks. It can be confusing to hear or see a phone number presented differently. For example, 55-523-11002 is the same number, but it looks and sounds different and seems unwieldy. Learn to see and hear numbers in chunks that make sense for you.

exercises

If you don't work with numbers in your job, then you probably don't get enough of a chance to become comfortable with them. This is a relatively easy memory category, quite amenable to improvement. But it is also the one area that can evoke strong responses in some people. If you had bad experiences with math classes when you were in school, you may still be harboring some number phobia. Don't worry, you're not going to be tested—these exercises are for your benefit. Relax, take it slowly, and you'll be fine.

PIN MANIA

These days, most of us have far too many PINs (personal identification numbers) to remember. Take a look at each of the four PINs below, and try to make an association with the number to help you remember it. Once you've thought of something solid, move on to the puzzle, "Words and Numbers" on page 253, then turn back to page 252 to see if you can write in the PIN numbers you memorized.

For example: 7613

A person familiar with the song "Seventy-Six Trombones" from *The Music Man* might think of that song for the first two digits. Someone with a 13-year-old child might use the child's age to remember the second two.

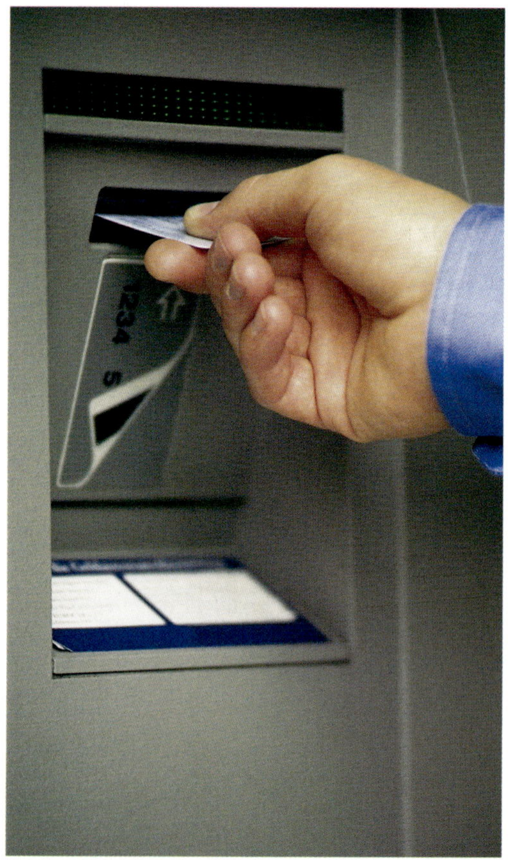

PIN Mania #1

Richard's ATM PIN: 4923

PIN Mania #2

Edwin's e-mail PIN: 403214

PIN Mania #3

Michelle's online banking PIN: 120489

PIN Mania #4

Eric's online travel site PIN: 52547

CALLER ID

Who's calling? Look at the names and phone numbers below. Try to remember which phone numbers are whose. Then turn to page 252 and see how well you do.

Caller ID #1

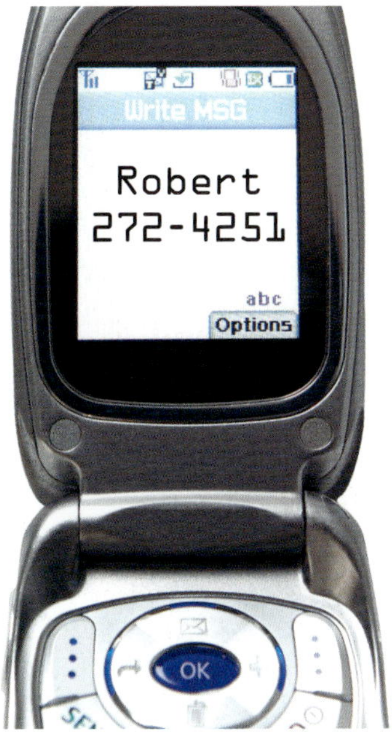
Write MSG
Robert
272-4251
abc
Options

Caller ID #2

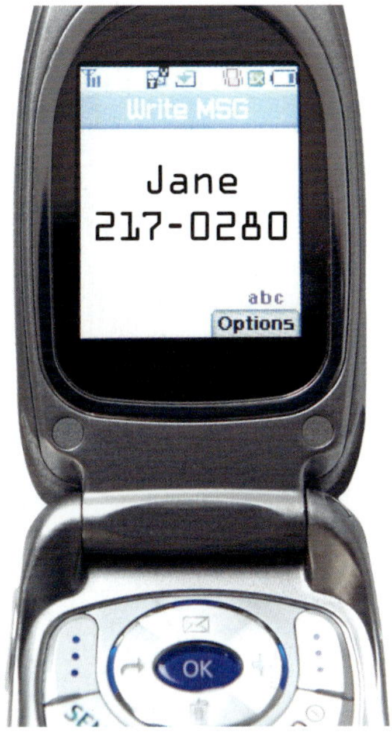
Write MSG
Jane
217-0280
abc
Options

Caller ID #3

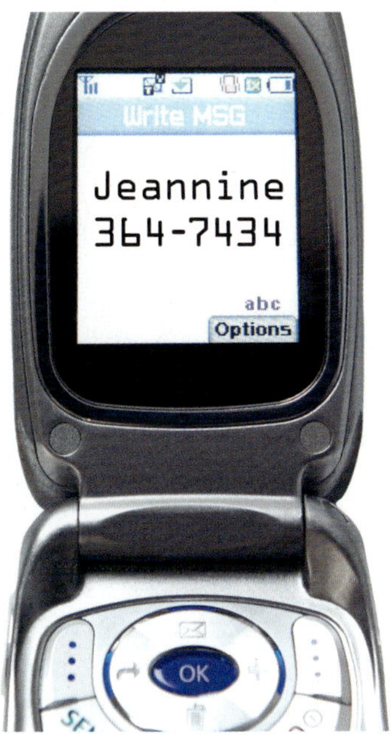
Write MSG
Jeannine
364-7434
abc
Options

Caller ID #4

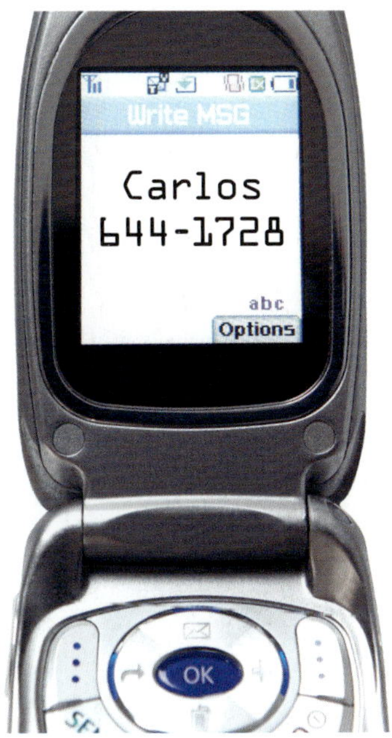

PIN MANIA (CONTINUED)

Write down the numbers you remember, then turn back to page 250 to see how you did.

PIN Mania #1

Richard's ATM PIN: ____________

PIN Mania #2

Edwin's e-mail PIN: ____________

PIN Mania #3

Michelle's online banking PIN: ____________

PIN Mania #4

Eric's online travel site PIN: ____________

CALLER ID (CONTINUED)

Circle the correct name for each the numbers, then turn back to page 251 to see how you did.

Caller ID #1

272-4251

A. Jane
B. Carlos
C. Robert
D. Jeannine

Caller ID #2

217-0280

A. Jane
B. Carlos
C. Robert
D. Jeannine

Caller ID #3

364-7434

A. Jane
B. Carlos
C. Robert
D. Jeannine

Caller ID #4

644-1728

A. Jane
B. Carlos
C. Robert
D. Jeannine

WORDS AND NUMBERS

These exercises will help you solve everyday problems involving numbers.

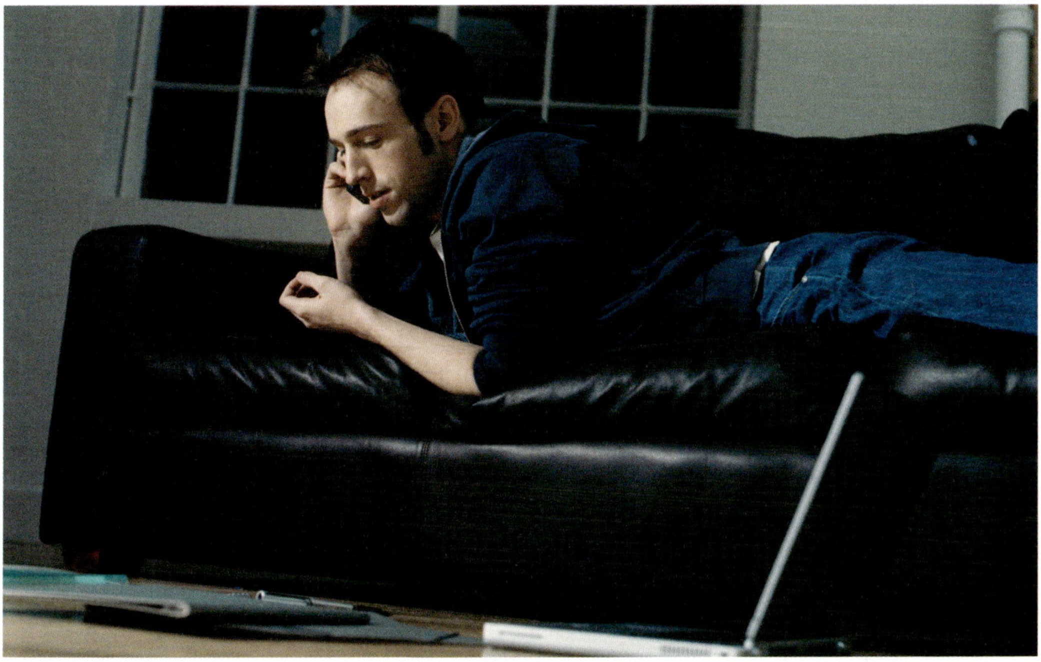

Words and Numbers #1

Dan is a full-time college student who has a part-time job. His girlfriend lives hundreds of miles away. On a particular day, his classes end at 4 p.m., after which he immediately drives to his job, arrives at 4:15 p.m., and works for 3 1/2 hours, plus a 45-minute break for dinner. After work, he drives straight home, immediately starts studying and continues studying for 2 hours and 10 minutes, and then telephones his girlfriend at 11 p.m. How long was Dan's drive from work to his home?

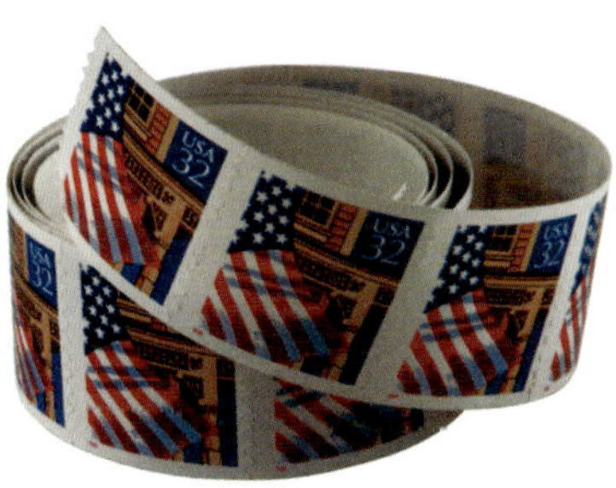

Words and Numbers #2

Dorothy loves entering contests by mail. She had an old roll of 100 42-cent stamps and used 55 of them before the rate went up to 44 cents per letter. If she already has 7 1-cent stamps and 8 2-cent stamps, how much does she have to spend on additional postage so she can use her remaining 42-cent stamps to mail her contest entries?

Answers on page 267

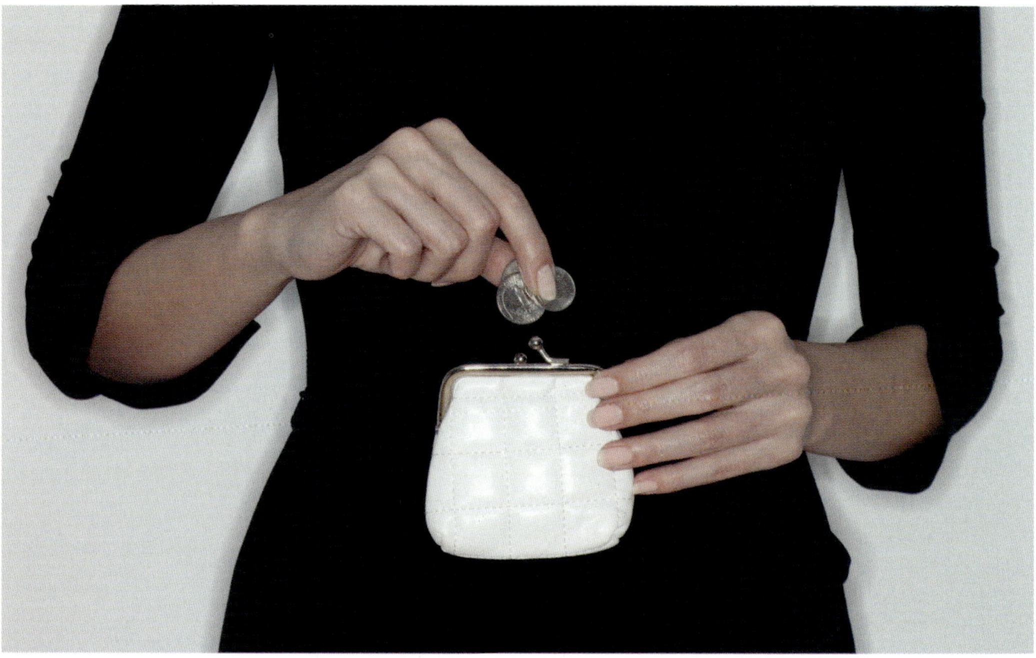

Words and Numbers #3

Jacqueline has 11 coins in her purse, all pennies, dimes, or quarters, and doesn't have any combination of coins that add up to exactly $1.00. If the total value of her coins is more than $1.00, how many each of pennies, dimes, and quarters does she have?

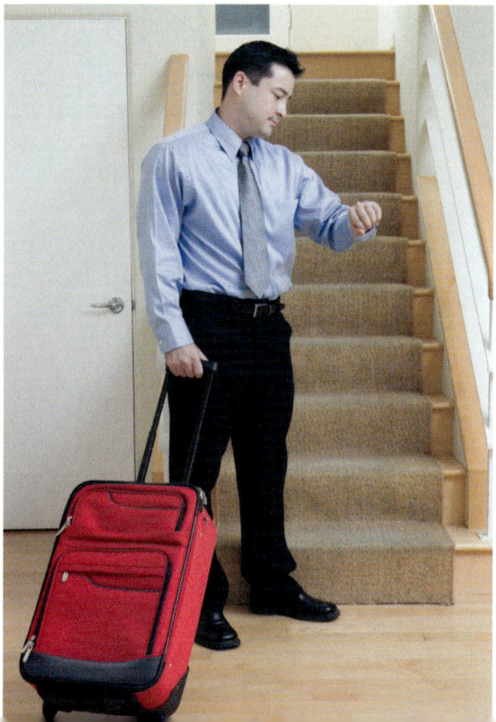

Words and Numbers #4

A certain airline has a weight limit of 20 pounds for a piece of carry-on baggage. Marc's empty suitcase weighs 1 pound, and he has these items that he'd like to put in it for his flight:

Jar of snacks: 2 pounds
Travel iron: 3 pounds
Crossword dictionary: 4 pounds
Gift for his mother: 7 pounds
Laptop computer: 9 pounds

Which of these items should he take, if he'd like to take as much (by weight) as possible?

Answers on page 267

HOW DOES IT ADD UP?

Place arithmetic symbols (plus, minus, times, or divided by) between the numbers in each group below to get the result asked for.

Example:
2, 3, 4, 5 to get 19

Answer:
2 x 3 x 4 – 5 = 19

1.

8, 6, 4, 11 to get 4

2.

10, 3, 8, 2 to get 30

3.

9, 2, 8, 4, 10 to get 50

4.

15, 5, 11, 6, 5 to get 100

5.

5, 4, 2, 4, 6 to get 6

6.

12, 2, 8, 4, 3, 4 to get 0

Answers on page 267

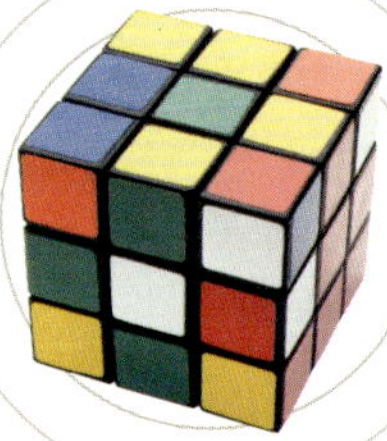

Improve your reasoning skills

Whether we realize it or not, we use reasoning skills every day. Reasoning actually involves various sets of skills, such as categorizing information (that animal looks feline, so it must be a cat), evaluating logic (if that man has only one arm, he could not have been the one to carry the heavy timber into the garage), extrapolation (if a robber robs one house on Monday, two houses on Tuesday, and three houses on Wednesday, he will probably rob four houses on Thursday), and good old problem solving.

From the time we are old enough to think, our brains start looking for patterns in the seemingly random events of life. We also amass information we can draw on later. Every fact we learn and every problem we solve improves our ability to reason. In that way—experience by experience, decision by decision—we make sense of the world.

The evidence isn't clear about whether we lose the power to think logically and solve difficult problems as we get older, but research shows that everyone—young and old alike—benefits from training and practice.

exercises

If you are not accustomed to doing brain gymnastics, then you may find this section particularly difficult. But remember that challenging your brain is the way to make it more capable. Think of these exercises as interesting puzzles to be solved. If you get tired or frustrated, stop and come back to it another day.

LOGICAL OR NOT?

This exercise requires that you pay attention to the story and follow the logic from sentence to sentence. First, read the paragraph and decide if all sentences are logical given the rest of the text. If not, underline the sentence or sentences that don't make sense.

Logical or Not #1

Betty and Bill were having Diane and Dave over that Wednesday evening to get the details on their recent vacation, so Bill put a $20 bill in his pocket and strolled over to Wally's, the local grocery store, to pick up a few things that they needed. But Wally's was closed when he got there—Bill had forgotten that Wally's closes early on weekends. So Bill had to walk clear across town, to the Mammoth Market, to get what he needed. He bought three varieties of cheese, corn chips, and a six-pack of cola. He paid the total cost of $19.75 with his credit card, put everything in his trunk, and went right home. As soon as he got home, Diane called to postpone dinner until the following week.

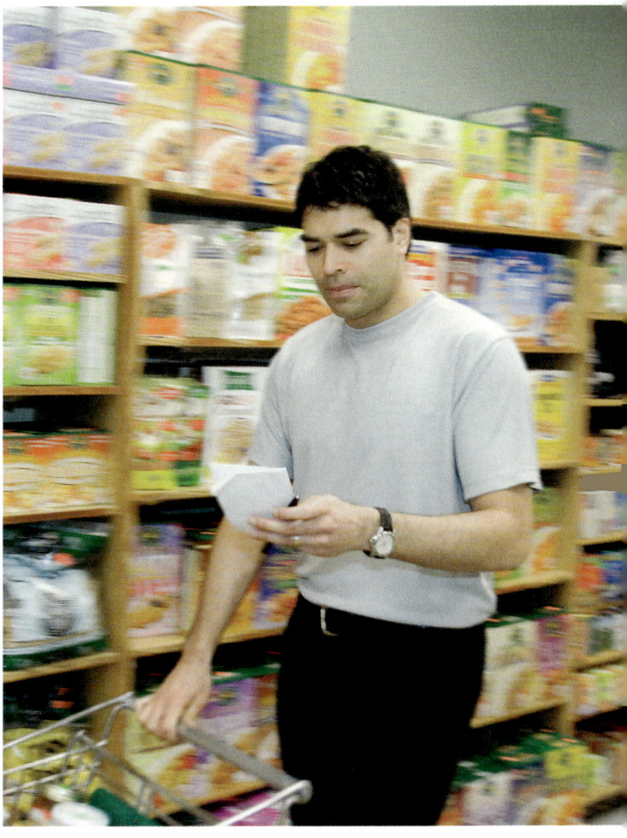

Answer on page 267

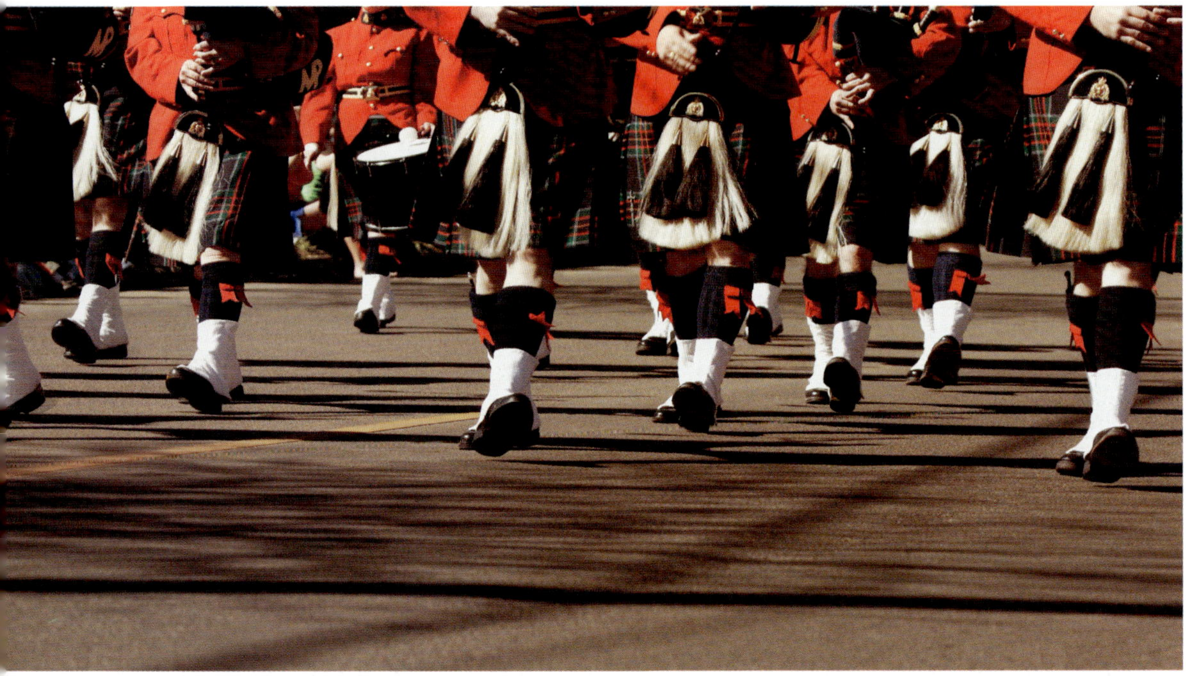

Logical or Not #2

The semiannual St. Patrick's Day celebration in our town is eagerly awaited by one and all. It doesn't matter if you're from Iceland or not, everyone joins in the festivities. The fun starts early in the morning, with the traditional green-egg breakfast (thanks to some food coloring!) served by our mayor in the town square. The parade starts at 10 a.m. and lasts for about 2 hours. There is the marching band, of course, with all the flutes, tubas, cellos, and trumpets, and elaborately constructed floats on which men in kilts play accordions. The nonmusical marchers include representatives from the public schools, civic associations, and the police and fire departments, with the Grand Marshall in his green limousine at the very end. Then, everyone rushes to McSweeney's restaurant for the traditional corned beef and cabbage dinner.

Logical or Not #3

Since I've retired, I've become a pretty active user of the Internet and get a lot of my news online, but I still like getting the newspaper every weekday morning (I'm much too busy on weekends to sit down with the paper). So my "newspaper week" starts every Monday morning. The paper arrives like clockwork at 6 a.m., which suits me fine since I'm an early riser. So, with my Monday morning cup of coffee in hand, I read the newspaper from Page 1 to the back cover, including the sports news, local and international news, stock-market listings, comic strips, and, of course, the daily crossword. After a quick breakfast, I kiss my wife good-bye and take the bus to the office.

Answers on page 267

Logical or Not #4

You know what a big tennis fan I am. So it was a happy coincidence that my husband and I arrived in Auckland on July 10th, the day before the Australian Open tennis tournament. As soon as we checked in at our hotel, I took a cab to the stadium, bought tickets for me and my wife, and hurried back to the hotel for dinner.

The tournament is held on two main courts. It's a good thing that they both have retractable roofs, so they can close them if there's rain or it gets too hot. Boy, can it get hot during the tournament! Nevertheless, when we went to bed, I was so excited about the tournament that I couldn't sleep.

Logical or Not #5

They call it the waiting room for a reason, you know. Waiting an hour or more to be seen by your doctor is most people's idea of fun. That's why I always bring lots of things to do. Usually, I fill a tote bag with stuff like knitting, magazines, candles, and stationery to catch up on my letter writing. Sometimes, thankfully not too often, there are actually more people waiting than there are seats in the waiting room. When that happens, I walk to the library just a block away and browse the fiction section for the newest books from my favorite authors. The last time I was there, I took out two whodunits, the latest John Grisham legal thriller, and a dieting book.

Answers on page 267

Logical or Not #6

Our neighbors recommended we try Mario's Italian restaurant, which just opened downtown. They raved about it: "Great food, great service, great prices—what more can you ask for?" So we had to check it out for ourselves. It really was everything they said it was. We were greeted warmly by Mario himself the moment we walked in the door: "Welcome back, Mr. and Mrs. Williams." The menu was enormous, with five pages of main courses alone. We finally decided what to order. Michele had the veal Marsala, and I decided on the moussaka. The food was great, the portions were huge, and the bill was really reasonable. So we've added Luigi's to our list of dining favorites.

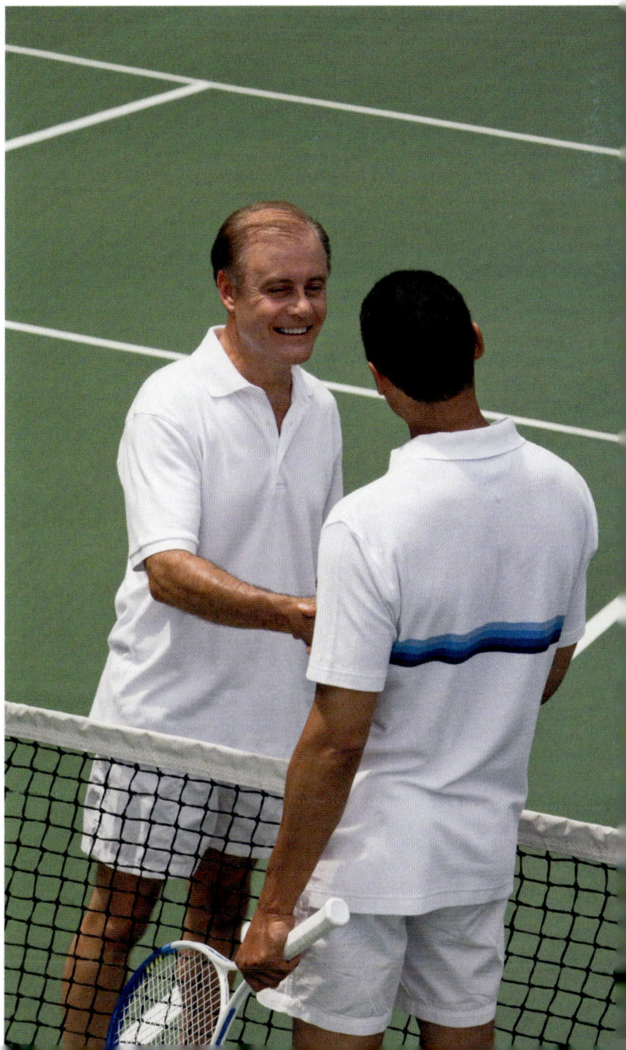

IF/THEN

You may have to strain your brain a bit to answer these word problems.

If/Then #1

Bill's sock drawer has eight pairs of socks in it, each pair has a different pattern, and they're scattered about individually in the drawer. There's a power failure in his home one night, just as he opens the drawer to take out a pair of socks. He takes nine socks out of the drawer, but he can't see them, since the room is dark. Does he have at least one matching pair of socks among the nine?

Answer:____________________________

If/Then #2

If in a yearly calendar of events National Egg Month comes before National Peanut Butter Month, National Strawberry Month comes after National Sweet Potato Month, and National Sweet Potato Month comes after National Egg Month, is National Egg Month before or after National Strawberry Month, or do we not have enough information to tell?

Answer:____________________________

If/Then #3

If we know that Brazil has more people than Russia, Russia has more people than Mexico, and Mexico has fewer people than Pakistan, does Brazil or Pakistan have more people, or do we not have enough information to tell?

Answer:____________________________

If/Then #4

If Amber's birthday is February 20, and her classmate Amanda was born 10 days later in the same year, do we know what Amanda's birthday is?

Answer:____________________________

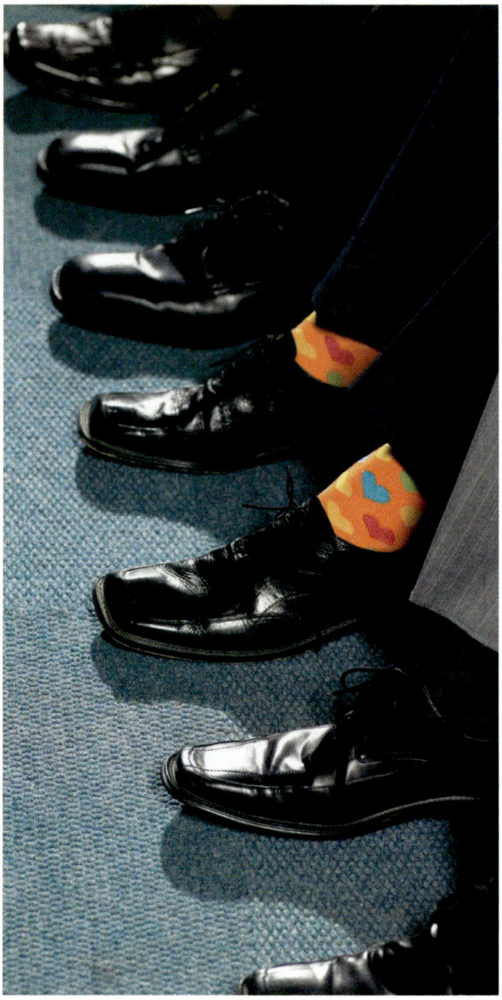

If/Then #5

If City B is due east of City A, City C is due north of city B, city D is due south of city B, and City E is due south of City A, what is the direction from City C to City D, or do we not have enough information to tell?

Answer:____________________________

Answers on page 267

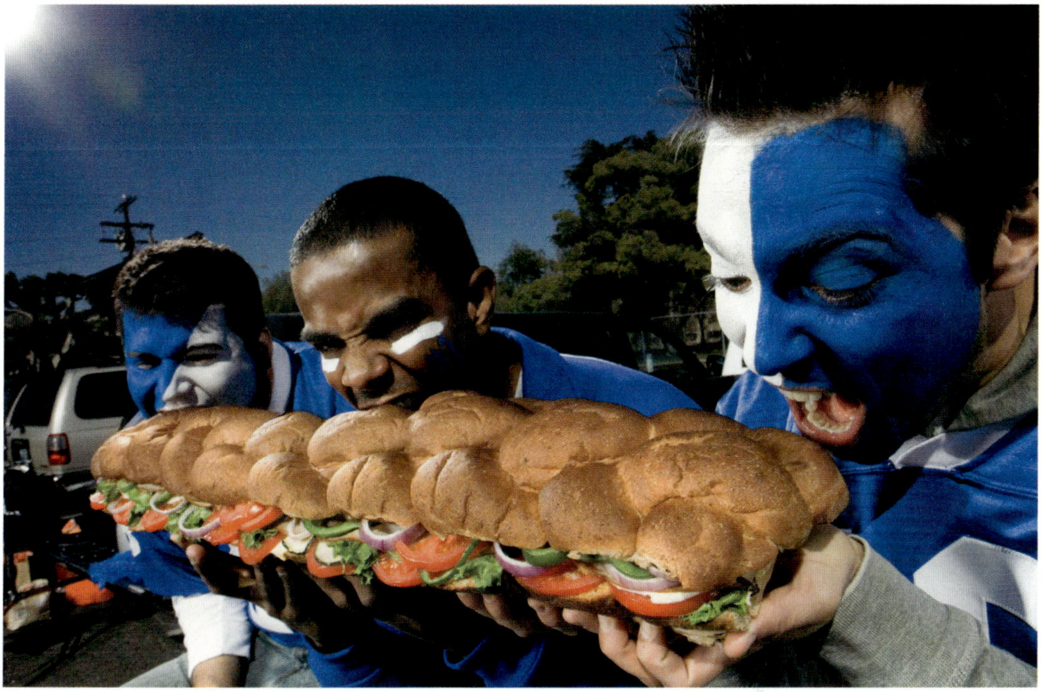

If/Then #6

A certain restaurant's lunch menu has three choices for sandwiches: tuna fish for $3, chicken salad for $4, and ham for $5. Three friends come into the restaurant for lunch, and each one orders a sandwich. If the total cost for the three sandwiches ordered is $10, do we know how many of each sandwich was ordered?

Answer:______________________________

If/Then #7

If we know that a bushel of wheat weighs more than a bushel of oats, a bushel of barley weighs less than a bushel of shelled corn, and a bushel of oats weighs more than a bushel of shelled corn, what weighs more, a bushel of wheat or a bushel of shelled corn, or do we not have enough information to tell?

Answer:______________________________

If/Then #8

The gas tank in Marie's car holds 20 gallons. Her car gets 15 miles per gallon in city driving and 25 miles per gallon in highway driving. If she drives 250 miles on a half-tank of gas, do we know how many highway miles and city miles she drove?

Answer:______________________________

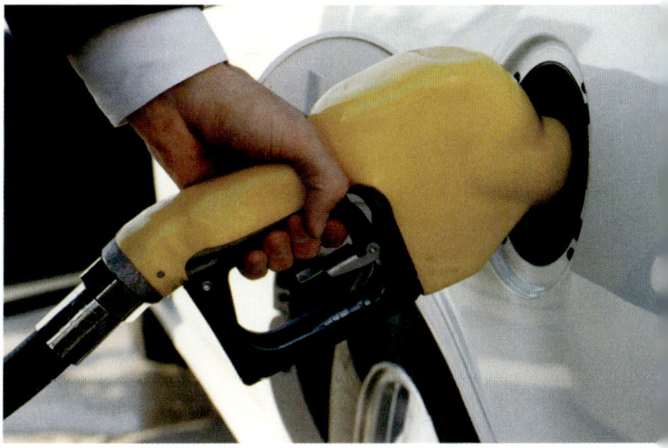

Answers on page 267

SEATING PLAN

Kate and Larry are getting married. It's your job to help them design a seating plan for the table at which their relatives will sit—but there are a few restrictions. See if you can figure out who should sit where.

People to seat:

Kate's Aunt Alice and Uncle Bob (married couple)

Larry's Cousin Carl

Kate's Cousin Dave

Larry's Aunt Ella and Uncle Frank (married couple)

Kate's Uncle George

Larry's Aunt Harriet

Kate's Cousin Ida

Larry's Uncle Jack

Seating restrictions (in order of importance)

1. All of Kate's relatives sit together, and all of Larry's relatives sit together
2. Married couples must sit together
3. Cousin Dave plays in a rock band and wants to sit as close to the band as possible
4. You're trying to get Cousin Carl to date Cousin Ida, so seat them together
5. Uncle Frank isn't talking to Uncle Jack, so they can't sit next to each other
6. Uncle George owes money to Cousin Dave, so he wants to sit as far from Dave as possible
7. Uncle Bob hasn't seen Uncle George for 20 years, and they have a lot to catch up on

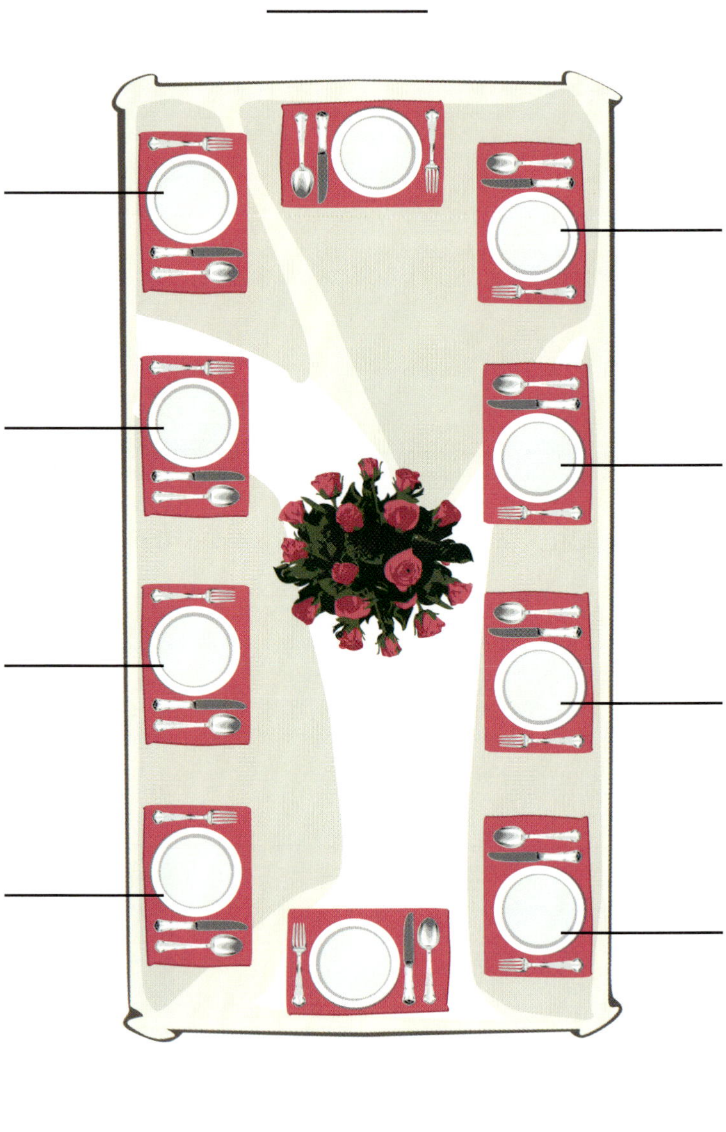

ROCK BAND

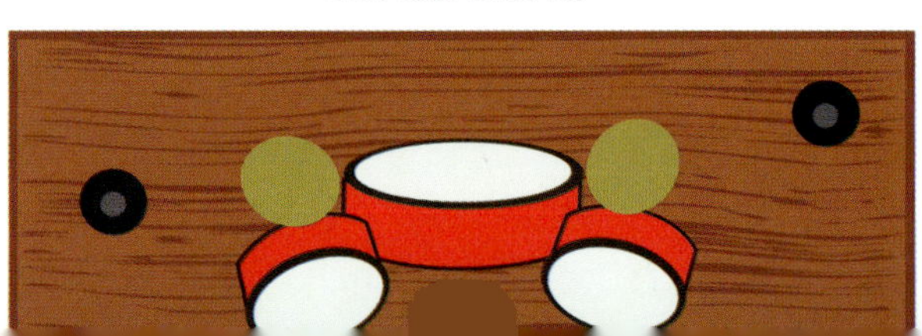

Answers on page 267

NEXT IN LINE

Study the sequence below and figure out which image should come next.

1.

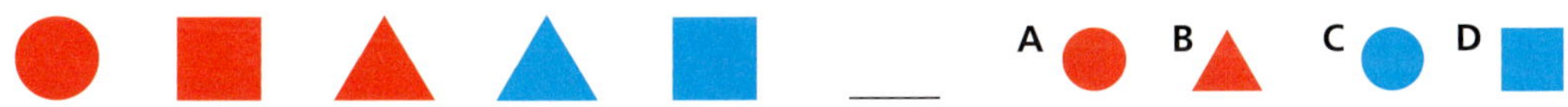

2.

3.

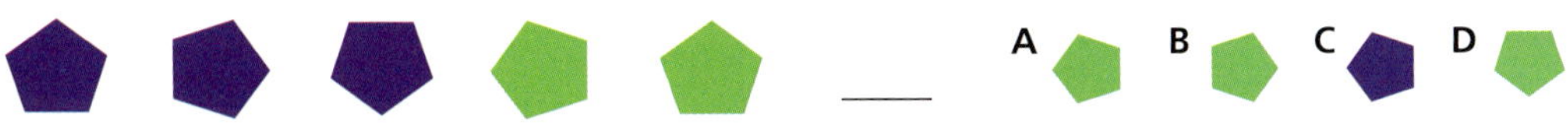

4.

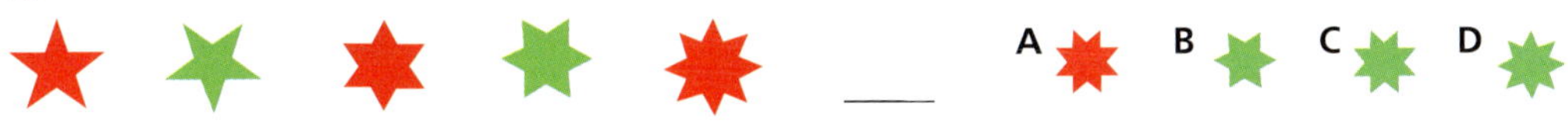

5.

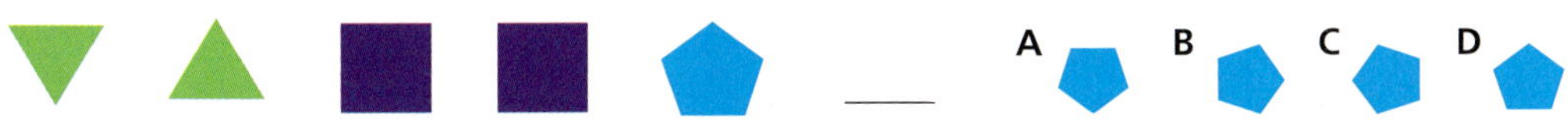

6.

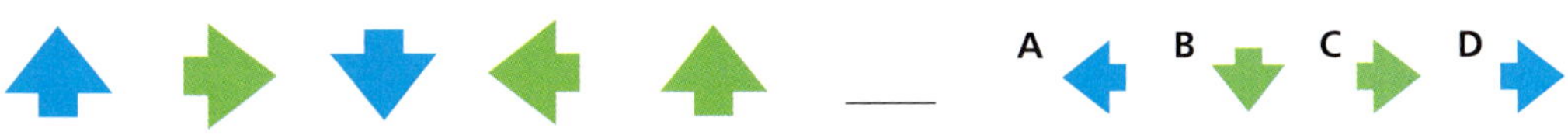

7.

8.

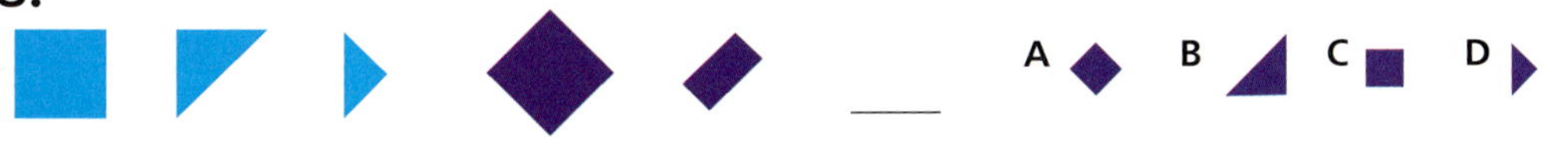

9.

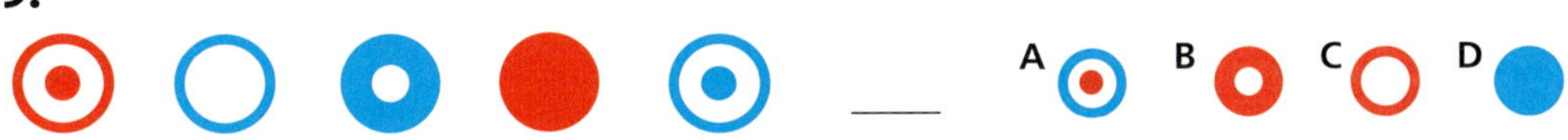

10.

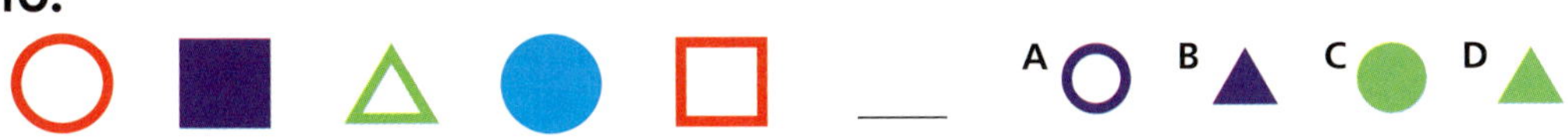

Answers on page 267

answers

Stack Tracking #1

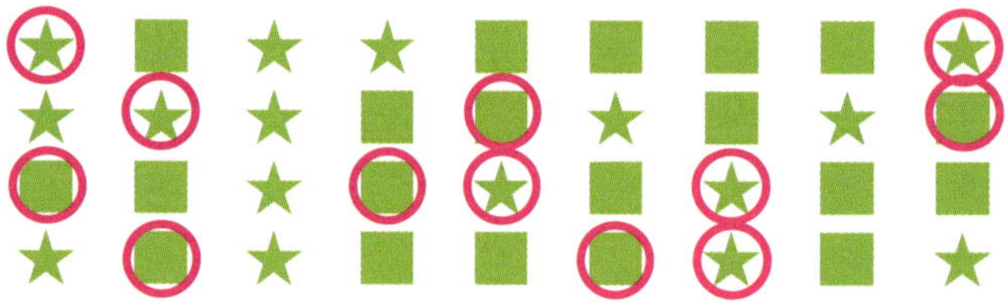

Stack Tracking #2

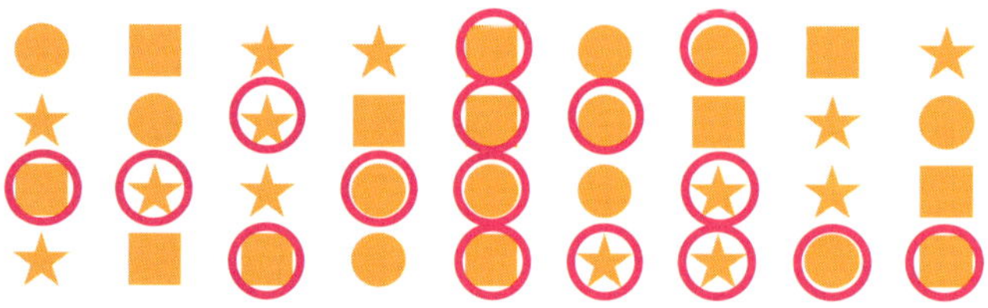

Stack Tracking #3

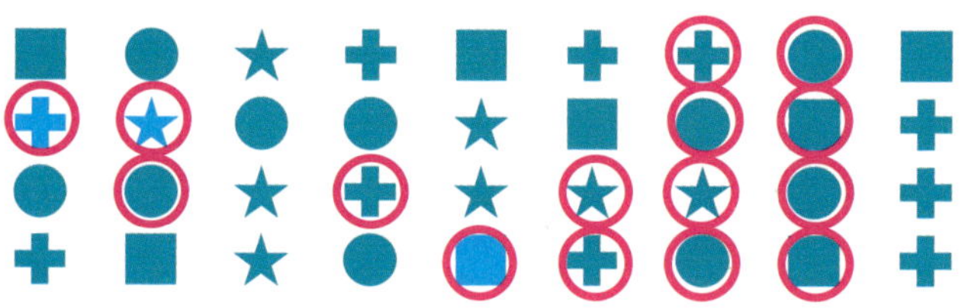

Stack Tracking #4

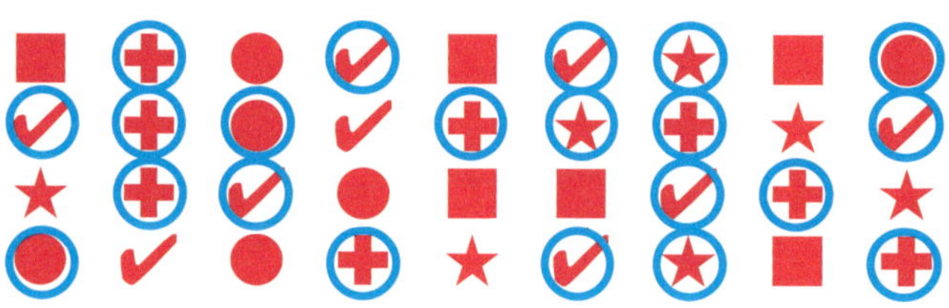

Stack Tracking #5

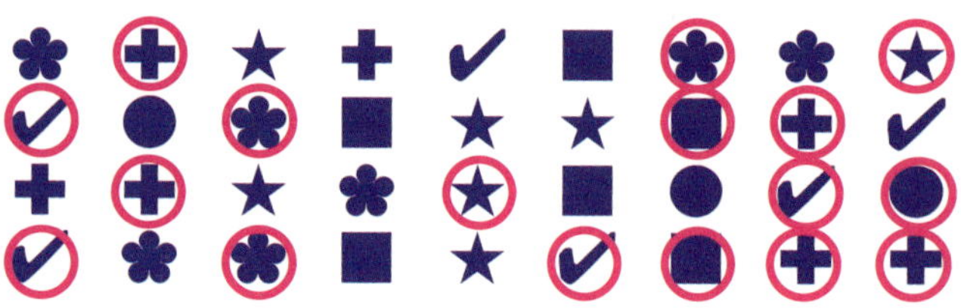

One Among Many #1

second row, third item:

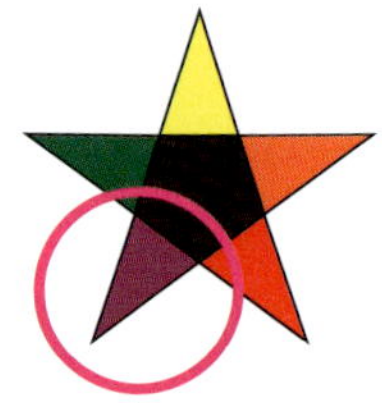

One Among Many #2

second row, fourth item:

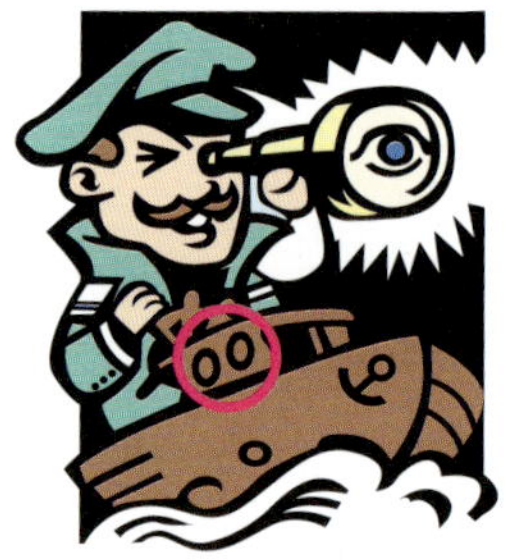

One Among Many #3

first row, third item:

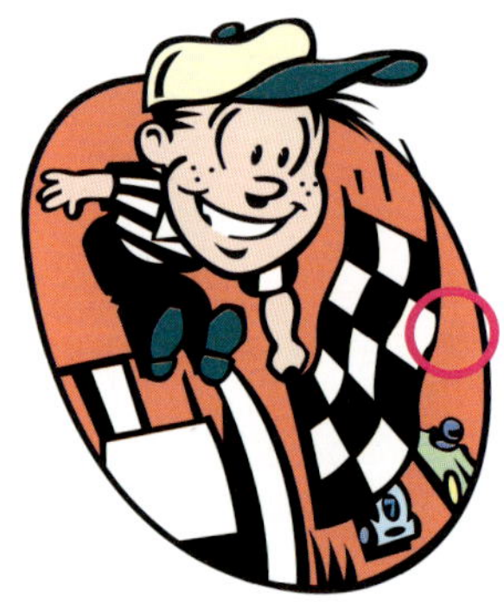

One Among Many #4

first row, second item:

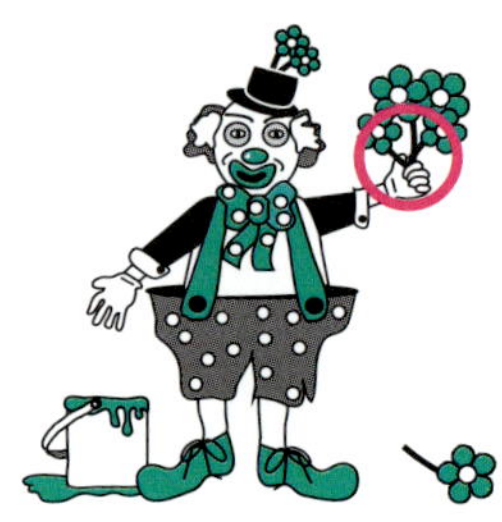

One Among Many #5

second row, second item:

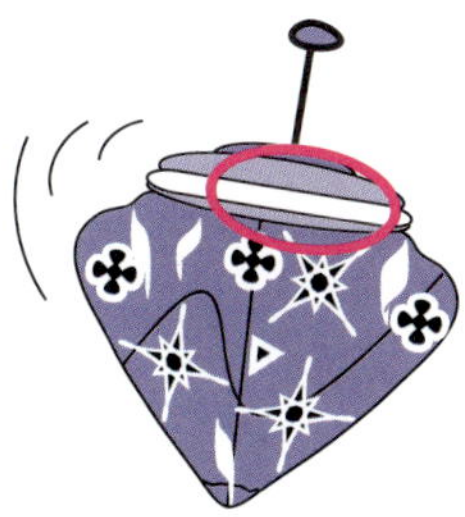

One Among Many #6

first row, third item:

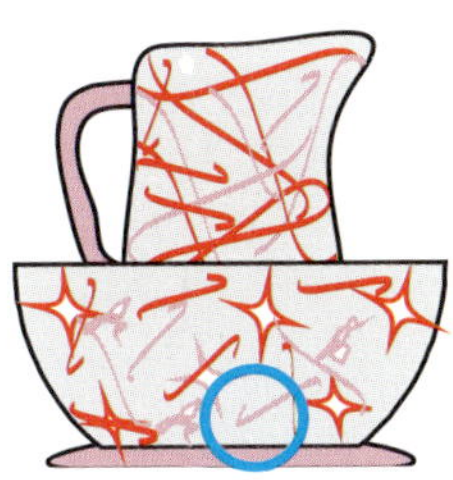

Picture Imperfect #1

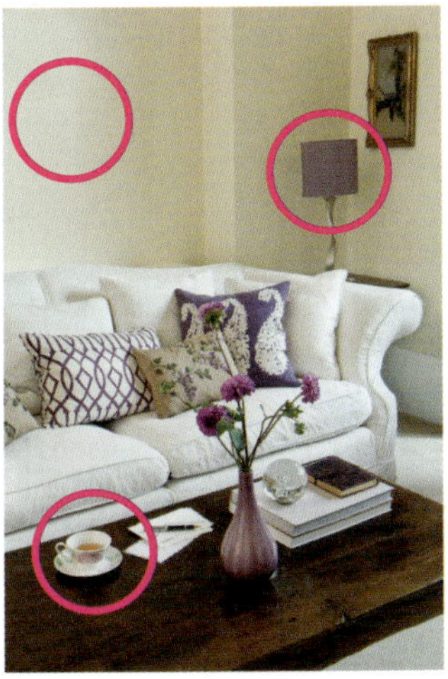

Picture Imperfect #2

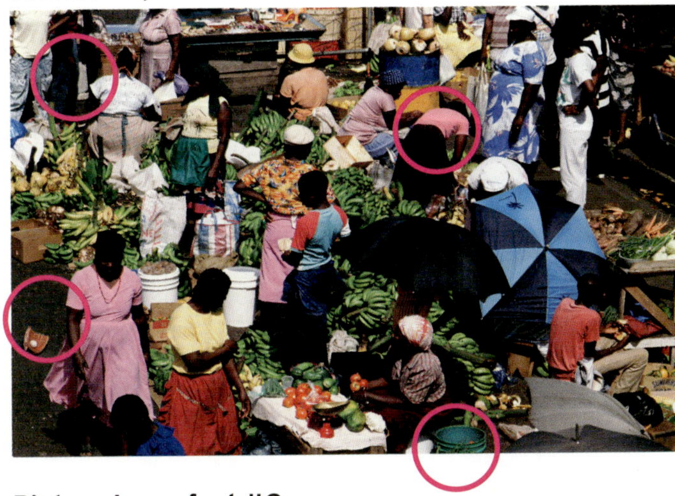

Picture Imperfect #3

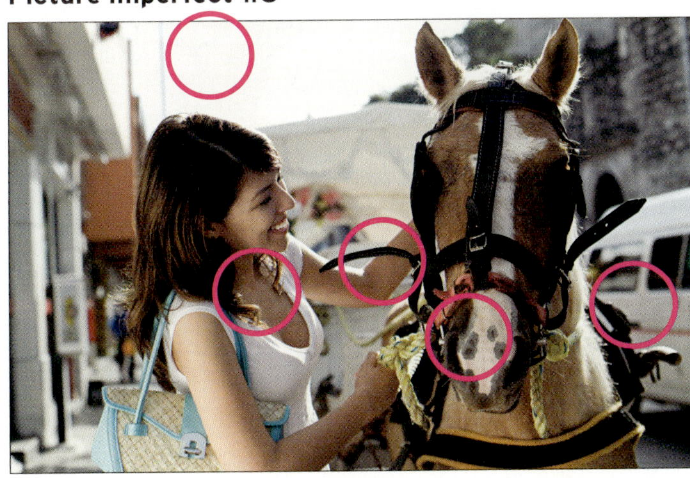

Picture Imperfect #4

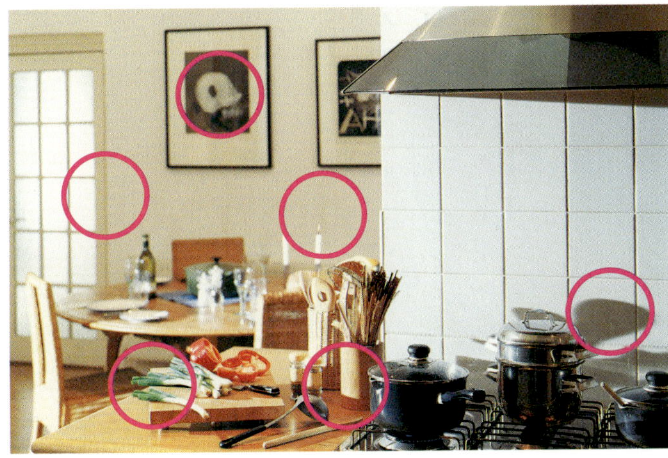

Picture Perfect #1

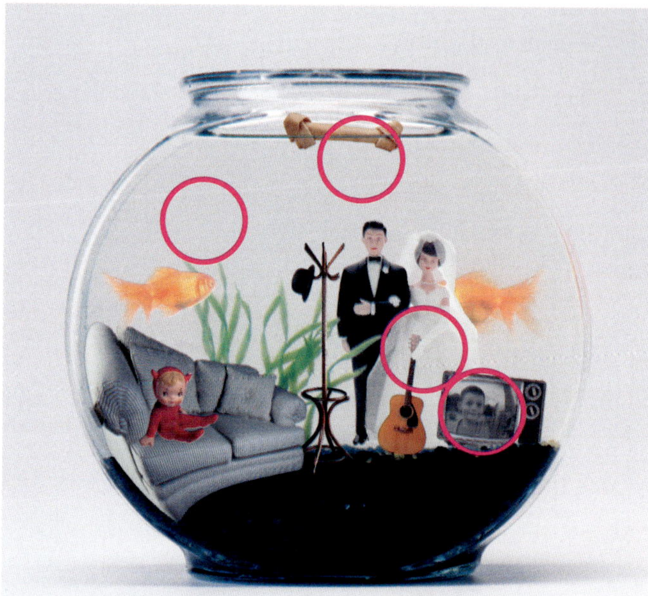

Picture Perfect #2

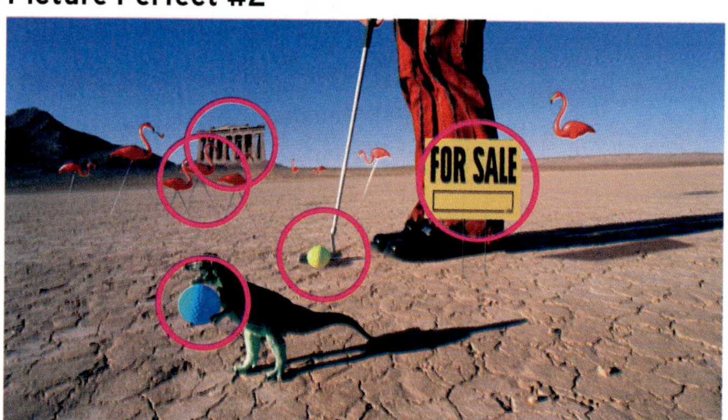

Picture Perfect #3

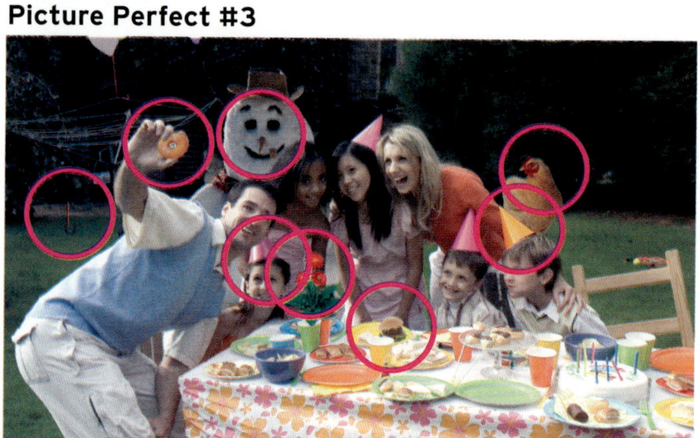

Letter Search #1

43 capitals, 33 lowercase, 6 red

Letter Search #2

28 capitals, 30 lowercase, 6 blue

Letter Search #3

10 capitals, 32 lowercase, 7 green

Irregular Words

1. Carrots (not green)
2. Wristwatch (not spherical)
3. Ostrich (can't fly)
4. Polo (not played with a net)
5. Inspire (not negative)
6. Zebras (don't have dots)
7. Camel (not a verb)
8. Watch (not four letters)
9. Money (the only word without the vowel "a")
10. Magazine (not something you watch)
11. Bathtub (doesn't make noise)
12. Pipe (doesn't grow)
13. Roller skates (aren't sharp)
14. Sunglasses (don't float)

Linkup

1. snow 2. year 3. atlas
4. racket 5. ruby 6. breach
7. colt 8. pothole 9. slither
10. rubber 11. chauffeur
12. geese 13. nucleus
14. fire 15. pupil 16. eagle
17. phone

Circle-Grams

1. quality 2. realize 3. deserve
4. pianist 5. cheeses
6. theater 7. hopeful
8. ominous 9. abdomen

Opposites Attract #1
1. e **2.** j **3.** f **4.** i **5.** a **6.** c
7. b **8.** d **9.** h **10.** g

Opposites Attract #2
1. g **2.** e **3.** h **4.** d **5.** a **6.** j
7. f **8.** i **9.** c **10.** b

Kissing Cousins #1
1. b **2.** h **3.** j **4.** i **5.** g **6.** d
7. e **8.** a **9.** f **10.** c

Kissing Cousins #2
1. f **2.** j **3.** h **4.** b **5.** c **6.** i
7. a **8.** d **9.** e **10.** g

Words and Numbers #1
20 minutes

Words and Numbers #2
67 cents

Words and Numbers #3
4 pennies, 4 dimes, 3 quarters

Words and Numbers #4
Travel iron, gift for mother, and laptop computer.
Total weight: 19 pounds.

How Does It Add Up?
1. $8 \times 6 - 4 \div 11 = 4$
2. $10 - 3 + 8 \times 2 = 30$
3. $9 - 2 \times 8 + 4 - 10 = 50$
4. $15 \div 5 + 11 + 6 \times 5 = 100$
5. $5 \times 4 \times 2 - 4 \div 6 = 6$
6. $12 \times 2 \div 8 \times 4 \div 3 - 4 = 0$

Logical or Not #1
The store closes early on weekends, but the dinner is on a Wednesday; Bill puts cash in his pocket but pays with a credit card; he walks to the store but puts the items in the car trunk.

Logical or Not #2
St. Patrick's Day is annual, not semiannual; it originated in Ireland, not Iceland; cellos are not marching band instruments; men in kilts would play bagpipes, not accordions.

Logical or Not #3
There are no stock-market listings on Mondays; the speaker is retired, so he would not go to the office.

Logical or Not #4
Auckland is in New Zealand, not Australia; the wife is speaking, yet she buys tickets for her and her wife; July is winter in Australia.

Logical or Not #5
"Is" instead of "isn't" most people's idea of fun; one can't use candles in a doctor's office; the diet book would not be found in the library's fiction section.

Logical or Not #6
The restaurant owner said "welcome back" but the couple had never eaten there before; moussaka is a Greek dish, not Italian; the restaurant name is Mario's, not Luigi's.

If/Then #1
Yes

If/Then #2
National Egg Month is before National Strawberry Month

If/Then #3
Not enough information to tell

If/Then #4
No. It could be March 1 (if a leap year) or March 2 (if not)

If/Then #5
City D is due south of City C

If/Then #6
Yes. Two tuna fish and one chicken salad.

If/Then #7
A bushel of wheat

If/Then #8
Yes. 250 highway miles.

Seating Plan
Clockwise from bottom center: Dave, Alice, Bob, George, Ida, Carl, Jack, Harriet, Frank, Ella

Next in Line
1. c **2.** b **3.** d **4.** c **5.** a
6. d **7.** b **8.** a **9.** c **10.** b

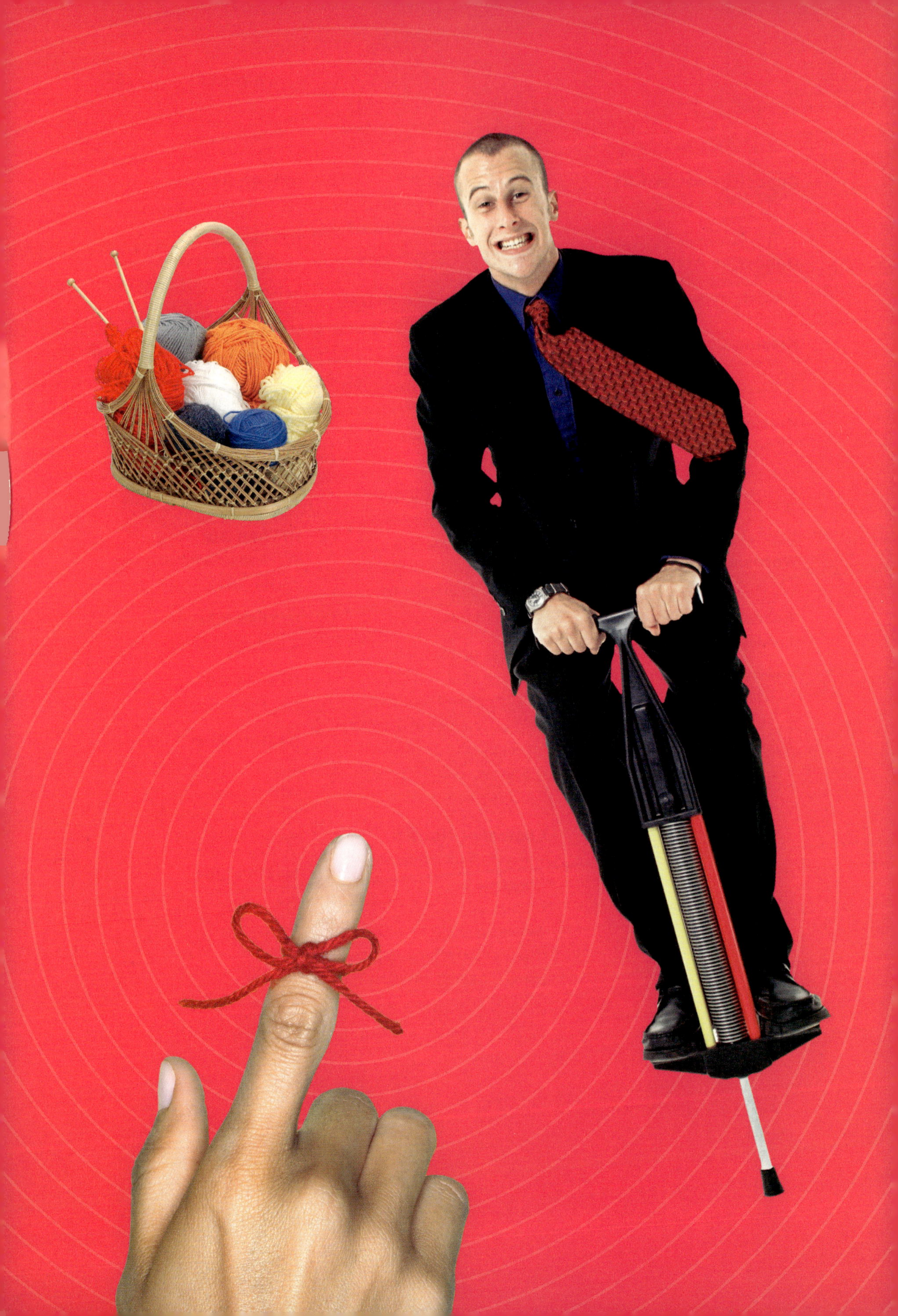

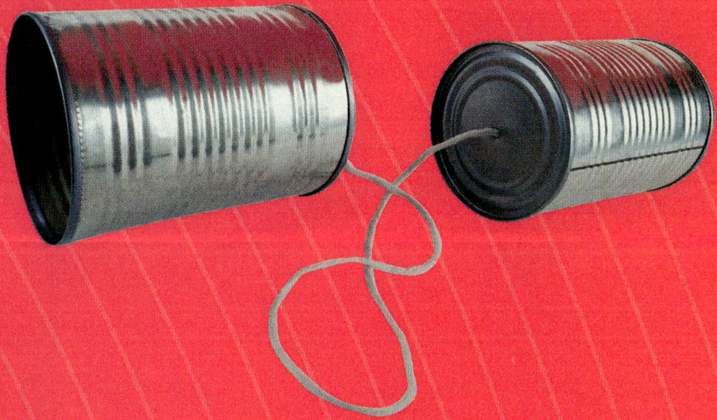

PART FIVE

resources

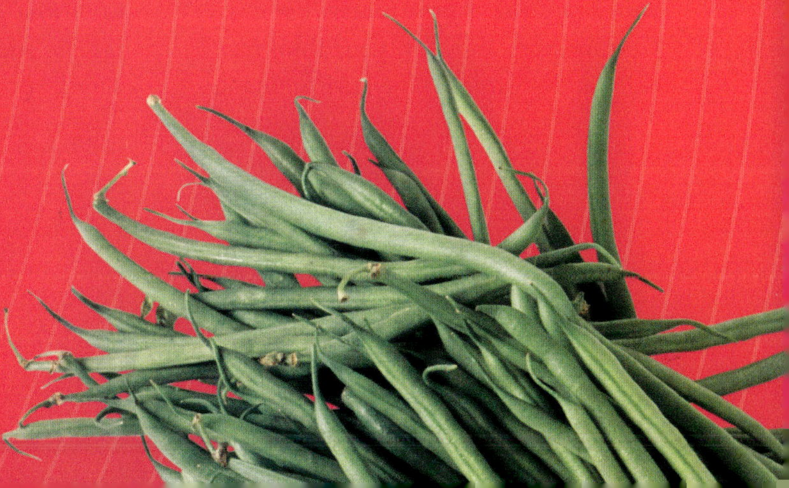

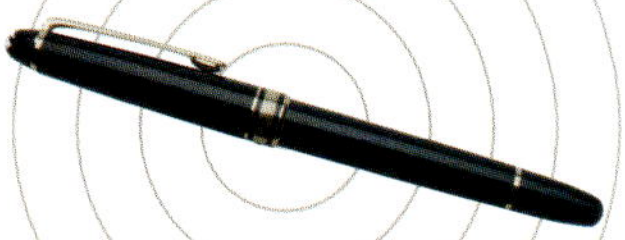

The 10-day jump-start plan

By now, your brain may be spinning with all the clever new ideas you've discovered on how to prevent brain drain. Maybe you've already tried a few. Every minute of every day presents a new opportunity to nourish, nurture, and grow your gray matter. How to put those opportunities to use? Check out this 10-day jump-start plan.

Blueberries on your breakfast cereal. A phone call to a friend. Bowling on Saturday instead of watching TV. Guarding your brain against the forces that drain your memory and slow your thinking skills is that simple! The key? Stepping outside your comfort zone just a little bit today...then choosing to do so over and over again in new and different ways. Protecting your "upstairs" also means indulging in tasty brain-healthy foods, luxurious sleep, fun with friends and family, and time in the great outdoors. Think you can handle it?

DAY 1

8 a.m.

Sprinkle a 1/2 cup of blueberries and a tablespoon of chopped nuts onto your breakfast cereal. Voilà! You've just added a heaping helping of brain-protecting antioxidants and good fats to your diet, in less than a minute! See how easy it is to prevent brain drain?

11 a.m.

Dial your doctor and make an appointment to review your meds. Is your allergy drug causing brain fog? Find out—and learn what you can do about it. Should you be taking a daily aspirin or fish oil for your heart and your brain? The appointment is your chance to ask. Prepare to bring the bottles of every pill—Rx, over-the-counter remedies, and supplements—that you take.

8 p.m.

Find your sneakers and put them where you'll see them first thing in the morning. You're going for a walk tomorrow!

Recipe of the Day

Angel Hair Pasta with Basil-and-Walnut Pesto, p. 295

DAY 2

9 a.m.

Lace up your walking shoes and head out the door. A 10- to 15-minute walk is all it takes to boost the flow of oxygen-rich blood to brain cells. And morning sun exposure will help you sleep better at night so new memories can be locked into place.

7 p.m.

Call up that longtime friend you haven't seen for awhile. Chat—and before you hang up, make a date for lunch or coffee sometime this week. Friendship is one of life's greatest joys … and it will make your heart sing and your brain thrive.

Recipe of the Day

Granola with Toasted Walnuts and Cranberries, p. 279

! Sweet fruit, crunchy nuts, and satisfying whole grains are part of the Mediterranean diet, which can help cut your risk for Alzheimer's disease by up to 68 percent.

DAY 3

Noon
Drizzle olive oil on your salad at lunch. The taste? Delicious. The brain bonus? Olive oil acts like aspirin, reducing inflammation in the brain. For "extra credit," make it a spinach salad.

4 p.m.
Do a household chore that you always leave to your spouse or that rarely gets done. Mow the lawn if you normally scrub the pots; weed the garden if you normally dust the furniture. Cross-training your brain builds new connections between brain cells—and it's so simple to do at home.

10:15 p.m.
Hit the hay 15 minutes earlier than usual, then stick with your new bedtime all week. A good night's sleep is spa time for your mind, regenerating brain tissue, preserving memories, and even boosting your IQ.

Recipe of the Day
Spinach, Sweet Potato, and Shiitake Salad, p. 284

DAY 4

8 a.m.
Get out a tape measure and measure your waistline. If your number (see page 160) puts you in the danger zone, plan to make exercise a front-and-center strategy for preventing brain drain.

10 a.m.
Take your prettiest large bowl or fruit plate and place it prominently on the kitchen table or counter. Fill it with fruit, such as bananas, oranges, and rinsed apples and pears. This pretty-as-a-picture centerpiece is your new go-to spot for antioxidant-packed, brain-nourishing snacks.

8 p.m.
Indulge yourself. Take a bubble bath, ask your partner for a foot massage, have sex, or savor a square of luscious dark chocolate. Pleasure raises levels of dopamine, an attention-focusing brain chemical.

Recipe of the Day
Quinoa Pilaf with Cherries and Walnuts, p. 297

! Does walking make you smarter? Yes! Exercise is like "Miracle-Gro" for your mind—just a few minutes a day spurs brain cell growth.

DAY 5

7:30 a.m.
Toss a handful of walnuts into a resealable bag and tuck it into your purse or briefcase as your mid-morning snack. Walnuts are chock-full of good fats that improve cell-to-cell communication in the brain.

10 a.m.
Make "face time" your rule today: Talk to co-workers, neighbors, and friends in person instead of by e-mail or phone. Go to the bank teller instead of the ATM, and chat up any shopkeepers you encounter. Even brief conversations boost brain power.

6 p.m.
Serve fish, the ultimate brain food, for dinner. Go for salmon, tilapia, haddock, mackerel, or even anchovies. All are rich in DHA, the omega-3 fat critical for clear thinking, organization, alertness, learning, and reasoning.

Recipe of the Day
Mustard-Glazed Salmon with Lentils, p. 289

DAY 6

7 a.m.
Let the sun shine in! Throw open the curtains and pull up the shades first thing this morning. A dose of early-morning sunlight resets your body clock, boosting mental alertness—and improving your sleep tonight.

11 a.m.
Shop at a farmers' market or at a nearby supermarket with the biggest, freshest produce department. Stock up on a rainbow of brain-friendly and mouth-watering veggies and fruits—then reward yourself with a gourmet lunch salad.

7 p.m.
Gather your family or close friends around the dining room table for game night. Brain-teasers like Scrabble build extra connections in the brain that protect you from brain drain. Serve a fruity dessert or a platter of sliced fruit and nuts for even more brain benefits.

Recipe of the Day
Spiced Apple and Blueberry Tart, p. 301

! Your brain loves company. Fun with friends feels great—and people with active social lives tend to suffer less cognitive decline later in life.

DAY 7

7 a.m.
Cuddle with your honey this morning before you get out of bed. Intimate touch delights neurons and forges new brain cell links. But just think of it as pure bliss.

8 a.m.
Today is "opposite" day, so step outside your usual routine. Brush your teeth with your nondominant hand, take a different route to work, or stand when you normally sit. Shaking things up keeps your brain active—and takes it off autopilot.

8 p.m.
Watch a comedy or a foreign movie. A comedy induces brain-healthy laughter, while foreign movies challenge your brain to watch the action and read the subtitles at the same time.

Recipe of the Day
Braised Pork with Cranberries, p. 294

DAY 8

7:30 a.m.
Savor a hot cup of java. Studies show that coffee sharpens alertness and boosts processing speed. Not a coffee-drinker? No worries; tea also confers brain benefits.

12:30 p.m.
Go to a park and pay close attention to everything you see (beautiful leaves), smell (grass), feel (the wind on your face), and hear (birds chirping). Flooding your brain with sensory data keeps your gray matter on its toes.

8 p.m.
Brainstorm a "call list" of friends, old and new. Starting tonight, catch up with one every day by phone or e-mail. Widening your social circle significantly lowers your risk for brain drain.

Recipe of the Day
Mackerel Tandoori-Style, p. 291

! Challenging your brain with new experiences keeps it young—and the pleasure and surprise puts a sparkle in your eye and a spring in your step.

DAY 9

12:30 p.m.
Add 5 more minutes to your daily walk. From now on, plan to increase your walking time by an additional 5 minutes each week until you're moving for 30 minutes. See how easy it is to become active?

7:30 p.m.
Turn off the TV and call a friend or start a project (get out your knitting needles, a puzzle, or a new book).

10 p.m.
Write in your gratitude journal. Spending more of your mental energy on gratitude than on worry will help you reduce brain-draining stress.

Recipe of the Day
Steamed Sesame Spinach, p. 298

DAY 10

11 a.m.
Buy some new plants for your kitchen, living room, or office. Studies show that exposure to greenery fosters sharper recall, quicker reactions, and creativity.

7 p.m.
Sit in a comfortable chair in a quiet room for 10 minutes. Close your eyes, pay attention to your breath as it flows in and out, and let your muscles relax. You'll feel refreshed and reduce levels of stress hormones that are toxic to your brain.

10 p.m.
Turn back your bedtime another 15 minutes tonight, and keep it there. Your mind thrives on a good night's sleep

Recipe of the Day
Country Vegetable Soup with Pesto, p. 283

! Gentle stress-busters—hugging, laughter, relaxation—do more than shield your brain from tension's corrosive effects. They boost happiness, right now. Ahhhhh!

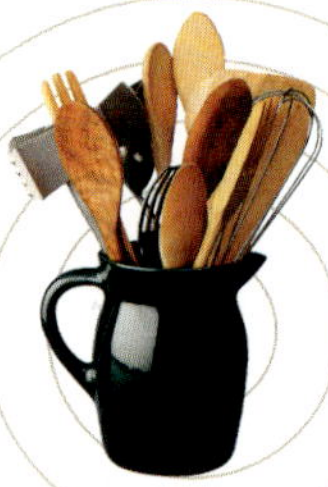

HEALTHY BRAIN recipes

Craving a better memory or a sharper mind? Grab a fork! Science proves that putting the right foods on your plate can armor your brain against the effects of age, toxins, and disease and protect the neuronal networks that let you think, process, plan, decide, and dream.

Think of every meal as a new and precious opportunity to slow or reverse brain drain. The recipes that follow were designed to help you get the most-protective foods into each one—foods like salmon and other fatty fish, olive oil, garlic, whole grains, nuts and flaxseeds, and antioxidant-rich vegetables and fruits (especially berries). Many of the recipes are also rich in anti-inflammatory spices, such as turmeric and ginger. Look for these and other brain-healthy ingredients in orange type.

How much of a difference can your diet make? Plenty. Eating more of certain foods (and less of others) can significantly improve your memory and thinking skills and even reduce your risk of Alzheimer's disease by a staggering percentage, not to mention lower your risk of a brain-damaging stroke. Best yet, these recipes taste as good as their benefits sound. *Bon appétit!*

BREAKFAST

Toasted Oat-and-Bran Tea Bread

SERVES 12

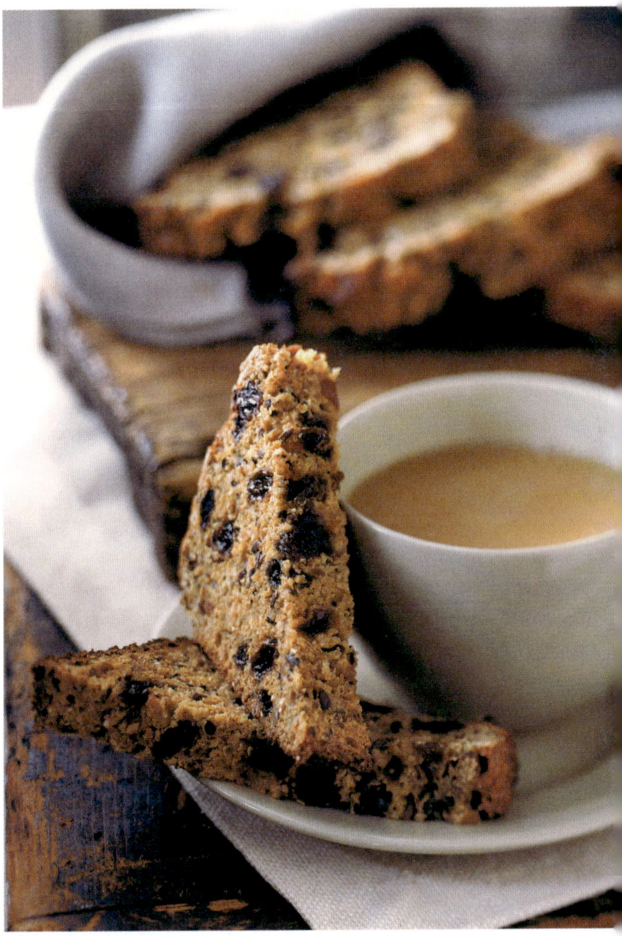

1 1/2 cups old-fashioned rolled **oats**
1/2 cup **flaxseeds**
1/2 cup **wheat bran**
1 cup flour
1/2 cup firmly packed light brown sugar
2 teaspoons baking powder
3/4 teaspoon salt
1 1/2 cups plain low-fat yogurt
2/3 cup honey
1 large egg
1 cup dark **raisins**

1. Preheat the oven to 350°F. Lightly grease a 9 x 5-inch metal loaf pan.

2. Place the oats, flaxseeds, and wheat bran on a baking sheet, and bake until the oats are golden brown, 7 to 9 minutes. Transfer to a food processor and process until finely ground.

3. Transfer the oat mixture to a large bowl. Stir in the flour, brown sugar, baking powder, and salt.

4. In a separate bowl, whisk together the yogurt, honey, and egg. Make a well in the center of the dry ingredients and fold in the yogurt mixture until just combined. Fold in the raisins.

5. Spoon the batter into the prepared loaf pan, smoothing the top. Bake for 1 hour, 20 minutes, or until a cake-tester inserted in the center of the loaf comes out clean. Cool for 5 minutes in the pan, then invert the loaf onto a wire rack to cool completely.

Per serving: 276 calories, 7 g protein, 57 g carbohydrates, 4.9 g fiber, 4.3 g total fat, 0.8 g saturated fat, 20 mg cholesterol, 261 mg sodium.

BRAIN FOOD

Whole grains like **oats** and **bran** help you avoid blood-sugar surges that are toxic to the brain.

Fruit Boats with Orange-Balsamic Glaze

SERVES 4

Glaze

1/4 cup balsamic vinegar
1/4 teaspoon freshly grated orange zest
2 tablespoons fresh orange juice
2 teaspoons brown sugar

Fruit

1 large **cantaloupe**
1 pint **strawberries**, hulled and quartered
1/2 pint **blueberries**
1/2 pint **raspberries**
2 **kiwifruits**, peeled, halved, and cut into thin wedges

1. *To make the glaze:* Combine the vinegar, orange zest and juice, and brown sugar in a microwavable dish. Microwave on High until syrupy, 2 to 3 minutes. Or, cook over medium-high heat in a small saucepan, 4 to 5 minutes. Set aside.

2. *To prepare the fruit:* Cut the cantaloupe lengthwise in half. Discard the seeds. Cut each melon half crosswise to form triangular "boats." Scoop out cantaloupe with a melon baller, leaving a thin layer of flesh on the rind. Put cantaloupe balls, strawberries, blueberries, raspberries, and kiwis in a large bowl.

3. Drizzle fruit with glaze. Toss to coat evenly. Spoon into cantaloupe boats and serve.

Per serving: 180 calories, 3 g protein, 43 g carbohydrates, 8 g fiber, 1 g total fat, 0 g saturated fat, 0 mg cholesterol, 24 mg sodium.

cooking tip

To keep the juice of dark fruits (such as blueberries and raspberries) from coloring paler fruits (including melons, pears, and peaches), wait to mix them until just before serving.

Berry-Flaxseed Smoothie

SERVES 2

2 tablespoons whole **flaxseeds**
1/2 cup fresh orange juice
1/2 cup vanilla nonfat yogurt
1 cup unsweetened frozen mixed **berries** or **blueberries**
1 small **banana**, sliced

1. Place the flaxseeds in a blender, cover, and blend until ground into a fine powder.

2. Add the orange juice, yogurt, berries, and banana. Cover and blend until smooth and creamy.

Per 1-cup serving: 200 calories, 5 g protein, 36 g carbohydrates, 7 g fiber, 5 g total fat, 0 g saturated fat, 1 mg cholesterol, 33 mg sodium.

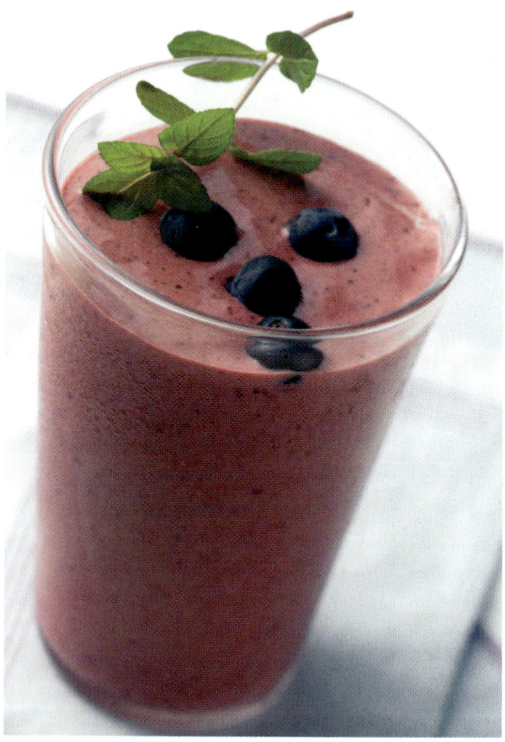

Granola with Toasted Walnuts and Cranberries

MAKES 5 CUPS

- 3 cups old-fashioned or quick-cooking **oats**
- 1/2 cup coarsely chopped **walnuts**
- 2 tablespoons **wheat germ**
- 2 tablespoons **sesame seeds**
- 1/4 teaspoon salt
- 1/3 cup honey
- 1 tablespoon light brown sugar
- 1 tablespoon extra-light **olive oil**
- 1 teaspoon vanilla extract
- 1 cup dried **cranberries**

1. Preheat oven to 300°F. Combine oats, walnuts, wheat germ, sesame seeds, and salt in a 13 x 9-inch baking pan. Bake until oats and nuts are toasted and fragrant, about 30 minutes. Remove pan from oven. Increase oven temperature to 350°F.

2. Meanwhile, combine the honey, brown sugar, and oil in a small skillet over medium heat. Cook until the sugar has melted, about 1 minute. Remove from the heat and stir in the vanilla.

3. Drizzle the honey mixture over the oat mixture and stir to coat. Return to oven and bake, stirring occasionally, until the oats are crispy, about 10 minutes.

4. With a spoon, break up any clumps. Stir in the cranberries. Let cool. Store in an airtight container.

Per 1/3-cup serving: 154 calories, 4 g protein, 25 g carbohydrates, 3 g fiber, 5 g total fat, 0.5 g saturated fat, 0 mg cholesterol, 41 mg sodium.

Oatmeal with Apple and Flaxseeds

SERVES 4

- 2 cups low-fat (1%) milk or vanilla soy milk
- 3/4 cup old-fashioned rolled **oats**
- 1 medium **apple**, peeled, cored, and chopped
- 1/3 cup dried **cranberries** or **raisins**
- 1/2 teaspoon ground cinnamon
- 1/4 cup whole **flaxseeds**, ground, or 1/3 cup flaxseed meal
- 1/4 cup plain or vanilla nonfat yogurt
- 1/4 cup maple syrup, warmed, or 2 tablespoons brown sugar

1. Combine the milk, oats, apple, cranberries or raisins, and cinnamon in a heavy medium saucepan. Bring to a simmer over medium-high heat, stirring almost constantly.

2. Reduce the heat to medium-low and cook, stirring often, until creamy and thickened, 3 to 5 minutes.

3. Stir in the flaxseed. Spoon the cereal into individual bowls and top each serving with a dollop of yogurt and a drizzle of maple syrup or a sprinkle of brown sugar.

Per serving: 282 calories, 10 g protein, 47 g carbohydrates, 6 g fiber, 7 g total fat, 1 g saturated fat, 8 mg cholesterol, 84 mg sodium.

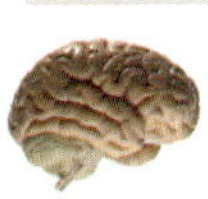

BRAIN FOOD

Crunchy, nutty **flaxseed** is rich in protein, fiber, and "good" fats like those in fish—everything your brain could ask for.

SOUP, SALAD, AND LIGHT BITES

Hot and Spicy Tomato-Apple Gazpacho

SERVES 4

- 3 cups tomato juice
- 3 tablespoons tomato paste
- 1 large apple (unpeeled), cut into chunks
- 3/4 cup finely chopped red onion (about 1 medium)
- 2 cloves garlic, peeled
- 1/3 cup natural (unblanched) almonds
- 1/4 cup red-wine vinegar
- 2 teaspoons Louisiana-style red pepper sauce
- 1 teaspoon chili powder
- 3/4 teaspoon ground coriander
- 1/4 teaspoon salt
- 1/2 cup water
- 4 plum tomatoes, cut into 1/2-inch chunks
- 1 Hass avocado, peeled, pitted, and cut into 1/2-inch chunks

1. In a blender, combine the tomato juice, tomato paste, apple, 1/2 cup of the onion, the garlic, almonds, vinegar, red pepper sauce, chili powder, coriander, and salt; process until blended but not pureed (it should still have a chunky texture).

2. Pour into a serving bowl and stir in the water and the tomato chunks; chill.

3. Serve the gazpacho topped with the remaining 1/4 cup onion and the avocado.

Per serving: 213 calories, 6 g protein, 26 g carbohydrates, 5.4 g fiber, 12 g total fat, 1.4 g saturated fat, 0 mg cholesterol, 985 mg sodium.

Spiced Moroccan Carrot Soup

SERVES 4

- 1 tablespoon olive oil
- 1 medium onion, thinly sliced
- 3 cloves garlic, thinly sliced
- 1 pound carrots, thinly sliced
- 3/4 teaspoon ground cinnamon
- 3/4 teaspoon ground ginger
- 3/4 teaspoon turmeric
- 1/2 teaspoon paprika
- 1 cup carrot juice
- 2 tablespoons tomato paste
- 3 tablespoons rice
- 3/4 teaspoon salt
- 1/2 teaspoon black pepper
- 2 cups water
- 1/2 cup chopped cilantro

1. In a medium saucepan, heat the oil over medium heat. Add the onion and garlic, and cook, stirring frequently, until the onion is golden, about 5 minutes.

2. Stir in the carrots, cinnamon, ginger, turmeric, and paprika, and cook for 1 minute. Stir in the carrot juice, tomato paste, rice, salt, pepper, and water; bring to a boil. Reduce to a simmer; cover and cook until the carrots and rice are tender, about 20 minutes.

3. Transfer the mixture to a food processor and puree until smooth. Sprinkle the soup with the cilantro when serving.

Per serving: 167 calories, 4 g protein, 31 g carbohydrates, 4.9 g fiber, 4 g total fat, 0.5 g saturated fat, 0 mg cholesterol, 562 mg sodium.

Curried Red Lentil Soup

SERVES 8

2 teaspoons canola oil
2 cups chopped **onions** (2 medium)
4 cloves **garlic**, minced
4–5 teaspoons **curry powder**
1 1/2 cups red **lentils**, rinsed and sorted
6 cups reduced-sodium chicken broth or vegetable broth
3/4 cup water
2 tablespoons **tomato** paste
1/4 teaspoon ground cinnamon
2 tablespoons fresh **lemon juice**
1/4 teaspoon salt, or to taste
Freshly ground black pepper, to taste
1/2 cup plain nonfat yogurt
1/4 cup chopped **scallion** greens

1. Heat the oil in a 4- to 6-quart (4- to 6-liter) soup pot over medium heat. Add the onions and cook, stirring frequently, until softened, 2 to 3 minutes.

2. Add the garlic and curry powder. Cook, stirring, for 30 seconds. Add the lentils and stir to coat. Add the broth, water, tomato paste, and cinnamon. Bring to a simmer, reduce heat to low, cover, and simmer until the lentils are very tender, about 20 minutes.

3. In batches, transfer the soup to a food processor or blender and puree. (Use caution when blending hot liquids.) Return the puree to the soup pot and heat through. Season with lemon juice, salt, and pepper.

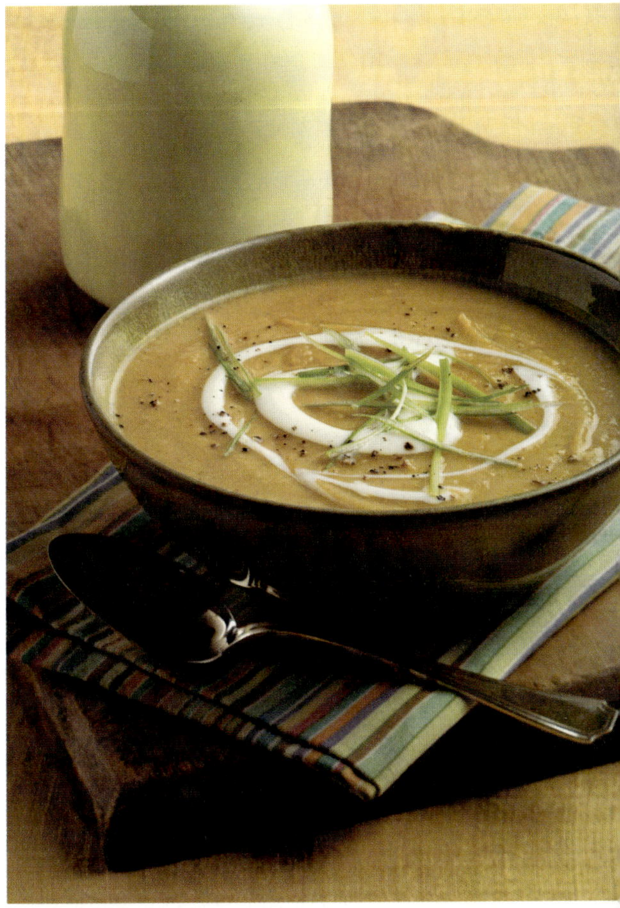

4. Garnish each serving with a dollop of yogurt and a sprinkling of scallion greens.

Per 1-cup serving: 187 calories, 14 g protein, 29 g carbohydrates, 12 g fiber, 2 g total fat, 1 g saturated fat, 4 mg cholesterol, 199 mg sodium.

BRAIN FOOD

Curry powder fights "rust" and inflammation in the brain and may help lower the risk of Alzheimer's disease.

Chicken-Kale Soup with Roasted Pepper Puree

SERVES 4

- 4 cups water
- 1 1/4 pounds skinless, boneless chicken thighs, cut into 1-inch chunks
- 4 carrots, thinly sliced
- 3 large red onions, cut into 1/2-inch chunks
- 5 cloves garlic, minced
- 2 tablespoons finely chopped fresh ginger
- 1 teaspoon cayenne pepper
- 1 teaspoon salt
- 2 red bell peppers, seeded and cut lengthwise into flat panels
- 1 tablespoon hulled roasted pumpkin seeds
- 1 tablespoon flaxseed oil
- 1 clove garlic, peeled
- 1/4 cup orzo pasta
- 8 cups shredded kale

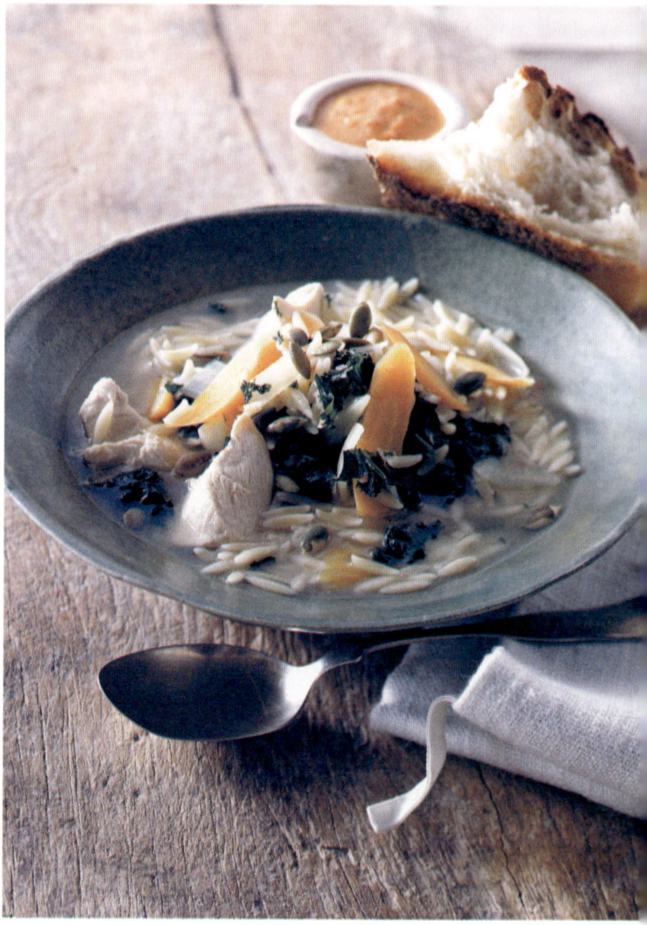

1. In a large saucepan or stockpot, combine the water, chicken, carrots, onions, minced garlic, ginger, cayenne, and salt; bring to a boil over high heat. Reduce to a simmer; partially cover, and cook for 25 minutes.

2. Meanwhile, preheat the broiler. Place the pepper pieces, skin-side up, on a broiler pan and broil 6 inches from the heat until the skin is well-charred, about 10 minutes. When cool enough to handle, peel the peppers and transfer them to a food processor along with the pumpkin seeds, oil, and garlic clove; process until pureed.

3. Add the orzo to the soup, and cook, uncovered, for 5 minutes. Stir in the kale, and cook until the kale and orzo are tender, about 5 minutes.

4. Serve the soup with the roasted pepper puree.

Per serving: 433 calories, 38 g protein, 48 g carbohydrates, 9.1 g fiber, 12 g total fat, 2.2 g saturated fat, 118 mg cholesterol, 649 mg sodium.

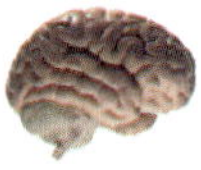

BRAIN FOOD

A Harvard study found that women who frequently ate **cruciferous vegetables** including kale had fewer memory problems than women who rarely ate them.

Country Vegetable Soup with Pesto

SERVES 4

- 1 onion, chopped
- 1 carrot, chopped
- 1 celery rib, sliced
- 2 cloves garlic, finely chopped
- 1 pound plum tomatoes, peeled seeded, and chopped
- 1 medium yellow squash, sliced
- 1 medium zucchini, sliced
- 1 can (14 1/2 ounces) reduced-sodium chicken broth
- 1 can (14 1/2 ounces) vegetable broth
- 1 cup loosely packed fresh basil leaves
- 2 1/2 tablespoons prepared pesto sauce

1. Coat a large saucepan with nonstick cooking spray and set over medium-high heat. Sauté the onion, carrot, celery, and garlic until soft, about 5 minutes.

2. Add the tomatoes, squash, and zucchini. Sauté until soft, about 8 minutes. Stir in the chicken and vegetable broth, and bring to a boil. Reduce heat and simmer, uncovered, until the flavors are blended, about 20 minutes.

3. Put the basil and pesto sauce in a food processor and pulse until the basil is chopped. Process until thick and creamy.

4. Ladle soup into bowls and top with the pesto.

Per serving: 110 calories, 5 g protein, 18 g carbohydrates, 5 g fiber, 3.5 g total fat, 0 g saturated fat, 0 mg cholesterol, 523 mg sodium.

Greek Lentil Salad

SERVES 6

- 1 cup dried green or brown lentils, rinsed
- 1 teaspoon salt
- 3 tablespoons fresh lemon juice
- 2 tablespoons extra-virgin olive oil
- 1 clove garlic, minced
- Freshly ground black pepper, to taste
- 1 cup chopped scallions (1 bunch)
- 1 cup (12 ounces) roasted red peppers from a jar, rinsed and diced
- 1/2 cup (2 ounces) crumbled feta cheese
- 1/3 cup chopped fresh dill
- 6 cups trimmed arugula or watercress, washed, dried, and torn

1. Place the lentils in a large saucepan and cover with water. Bring to a simmer. Reduce the heat to medium-low, partially cover, and simmer for 15 minutes. Add 1/2 teaspoon of the salt and cook until the lentils are tender but not broken down, 10 to 15 minutes longer. Drain and let cool slightly.

2. Whisk the lemon juice, oil, garlic, the remaining 1/2 teaspoon salt, and the pepper in a large bowl. Add the lentils and toss gently to mix. Add the scallions, red peppers, feta, and dill. Toss again.

3. To serve, mound lentil mixture on a bed of arugula.

Per 3/4-cup serving: 160 calories, 10 g protein, 13 g carbohydrates, 10 g fiber, 7 g total fat, 2 g saturated fat, 5 mg cholesterol, 700 mg sodium.

cooking tip

Common brown lentils are fine for this recipe, but small green lentils from France (known as Le Puy lentils) are preferred for salads because they retain their shape and have an appealing chewy texture. Total cooking time is about 20 minutes for green lentils and 25 to 30 minutes for brown lentils.

Spinach, Sweet Potato, and Shiitake Salad

SERVES 4

Salad

1 pound sweet potatoes, peeled, halved lengthwise, and cut crosswise into 1/2-inch slices
1/3 cup walnuts
1 tablespoon olive oil
2 cloves garlic, slivered
12 ounces fresh shiitake mushrooms, stems discarded and caps thickly sliced
1/2 teaspoon salt
12 cups spinach leaves

Dressing

1/2 cup red-wine vinegar
1 tablespoon Dijon mustard
4 teaspoons olive oil

1. *To make the salad:* Preheat the oven to 400°F. Place the sweet potatoes on a lightly oiled baking sheet, and bake until tender, 15 to 20 minutes.

2. Toast the walnuts on a separate pan in the oven until crisp, 5 to 7 minutes. When cool enough to handle, coarsely chop the nuts.

3. In a large skillet, heat the oil over medium heat. Add the garlic and until fragrant, about 30 seconds. Add half the mushrooms, sprinkle with 1/4 teaspoon of the salt, and cook until they begin to soften, about 4 minutes. Add the remaining mushrooms and the remaining 1/4 teaspoon salt, and cook until all the mushrooms are tender, about 5 minutes.

4. Place the spinach in a large bowl. Add the sweet potatoes and walnuts. Remove the mushrooms from the skillet with a slotted spoon, and add them to the bowl with the spinach.

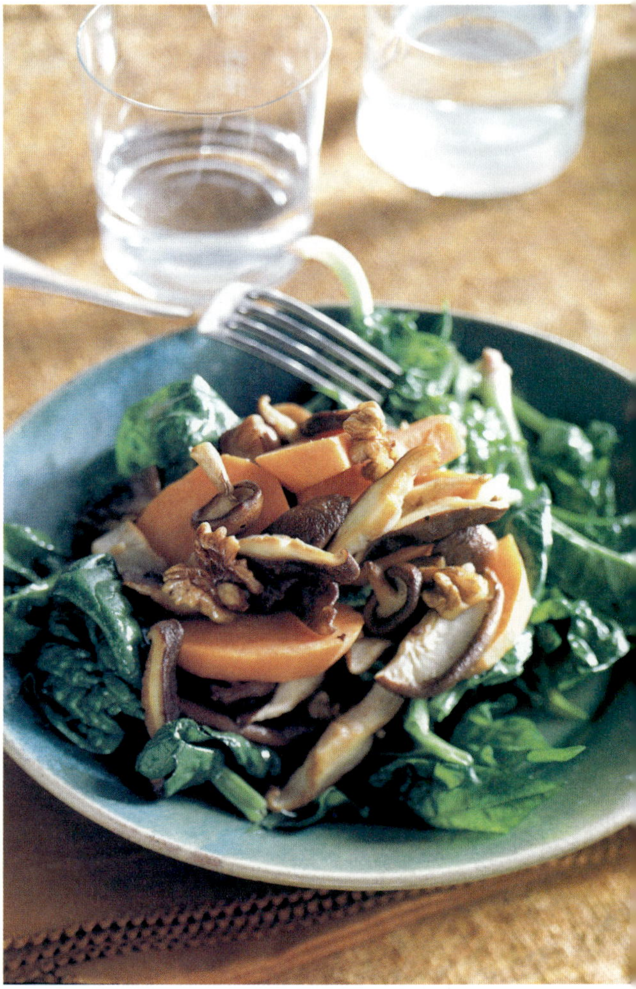

5. *To make the dressing:* Add the vinegar, mustard, and oil to the skillet, and whisk over high heat until warm. Pour the dressing over the salad, and toss to combine.

Per serving: 283 calories, 9 g protein, 32 g carbohydrates, 8.1 g fiber, 15 g total fat, 1.8 g saturated fat, 0 mg cholesterol, 524 mg sodium.

Tuna and Cannellini Salad with Lemon

SERVES 4

Dressing

- 3 tablespoons fresh lemon juice
- 1 clove garlic, minced
- 1/4 teaspoon salt, or to taste
- 1/8 teaspoon crushed red pepper
- 1/4 cup extra-virgin olive oil
- Freshly ground black pepper, to taste

Salad

- 1 can (19 or 15 ounces) cannellini beans, drained and rinsed
- 1 can (6 ounces) water-packed chunk light tuna, drained and flaked
- 1/3 cup finely diced red onion
- 2 teaspoons chopped fresh rosemary
- 1 1/2 teaspoons freshly grated lemon zest
- 6 cups arugula, washed, dried, and torn into bite-size pieces
- 1 cup cherry tomatoes, quartered

1. *To make the dressing:* Combine the lemon juice, garlic, salt, and crushed red pepper in a small bowl. Gradually whisk in the oil. Season with pepper.

2. *To make the salad:* Combine the beans, tuna, onion, rosemary, and lemon zest in a medium bowl. Add 1/4 cup of the lemon-garlic dressing (save remaining dressing for the arugula). Toss to coat well.

3. Just before serving, place the arugula in a large bowl. Add the reserved lemon-garlic dressing and toss to coat well. Divide the arugula mixture among 4 plates. Top with tuna-bean salad and garnish with cherry tomatoes.

Per serving: 305 calories, 18 g protein, 25 g carbohydrates, 7 g fiber, 15 g total fat, 2 g saturated fat, 26 mg cholesterol, 500 mg sodium.

Bulgur Salad with Tangerine-Pomegranate Dressing

SERVES 4

Dressing

- 1 teaspoon freshly grated tangerine or orange zest
- 1 cup fresh tangerine or orange juice
- 2 tablespoons tomato paste
- 2 tablespoons pomegranate molasses
- 2 tablespoons olive oil
- 1 teaspoon salt

Salad

- 1 cup medium-grain bulgur
- 2 1/2 cups boiling water
- 1 1/2 cups corn kernels
- 2/3 cup dried cherries (3 ounces)
- 2/3 cup thinly sliced scallions
- 1/3 cup roasted peanuts, coarsely chopped

1. In a large heat-proof bowl, combine the bulgur and the water. Let stand for 30 minutes at room temperature. Drain well.

2. *To make the dressing:* In a large bowl, whisk together the zest, juice, tomato paste, molasses, oil, and salt.

3. *To make the salad:* Add the bulgur to the liquid, and fluff with a fork. Add the corn, cherries, scallions, and peanuts, tossing to combine. Serve at room temperature or chilled.

Per serving: 414 calories, 10 g protein, 69 g carbohydrates, 10 g fiber, 14 g total fat, 2 g saturated fat, 0 mg cholesterol, 520 mg sodium.

cooking tip

Pomegranate molasses—a sweet-sour pomegranate concentrate—is available in Middle Eastern and some specialty food stores. If you can't find pomegranate molasses, substitute a mixture of currant jelly (2 tablespoons) and fresh lemon or lime juice (1 tablespoon).

Guacamole with a Kick

SERVES 16

- 1/2 cup plain low-fat yogurt
- 2 small jalapeño peppers
- 2 plum **tomatoes**, finely chopped
- 1 small white **onion**, finely chopped
- 2 tablespoons minced cilantro
- 1/2 teaspoon salt
- 1/2 cup nonfat sour cream
- 2 large **avocadoes**, peeled, halved, and pitted
- 2 tablespoons fresh lime juice
- 3 ounces baked tortilla chips

1. Line the bottom of a mesh strainer with cheesecloth, a coffee filter, or a paper towel and set over a medium bowl (strainer should not touch bottom of bowl). Spoon in yogurt, cover, and refrigerate at least 8 hours or overnight, until yogurt cheese is thick and creamy.

2. Remove the seeds and ribs from the jalapeños with a melon baller (wear gloves when handling, as the peppers can burn); mince. Mix jalapeños, tomatoes, onion, cilantro, and salt in a large bowl. Fold in the yogurt cheese and sour cream.

3. Mash the avocado with a potato masher and sprinkle with the lime juice. Quickly fold into the tomato mixture. Serve with chips.

Per 3-ounce serving: 72 calories, 2 g protein, 8 g carbohydrates, 2 g fiber, 4 g total fat, 0.75 g saturated fat, 0 mg cholesterol, 124 mg sodium.

cooking tip

Choose a yogurt that does not contain gelatin, as this holds onto the whey, hampering the draining process.

Chicken Waldorf Salad with Toasted Walnuts

SERVES 4

- 1/3 cup **walnuts**
- 1 pound skinless, boneless chicken breasts
- 1/2 teaspoon salt
- 1/2 teaspoon black pepper
- 3/4 cup plain low-fat yogurt
- 3 tablespoons prepared **horseradish**
- 2 tablespoons light mayonnaise
- 2 tablespoons fresh **lemon juice**
- 2 cups seedless red **grapes**, halved
- 1 1/2 cups thinly sliced **celery** (about 3 stalks)
- 2 medium red **apples** (unpeeled), cut into 1/2-inch cubes
- 4 cups shredded romaine **lettuce**

1. Preheat the oven to 350°F. Place the walnuts on a baking sheet, and bake until slightly crisped and fragrant, about 7 minutes. When cool enough to handle, coarsely chop.

2. Preheat the broiler. Sprinkle the chicken with 1/4 teaspoon of the salt and 1/4 teaspoon of the pepper. Broil 6 inches from the heat until cooked through, 4 to 5 minutes per side. Cool to room temperature, then cut into 1-inch chunks.

3. In a large bowl, whisk together the yogurt, horseradish, mayonnaise, lemon juice, and the remaining 1/4 teaspoon salt and 1/4 teaspoon pepper.

4. Add the walnuts, chicken, grapes, celery, and apples; toss to coat. Add the romaine and toss again.

Per serving: 351 calories, 32 g protein, 35 g carbohydrates, 5 g fiber, 11 g total fat, 2 g saturated fat, 71 mg cholesterol, 508 mg sodium.

Roasted-Vegetable Wraps with Chive Sauce

SERVES 8

- 3/4 cup plain low-fat yogurt
- 1 tablespoon olive oil
- 1 tablespoon rice wine vinegar
- 1 teaspoon chopped fresh rosemary
- 1 clove garlic, minced
- 1/4 teaspoon salt
- 2 medium zucchini (8 ounces each)
- 2 large red bell peppers, each seeded and cut into 8 strips
- 1 large red onion, cut into 16 wedges
- 8 98% fat-free flour tortillas (7-inch)
- 1/4 teaspoon onion salt
- 1 tablespoon snipped fresh chives

1. Line the bottom of a mesh strainer with cheesecloth, a coffee filter, or a paper towel and set over a medium bowl (strainer should not touch bottom of bowl). Spoon in yogurt, cover, and refrigerate at least 8 hours or overnight, until yogurt cheese is thick and creamy.

2. Place an oven rack in the upper third of the oven and preheat the oven to 450°F. Lightly coat a jelly-roll pan with nonstick cooking spray.

3. Whisk the oil, vinegar, rosemary, garlic, and salt in a small bowl.

4. Cut each zucchini in half crosswise, then lengthwise into 1/4-inch slices. Place on the jelly-roll pan along with the peppers and onion. Add the oil mixture and toss to coat.

5. Roast, tossing frequently, until the vegetables are brown and tender, about 30 minutes.

6. Sprinkle the tortillas with a little water, wrap in foil, and place in the oven with the vegetables during the last 5 minutes of cooking time.

7. Meanwhile, combine the yogurt, onion salt, and chives in a small bowl.

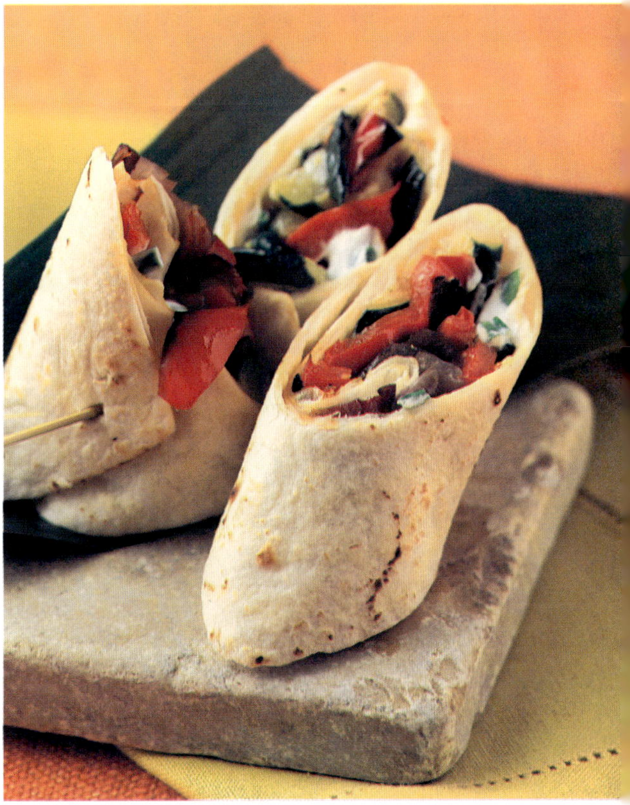

8. Remove the tortillas from the oven. Spread the chive sauce evenly on the tortillas and top with the vegetables. Fold in the sides of the tortillas and roll up. Cut each wrap into 3 pieces on the diagonal.

Per serving: 120 calories, 5 g protein, 24 g carbohydrates, 7 g fiber, 2 g total fat, 0.5 g saturated fat, 1 mg cholesterol, 435 mg sodium.

cooking tip

Roasting vegetables at high heat caramelizes them—it enhances their flavor by concentrating their sugars. For best results, use a shallow pan, arrange the vegetables in a single layer, and put the pan in the hottest part of the oven (usually the top third). To ensure even browning, toss the vegetables frequently until they turn a deep caramel color.

DINNER

Salmon on a Bed of Greens

SERVES 4

- 1/4 cup grapefruit juice
- 1 1/2 tablespoons mustard
- 1 1/2 tablespoons honey
- 1/4 teaspoon red-pepper flakes
- 4 **salmon** fillets (6 ounces each)
- 1 1/2 pounds **kale**, large stems removed and leaves chopped
- 3 tablespoons **olive oil**
- 1/2 red **bell pepper**, seeded and finely chopped
- 1/2 yellow **bell pepper**, seeded and finely chopped

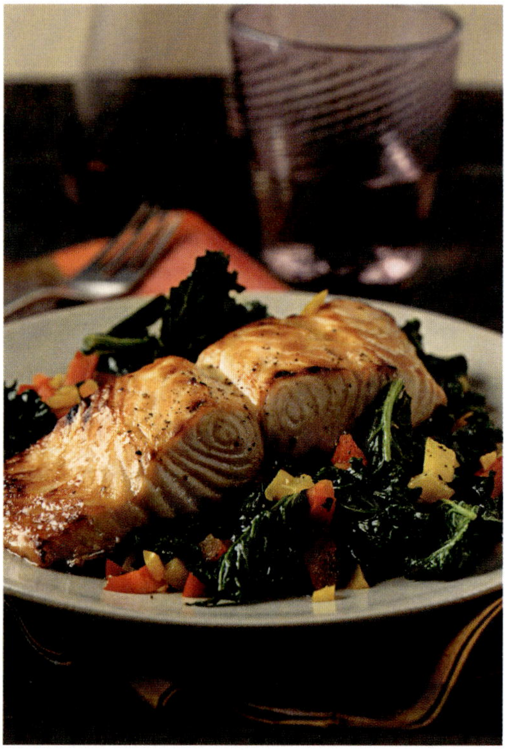

1. In baking dish large enough to hold fish fillets in a single layer, combine the grapefruit juice, mustard, honey, and pepper flakes. Add the salmon, turning to coat both sides with marinade. Refrigerate, covered, for 30 minutes.

2. Preheat the broiler.

3. Meanwhile, in a large pot, bring 2 quarts of water to a boil. Add the kale. Return the water to a boil and cook for 5 minutes. Drain well. Squeeze out excess water.

4. Heat the oil in a large skillet over medium heat. Add the peppers. Sauté for 1 minute. Add the kale and sauté until the kale and peppers are tender, about 3 minutes. Remove the skillet from the heat.

5. Remove the salmon from the marinade (reserve marinade). Place the salmon, skin-side down, on the rack in a foil-lined broiler pan. Broil 4 inches from heat for 3 minutes. Brush on the remaining marinade. Broil until the fish is opaque and flakes when touched with a knife, 3 to 4 minutes. (If fish begins to brown too much, move it to a lower rack.)

6. Spoon the kale and pepper mixture onto plates and top each serving with a piece of salmon.

Per serving: 402 calories, 41 g protein, 21 g carbohydrates, 3 g fiber, 18 g total fat, 3 g saturated fat, 97 mg cholesterol, 233 mg sodium.

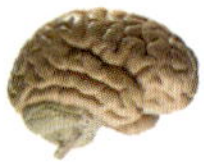

BRAIN FOOD

Salmon is nature's ultimate brain food; its **omega-3 fats** help brains cells deliver signals efficiently and may even spur the growth of new cells.

Mustard-Glazed Salmon with Lentils

SERVES 4

- 2 cans (19 ounces) lentil soup
- 1 pound salmon fillet, cut into 4 pieces
- Freshly ground black pepper, to taste
- 3 tablespoons coarse-grain or Dijon mustard
- 2 teaspoons olive oil
- 2/3 cup scallions, trimmed and chopped (1 bunch)
- 1/2 teaspoon dried thyme
- 1 tablespoon fresh lemon juice
- Lemon wedges

1. Preheat the oven to 450°F. Line a small baking pan with aluminum foil and coat it with nonstick spray.

2. Place the lentil soup in a mesh strainer set over a bowl. Let drain for several minutes.

3. Place the salmon, skin-side down, in the baking pan. Season with pepper and spread with the mustard. Bake the salmon until opaque in the center, 12 to 15 minutes.

4. Meanwhile, heat the oil in a medium saucepan over medium heat. Add the scallions and cook, stirring, until softened, 1 to 2 minutes.

5. Add the drained lentil soup and thyme. Heat through.

6. Stir in the lemon juice. Spoon the lentil mixture onto plates and top each serving with a piece of salmon. Garnish with lemon wedges.

Per serving: 330 calories, 34 g protein, 28 g carbohydrates, 9 g fiber, 10 g total fat, 1 g saturated fat, 59 mg cholesterol, 981 mg sodium.

cooking tip

To cook salmon in the microwave, place in a microwave-safe dish, cover with wax paper, and microwave on high for 5 to 7 minutes.

Broiled Salmon with Avocado-Mango Salsa

SERVES 4

- 2 1/2 teaspoons paprika
- 2 teaspoons ground coriander
- 3/4 teaspoon salt
- 4 skinless, boneless salmon fillets (about 6 ounces each)
- 1 large mango, peeled and cut into 1/2-inch chunks (about 1 1/2 cups)
- 1 Hass avocado, peeled, pitted, and cut into 1/2-inch chunks
- 1 cup canned chickpeas, drained and rinsed
- 1/3 cup chopped cilantro
- 1 teaspoon freshly grated lemon zest
- 2 tablespoons fresh lemon juice
- 2 teaspoons olive oil
- 6 cups mesclun or frisée lettuce, torn into bite-size pieces

1. In a large bowl, stir together the paprika, coriander, and salt. Measure out 2 teaspoons of the mixture and sprinkle it over the salmon, rubbing it into the fish. Place the salmon on a broiler pan.

2. To the spice mixture remaining in the bowl, add the mango, avocado, chickpeas, cilantro, lemon zest, lemon juice, and oil; toss to combine.

3. Broil the salmon 6 inches from the heat for 5 minutes for medium. Serve the salmon and salsa on a bed of lettuce.

Per serving: 551 calories, 42 g protein, 35 g carbohydrates, 7.8 g fiber, 29 g total fat, 5.2 g saturated fat, 100 mg cholesterol, 745 mg sodium.

Crispy Tuna Steaks in Citrus Sauce

SERVES 4

Sauce

- 1 1/2 cups fresh orange juice
- 2 tablespoons dry white wine (optional)
- 2 tablespoons cornstarch
- 2 large oranges, peeled and sectioned

Tuna

- 2 tablespoons chopped fresh cilantro
- 2 tablespoons cornmeal
- 1/2 teaspoon salt
- 1/4 teaspoon black pepper
- 4 tuna steaks (1/2 inch thick, 6 ounces each)
- 4 teaspoons olive oil

1. *To make the sauce:* Whisk the orange juice, wine (if using), and cornstarch in small saucepan until smooth. Bring to a boil over medium-high heat and cook, stirring, until it boils and thickens, about 2 minutes. Remove from heat and stir in the orange sections. Keep warm.

2. *To make the tuna:* Mix the cilantro, cornmeal, salt, and pepper in a pie plate. Coat both sides of the tuna steaks with the cornmeal mixture, pressing firmly so the mixture adheres.

3. Heat 2 teaspoons of the oil in a large cast-iron skillet over medium-high heat until hot but not smoking. Sear the tuna for 2 to 3 minutes on each side for medium-rare. Add the remaining 2 teaspoons oil just before turning fish. Serve with the sauce.

Per serving: 338 calories, 41 g protein, 28 g carbohydrates, 3 g fiber, 6 g total fat, 1 g saturated fat, 76 mg cholesterol, 355 mg sodium.

Sardines in a Peppercorn Crust

SERVES 4

- 8 large, fresh sardines (about 1 pound)
- 1 teaspoon mixed peppercorns
- Small bunch of fresh dill, rinsed, dried and chopped
- 1 clove garlic, crushed
- 2 lemons
- Salt
- 3 tablespoons olive oil
- 8 small sprigs of fresh rosemary, rinsed
- 4 lettuce leaves, rinsed, dried, and finely shredded
- 8 sprigs of watercress, rinsed and dried

1. Preheat the grill to the highest setting. Cut along the belly of each sardine with kitchen scissors, then pull out the insides. Rinse the fish inside and out, rubbing off the scales with your fingers. Dry on paper towels.

2. Crush the peppercorns with a mortar and pestle or rolling pin and put them into a small bowl. Add the dill and garlic. Finely grate the rind of 1 lemon into the bowl. Add some salt and the olive oil and mix.

3. Place the fish in a shallow pan. Put a sprig of rosemary inside each fish, then spoon some of the dill mixture on each piece. Turn and coat the other side, reserving any leftover mixture. Marinate for 5 to 10 minutes.

4. Meanwhile, arrange the lettuce and watercress on plates. Cut four wedges from the other lemon, remove any seeds, and put one wedge on each plate.

5. Thread each sardine lengthwise onto a metal skewer, then grill for 2 to 3 minutes on each side.

6. Slide the sardines off the skewers and put 2 on each plate on top of the salad. Spoon the reserved dill mixture over them and the salad leaves and serve.

Per serving: 234 calories, 16 g protein, 2 g carbohydrates, 1 g fiber, 18 g total fat, 3 g saturated fat, 51 mg cholesterol, 120 mg sodium.

Mackerel Tandoori-Style

SERVES 4

- 1 teaspoon ground cumin
- 1/4 cup plain low-fat yogurt
- 1 tablespoon fresh lemon juice
- 2 teaspoons minced fresh **ginger**
- 1 clove **garlic**, peeled
- 2 teaspoons paprika
- 1/2 teaspoon salt
- 1/4 teaspoon ground cardamom
- 1/4 teaspoon cayenne pepper
- 4 **mackerel** fillets (about 6 ounces each), skin on, each halved crosswise
- 1 tablespoon plus 2 teaspoons **olive oil**
- 2 large **onions**, halved and thinly sliced
- 1 1/2 teaspoons sugar
- 1 large red **bell pepper**, seeded and cut into matchsticks

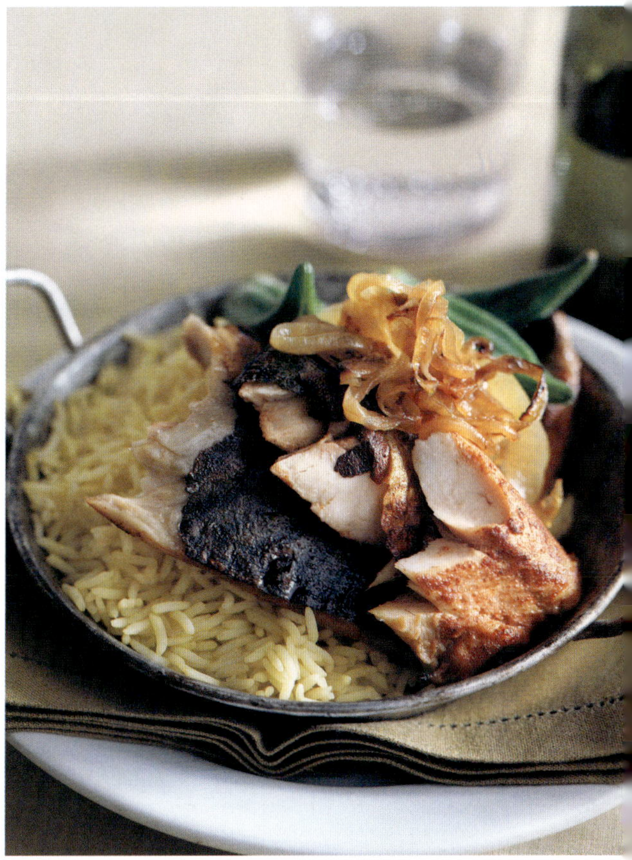

1. In a small skillet, toast the cumin over low heat until fragrant, about 2 minutes. Transfer to a blender along with the yogurt, lemon juice, ginger, garlic, paprika, salt, cardamom, and cayenne; puree.

2. Place the mackerel, skin-side down, in a shallow ovenproof pan and make several diagonal slashes in the flesh. Spread the yogurt mixture over the fish. Refrigerate for at least 2 hours, or overnight.

3. About 30 minutes before serving time, remove the fish from the refrigerator. In a large skillet, heat 1 tablespoon of the oil over medium heat. Add the onions and sugar; cook, stirring frequently, until the onions are lightly browned, about 20 minutes. Add the bell peppers, and cook until they are crisp-tender, about 5 minutes; set aside.

4. Meanwhile, preheat the oven to 450°F. Sprinkle the mackerel with the remaining 2 teaspoons oil, and bake until cooked through, about 12 minutes. Serve the mackerel topped with the caramelized onion mixture.

Per serving: 414 calories, 29 g protein, 16 g carbohydrates, 2.3 g fiber, 26 g total fat, 5.5 g saturated fat, 100 mg cholesterol, 432 mg sodium.

BRAIN FOOD

Like salmon, **mackerel** is a superb source of omega-3s, perhaps the single most important nutrient for your brain.

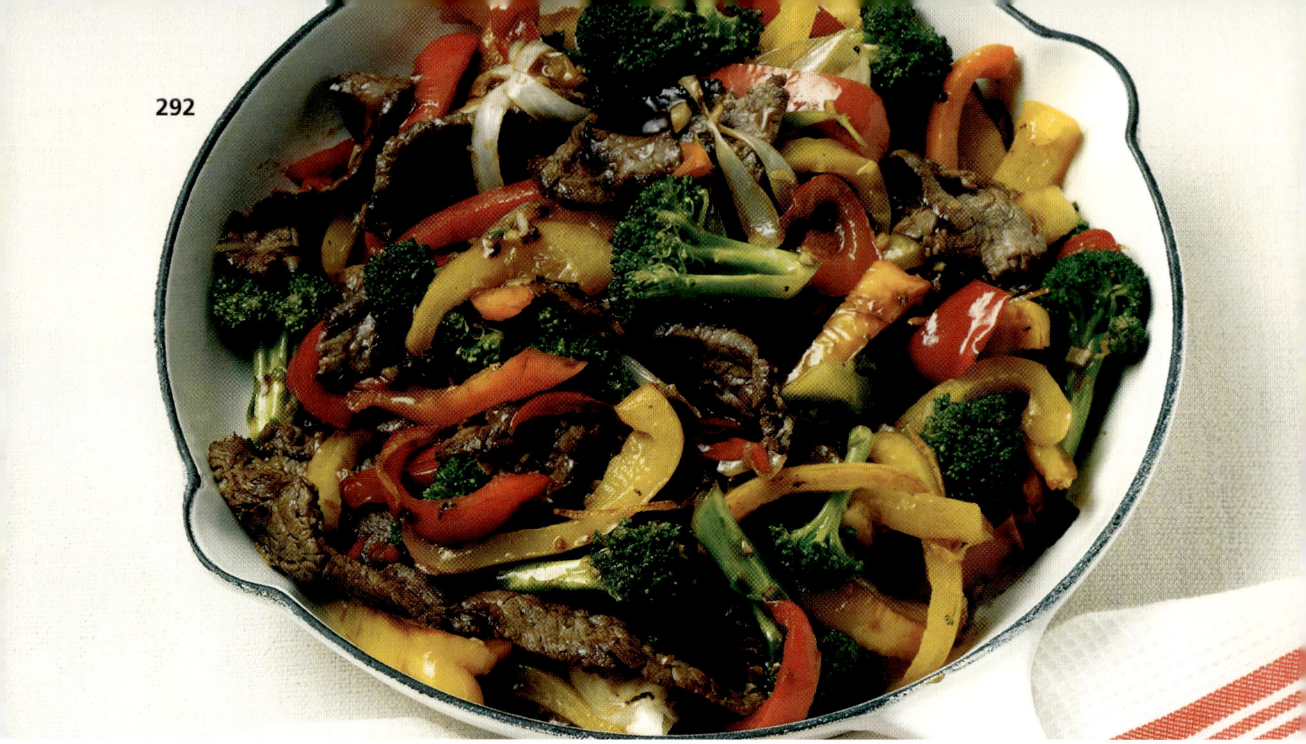

Orange Beef Stir-Fry with Broccoli and Peppers

SERVES 4

- 1/2 cup fresh orange juice
- 2 tablespoons reduced-sodium soy sauce
- 1 tablespoon oyster sauce
- 1 tablespoon rice-wine vinegar
- 1 1/2 teaspoons chile-garlic sauce or hot red pepper sauce
- 1 1/2 teaspoons cornstarch
- 1 tablespoon canola oil
- 12 ounces flank steak, trimmed, halved lengthwise, and cut into 1/4-inch-thick slices
- 1 tablespoon minced fresh **ginger**
- 2 teaspoons freshly grated orange zest
- 3 cloves **garlic**, minced
- 1 cup sliced **onion** (1 medium)
- 1 pound **broccoli** crowns, cut into 1-inch florets (4 cups)
- 1 red or yellow **bell pepper**, seeded and cut into 2- x 1/4 -inch slivers
- 1/4 cup water

1. In a small bowl, whisk together the orange juice, soy sauce, oyster sauce, vinegar, chile-garlic sauce or red pepper sauce, and cornstarch; set aside.

2. Heat 1 teaspoon of the oil in a large non-stick skillet or stir-fry pan over high heat. Add half of the steak and cook, without stirring or turning, until browned on the underside, about 1 minute. Stir and turn the slices, then cook just until browned on the other side, about 30 seconds more. Transfer to a plate. Add another 1 teaspoon oil and repeat with the remaining steak, and transfer to the plate.

3. Add the remaining 1 teaspoon oil to the skillet, then add the ginger, orange zest, and garlic and stir-fry until fragrant, 10 to 20 seconds. Add the onion and stir-fry for 1 minute. Add the broccoli and peppers and stir-fry for 30 seconds. Add the water, cover, and cook just until crisp-tender, about 1 1/2 minutes.

4. Push the vegetables to the outside of the pan. Stir the orange sauce and then pour it into the center of the pan and cook, stirring, until glossy and thickened, about 1 minute. Stir the vegetables into the sauce, return the steak to the skillet, and turn to coat.

Per serving: 247 calories, 25 g protein, 17 g carbohydrates, 3 g fiber, 9 g total fat, 3 g saturated fat, 34 mg cholesterol, 655 mg sodium.

Rich Curried Chicken and Vegetables

SERVES 4

- 1 tablespoon **turmeric**
- 1 1/2 teaspoons ground **ginger**
- 1 teaspoon salt
- 1/2 teaspoon ground cinnamon
- 1/2 teaspoon sugar
- 1/2 teaspoon black pepper
- 1 1/4 pounds skinless, boneless chicken thighs, cut into 1-inch chunks
- 2 teaspoons **olive oil**
- 1 medium **onion**, halved and thickly sliced
- 4 cloves **garlic**, minced
- 2 1/2 cups water
- 3 **carrots**, thickly sliced
- 1 pound small red-skinned potatoes, quartered
- 2 teaspoons creamy **peanut butter**
- 4 cups **broccoli** florets

1. In a medium bowl, stir together the turmeric, ginger, 1/2 teaspoon of the salt, the cinnamon, sugar, and pepper. Add the chicken, tossing to coat.

2. In a nonstick Dutch oven, heat the oil over medium heat. Add the onion and garlic, and cook, stirring frequently, until the onion is tender, about 7 minutes.

3. Add 1/2 cup of the water, carrots, potatoes, peanut butter, and the remaining 1/2 teaspoon salt; bring to a boil. Cook until the carrots begin to soften, about 5 minutes.

4. Add the chicken, and cook until no longer pink, 2 minutes. Stir in the remaining 2 cups water and bring to a boil. Reduce to a simmer; cover and cook until the chicken is cooked through and the potatoes are tender, 15 minutes.

5. Add the broccoli; cover and cook until the broccoli is tender, about 5 minutes.

Per serving: 394 calories, 37 g protein, 38 g carbohydrates, 7.9 g fiber, 9.7 g total fat, 1.9 g saturated fat, 118 mg cholesterol, 789 mg sodium.

Chicken with Apples and Calvados

SERVES 4

- 2 medium **shallots**, finely chopped
- 2 tart **apples**, peeled and cut into 1/4-inch slices
- 1 cup apple juice
- 3/4 cup reduced-sodium chicken broth
- 1 tablespoon Calvados, applejack, or apple juice
- 1/4 cup all-purpose flour
- 1/2 teaspoon salt
- 1/2 teaspoon freshly ground black pepper
- 4 boneless, skinless chicken breast halves (5 ounces each)
- 2 tablespoons heavy cream

1. Lightly coat a large heavy nonstick skillet with nonstick cooking spray and set over medium-high heat. Sauté the shallots until soft, about 2 minutes. Add the apples and sauté until lightly browned, about 3 minutes. Add the apple juice, broth, and Calvados, applejack, or apple juice. Cook, stirring, until apples are tender, about 5 minutes. Transfer to a medium bowl. Wipe the skillet clean.

2. Combine the flour, salt, and pepper on a sheet of wax paper. Coat the chicken breasts with the flour, pressing with your hands so the flour adheres and the chicken is flattened evenly.

3. Lightly coat the skillet again with cooking spray and set over medium-high heat. Cook the chicken until browned and almost cooked through, about 3 minutes on each side.

4. Return the apple mixture and any juices to the skillet and bring to a boil. Reduce the heat and simmer for 2 minutes. Stir in the cream and remove from the heat.

Per serving: 300 calories, 35 g protein, 26 g carbohydrates, 2 g fiber, 5 g total fat, 2 g saturated fat, 93 mg cholesterol, 402 mg sodium.

Braised Pork with Cranberries

SERVES 4

- 1/2 cup sugar
- 1 teaspoon dried rosemary, minced
- 3/4 teaspoon salt
- 1/2 teaspoon black pepper
- 1/2 teaspoon ground **ginger**
- 1 pound well-trimmed pork tenderloin, halved crosswise
- 1 tablespoon **olive oil**
- 12 cloves **garlic**, peeled
- 8 **scallions**, cut into 2-inch lengths
- 4 **carrots**, cut into matchsticks
- 12 ounces fresh or frozen **cranberries**
- 2/3 cup fresh orange juice
- 1 bay leaf

1. Preheat the oven to 350°F. In a large bowl, stir together 1/4 cup of the sugar, the rosemary, salt, pepper, and ginger. Add the pork, and turn to coat.

2. In a nonstick Dutch oven or flameproof casserole, heat the oil over medium-high heat. Lift the pork from the spice mixture and add to the pan along with the garlic. Cook the pork until it is richly browned, 2 minutes per side. Transfer the pork to a plate.

3. Add the scallions and carrots to the pan, and cook until the carrots begin to color, about 3 minutes. Stir the remaining 1/4 cup sugar, the cranberries, orange juice, and bay leaf into the pan; bring to a boil.

4. Return the pork to the pan; reduce to a simmer, cover, and transfer to the oven. Bake until the pork is cooked through but still juicy, 30 minutes.

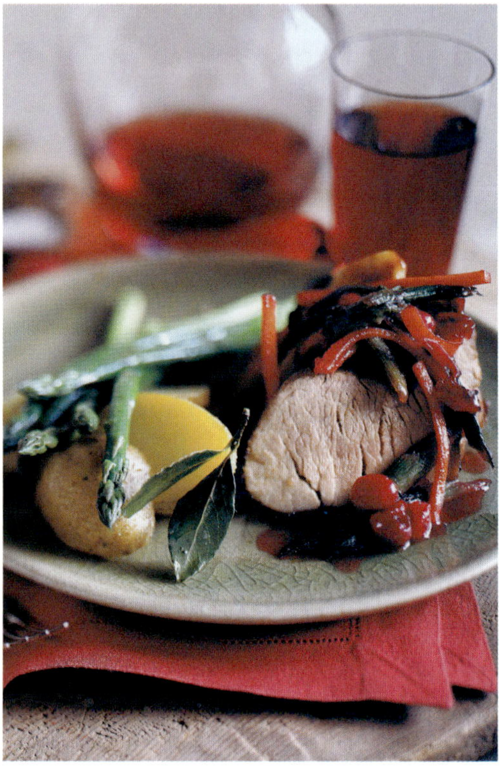

5. Lift the pork from the pan and slice. Remove and discard the bay leaf from the sauce. Serve the pork with the vegetables and sauce spooned on top.

Per serving: 380 calories, 26 g protein, 53 g carbohydrates, 6.6 g fiber, 7.7 g total fat, 1.8 g saturated fat, 74 mg cholesterol, 526 mg sodium.

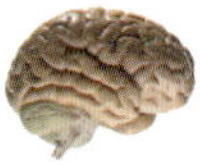

BRAIN FOOD

Cranberries are loaded with **antioxidants,** which help prevent oxidation, or "brain rust."

Angel Hair Pasta with Basil-and-Walnut Pesto

SERVES 4

- 4 ounces fresh basil leaves (2 cups)
- 4 ounces trimmed fresh **spinach** (2 cups)
- 2 ounces trimmed fresh **arugula** (1 cup)
- 1/3 cup **walnut** pieces
- 3 tablespoons grated Parmesan cheese
- 3 cloves **garlic**
- 1 teaspoon salt
- 1 tablespoon **olive oil**
- 12 ounces angel hair pasta or capellini
- 1 large **lemon**, halved
- Sprigs of fresh basil

1. Put basil, spinach, and arugula in a colander. Wash with cold running water. Shake to dry. Transfer to a food processor.

2. Add the walnuts, Parmesan, garlic, and salt and pulse until finely chopped. With the machine running, slowly drizzle the oil through feed tube, processing until thick.

3. Meanwhile, cook the pasta according to the package directions; drain.

4. Toss the pasta with the pesto in a large serving bowl until evenly coated. Squeeze lemon juice over the pasta and garnish with the basil.

Per serving: 446 calories, 15 g protein, 70 g carbohydrates, 4 g fiber, 12 g total fat, 2 g saturated fat, 3 mg cholesterol, 673 mg sodium.

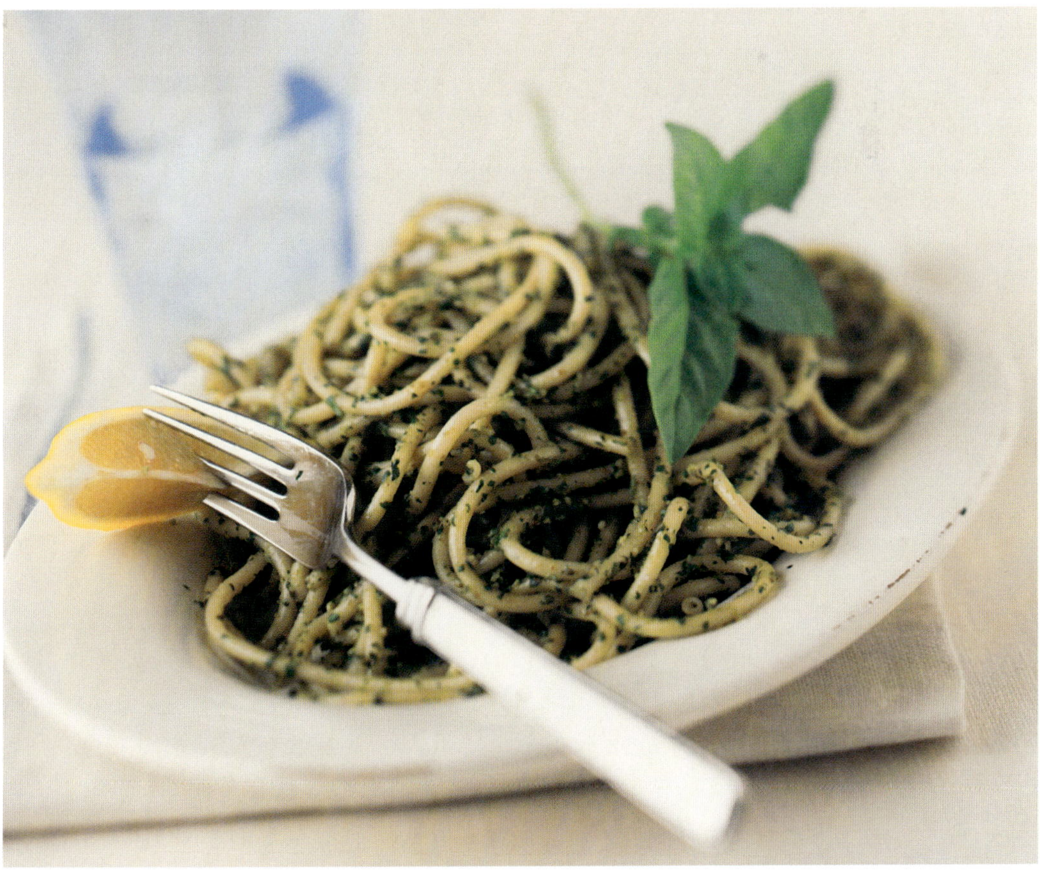

Barley Risotto with Asparagus and Mushrooms

SERVES 4

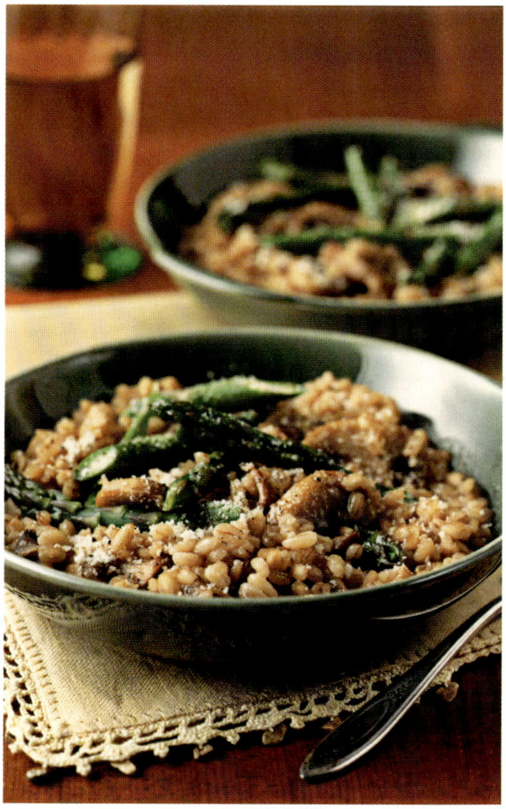

- 2 cans (14 1/2 ounces each) reduced-sodium, fat-free chicken broth
- 2 cups water
- 2 tablespoons olive oil
- 1 onion, finely chopped
- 8 ounces mushrooms (preferably wild varieties), coarsely chopped
- 2 cloves garlic, minced
- 1 cup pearl barley
- 8 ounces asparagus, stems cut into bite-size pieces (leave tips whole)
- 1/2 cup grated Parmesan cheese

1. In a medium saucepan, heat the broth and water to just below a simmer. Cover; keep at a simmer.

2. In a large deep nonstick skillet over medium heat, heat the oil. Sauté the onion until slightly softened, 3 minutes.

3. Add the mushrooms and garlic. Sauté until the mushrooms are softened, 5 minutes.

4. Stir in the barley and 2 cups of the hot broth mixture. Simmer, covered, for 15 minutes.

5. Meanwhile, blanch the asparagus tips in the pot of remaining hot broth for 2 minutes. Transfer them to a plate with a slotted spoon.

6. Add more hot broth to the barley mixture, 1/2 cup at a time, stirring frequently. Let each batch of liquid be absorbed before adding more. When adding the last batch of broth, stir in the asparagus stem pieces. Stir in the Parmesan.

5. Serve topped with the asparagus tips.

Per serving: 329 calories, 15 g protein, 49 g carbohydrates, 10 g fiber, 10 g total fat, 2 g saturated fat, 23 mg cholesterol, 743 mg sodium.

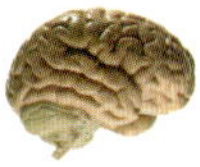

BRAIN FOOD

Chewy and satisfying, **barley** trumps rice because it's less likely to raise your blood sugar; high levels actually shrink the hippocampus.

SIDE DISHES

Barley Pilaf with Herbs

SERVES 6

- 2 teaspoons olive oil
- 2 slices turkey bacon, coarsely chopped
- 1 medium onion, finely chopped
- 3 cloves garlic, minced
- 2 carrots, thinly sliced
- 3/4 cup pearled barley
- 1 teaspoon salt
- 3/4 teaspoon rubbed sage
- 3/4 teaspoon thyme
- 3 1/4 cups water
- 1 teaspoon slivered lemon zest
- 3/4 teaspoon black pepper
- 1/4 cup grated Parmesan cheese

1. Heat the oil in a medium saucepan over medium heat. Add the bacon and cook for 2 minutes. Add the onion and garlic and cook until the onion is tender and golden brown, about 5 minutes.

2. Add the carrots to the pan and cook until tender, about 5 minutes.

3. Add the barley, stirring to combine. Add the salt, sage, thyme, and water to the pan and bring to a boil. Reduce to a simmer and cook, stirring frequently, until the barley is tender, about 45 minutes.

4. Stir in the lemon zest, pepper, and Parmesan until evenly combined.

Per serving: 153 calories, 6 g protein, 25 g carbohydrates, 5 g fiber, 4 g total fat, 1 g saturated fat, 7 mg cholesterol, 538 mg sodium.

Quinoa Pilaf with Cherries and Walnuts

SERVES 12

- 2 teaspoons olive oil
- 1 large onion, finely chopped
- 2 cups quinoa
- 2 cups boiling water
- 1 1/2 teaspoons salt
- 1 teaspoon black pepper
- 1/2 teaspoon dried thyme
- 1 cup dried cherries
- 1/2 cup walnuts, toasted and coarsely chopped

1. Heat the oil in a nonstick Dutch oven over medium heat. Add the onion and cook, stirring frequently, until golden brown, about 7 minutes.

2. Place the quinoa in a large ungreased skillet over medium heat and cook, stirring often, until lightly toasted, about 5 minutes.

3. Add the quinoa to the onion and stir in the water, salt, pepper, and thyme. Return to a boil, cover, and gently boil for 10 minutes. Uncover and cook, stirring occasionally, until the liquid has been absorbed and the quinoa is tender, 10 to 12 minutes.

4. Remove from the heat and stir in the cherries and walnuts. Serve hot, at room temperature, or chilled.

Per serving: 190 calories, 5 g protein, 31 g carbohydrates, 3 g fiber, 5 g total fat, 0.5 g saturated fat, 0 mg cholesterol, 300 mg sodium.

cooking tip

To turn this side dish into a meaty meal, just add some shredded leftover chicken breast, strips of roast pork tenderloin, or cubes of cooked lean beef.

Steamed Sesame Spinach

SERVES 4

1 pound fresh spinach, stems removed
1/8 teaspoon red-pepper flakes
1/2 teaspoon dark sesame oil
1 teaspoon salt
1 teaspoon fresh lemon juice
1 tablespoon toasted sesame seeds

1. Place a steamer basket in a medium saucepan with 2 to 3 inches of water. Add the spinach and pepper flakes and steam until tender, 3 to 5 minutes.

2. Transfer to a serving bowl. Add the oil, salt, and lemon juice and toss. Sprinkle with the sesame seeds.

Per serving: 35 calories, 3 g protein, 4 g carbohydrates, 3 g fiber, 2 g total fat, 0 g saturated fat, 0 mg cholesterol, 90 mg sodium.

Lemony Sugar Snaps

SERVES 4

1 1/2 pounds sugar snap peas
2 teaspoons olive oil
3 shallots, thinly sliced
1 clove garlic, minced
1 tablespoon freshly grated lemon zest
1 teaspoon salt

1. Remove strings from both sides of the sugar snap peas.

2. Heat the oil in large nonstick skillet over medium heat. Add the shallots and garlic and cook, stirring, until the shallots are softened, about 3 minutes.

3. Add the peas, lemon zest, and salt to the skillet and cook, stirring, until the peas are just tender, about 4 minutes.

Per serving: 99 calories, 4 g protein, 15 g carbohydrates, 5 g fiber, 2.5 g total fat, 0.5 g saturated fat, 0 mg cholesterol, 454 mg sodium.

Savory Cranberry Chutney

SERVES 6

2 teaspoons olive oil
1 large red onion, finely chopped
3 cloves garlic, minced
1 package (12 ounces) fresh or frozen cranberries
1/2 cup firmly packed light brown sugar
1/2 cup dried cherries
2 teaspoons freshly grated orange zest
1/2 cup fresh orange juice
1/4 teaspoon salt
1/2 teaspoon black pepper
1/8 teaspoon allspice

1. In a large saucepan, heat the oil over medium-low heat. Add the onion and garlic; cook, stirring frequently, until the onion is tender, 7 minutes.

2. Stir in the cranberries, brown sugar, cherries, orange zest, orange juice, salt, pepper, and allspice. Cook, stirring occasionally, until the berries have popped, 10 minutes. Cool to room temperature. Serve at room temperature or chilled.

Per serving: 175 calories, 1 g protein, 42 g carbohydrates, 2.8 g fiber, 1.7 g total fat, 0.2 g saturated fat, 0 mg cholesterol, 108 mg sodium.

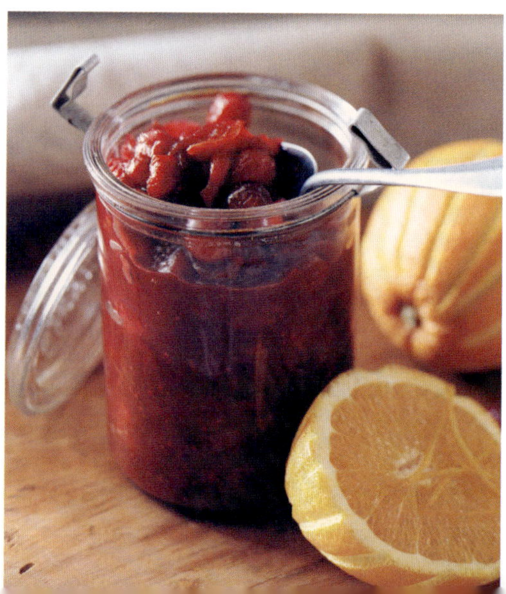

Asparagus with Confetti Vinaigrette

SERVES 4

1 1/2 pounds **asparagus**, woody stems peeled
1 1/4 teaspoons salt
2 large red **bell peppers**, seeded and finely chopped
2 large yellow **bell peppers**, seeded and finely chopped
4 **scallions**, thinly sliced
2 teaspoons fresh thyme or 1/2 teaspoon dried
1/3 cup reduced-sodium chicken broth
3 tablespoons white-wine vinegar
1/2 teaspoon black pepper

1. Bring 1/2 inch of water to a simmer in a large skillet over medium-high heat. Add the asparagus and 1 teaspoon of the salt. Simmer until the asparagus is tender, 3 to 4 minutes. Transfer to a platter and keep warm.

2. Wipe the skillet clean. Coat with nonstick cooking spray and set over medium-high heat. Sauté the bell peppers until tender, about 4 minutes.

3. Stir in the scallions and thyme and cook 1 minute longer.

4. Stir in the broth and vinegar and bring to a simmer.

5. Sprinkle with black pepper and the remaining 1/4 teaspoon of salt and pour over the asparagus.

Per serving: 90 calories, 6 g protein, 19 g carbohydrates, 6 g fiber, 1 g total fat, 0 g saturated fat, 0 mg cholesterol, 206 mg sodium.

Roasted Harvest Vegetables

SERVES 4

3 tablespoons **olive oil**
6 cloves **garlic**, thinly sliced
3 cups **butternut squash** chunks (1-inch)
10 ounces **Brussels sprouts**, trimmed and halved lengthwise
8 ounces fresh shiitake **mushrooms**, stems discarded and caps thickly sliced
2 large red **apples** (unpeeled), cut into 1-inch chunks
1/4 cup oil-packed sun-dried **tomatoes**, drained and thinly sliced
1 teaspoon dried rosemary, minced
1/2 teaspoon salt
1/4 cup grated Parmesan cheese

1. Preheat the oven to 400°F. In a large roasting pan, combine the olive oil and garlic. Heat in the oven for 3 minutes.

2. Add the squash, Brussels sprouts, mushrooms, apples, tomatoes, rosemary, and salt; toss to combine.

3. Roast until the vegetables are tender, about 35 minutes, tossing every 10 minutes.

4. Sprinkle the Parmesan over the vegetables, and roast 5 minutes longer.

Per serving: 292 calories, 8 g protein, 39 g carbohydrates, 9.3 g fiber, 14 g total fat, 2.4 g saturated fat, 4 mg cholesterol, 464 mg sodium.

BRAIN FOOD

Roasting brings out the sweetness in **vegetables,** which help fight dementia, including Alzheimer's disease.

DESSERT

Blueberry Bavarian

SERVES 6

- 1 cup low-fat (1%) milk
- 1/4 cup fat-free dry milk
- 2 packages (12 ounces each) thawed frozen **blueberries**
- 1/2 cup plus 1 tablespoon sugar
- 1/4 teaspoon salt
- 1 cup fat-free sour cream
- 1 packet unflavored gelatin
- 1/4 cup cold water
- 1/2 cup fresh **blueberries**

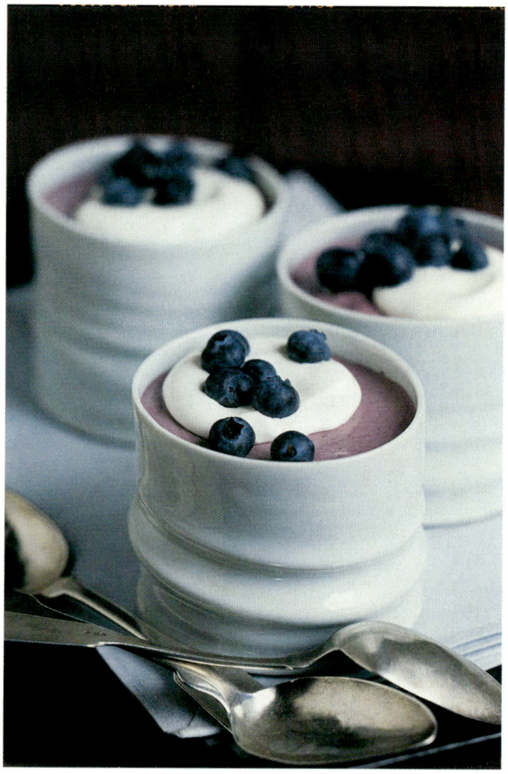

1. Combine the milk and dry milk in a small bowl and whisk until well-blended. Place in the freezer for up to 30 minutes.

2. Combine the blueberries, 1/2 cup sugar, and the salt in a medium saucepan over low heat. Bring to a simmer and cook until the sugar has dissolved, the berries have broken up, and the mixture has reduced to 2 1/4 cups, about 10 minutes. Let cool to room temperature.

3. Stir in 2/3 cup of the sour cream.

4. Sprinkle the gelatin over the water in a heatproof measuring cup. Let stand for 5 minutes to soften. Set the measuring cup in a small saucepan of simmering water and heat until the gelatin has melted, about 2 minutes. Let cool to room temperature.

5. With a hand mixer, beat the chilled milk until thick, soft peaks form. Beat in the remaining 1 tablespoon of sugar until stiff peaks form. Beat in the gelatin mixture.

6. Fold the milk mixture into the blueberry mixture.

7. Spoon into 6 dessert bowls or glasses. Chill until set, about 2 hours. At serving time, top each with a dollop of the remaining sour cream and some fresh blueberries.

Per serving: 202 calories, 7 g protein, 3 g carbohydrates, 3 g fiber, 1 g total fat, 0.5 g saturated fat, 2 mg cholesterol, 178 mg sodium.

cooking tip

For best results, chill the bowl and beaters before whipping the milk.

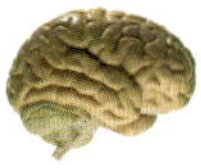

BRAIN FOOD

Blueberries may be the ultimate brain fruit, shown to rapidly improve memory in lab animals.

Spiced Apple and Blueberry Tart

SERVES 6

Pastry

- 1/3 cup all-purpose flour
- 1/3 cup **whole-wheat flour**
- 1 1/4 teaspoon allspice
- 1/3 cup cool unsalted butter, diced
- 2 tablespoons confectioner's sugar, sifted
- 1 egg yolk
- 1 tablespoon cold water
- 1 egg white, lightly beaten

Filling

- 3 large cooking **apples**
- 1/2 cup **blueberries**
- 1/4 cup light brown sugar
- 1 teaspoon ground cinnamon
- 1/2 teaspoon freshly grated nutmeg
- Vanilla frozen yogurt or Greek-style yogurt (optional)

1. *To make the pastry:* Sift the white and whole-wheat flours and the allspice into a medium bowl. Cut in the butter until the mixture resembles fine bread crumbs.

2. Stir in the sugar.

3. Mix the egg yolk with the water in a cup and add to the flour mixture. Mix to form a soft dough, adding a few drops more water, if needed. Wrap the dough in plastic wrap and chill for at least 30 minutes.

4. Preheat the oven to 375°F.

5. *To make the filling:* Peel and slice the apples, and mix with the blueberries in a large bowl. Stir together the brown sugar, cinnamon, and nutmeg in a small bowl. Reserve 1 tablespoon of the mixture, and stir the rest into the fruit to coat evenly.

6. Roll out the dough thinly on a nonstick baking sheet to make a 12-inch round. Brush the dough all over with egg white.

7. Pour the fruit mixture into the middle of the pastry round, then draw up the sides over the edge of the fruit filling, leaving the center open. Brush the outside of the packet with the remaining egg white and sprinkle with the reserved sugar mixture.

8. Bake until the pastry is golden brown and the apples are tender, 30 to 35 minutes. Serve warm with yogurt, if using.

Per serving: 265 calories, 3 g protein, 40 g carbohydrates, 5 g fiber, 12 g total fat, 7 g saturated fat, 62 mg cholesterol, 17 mg sodium.

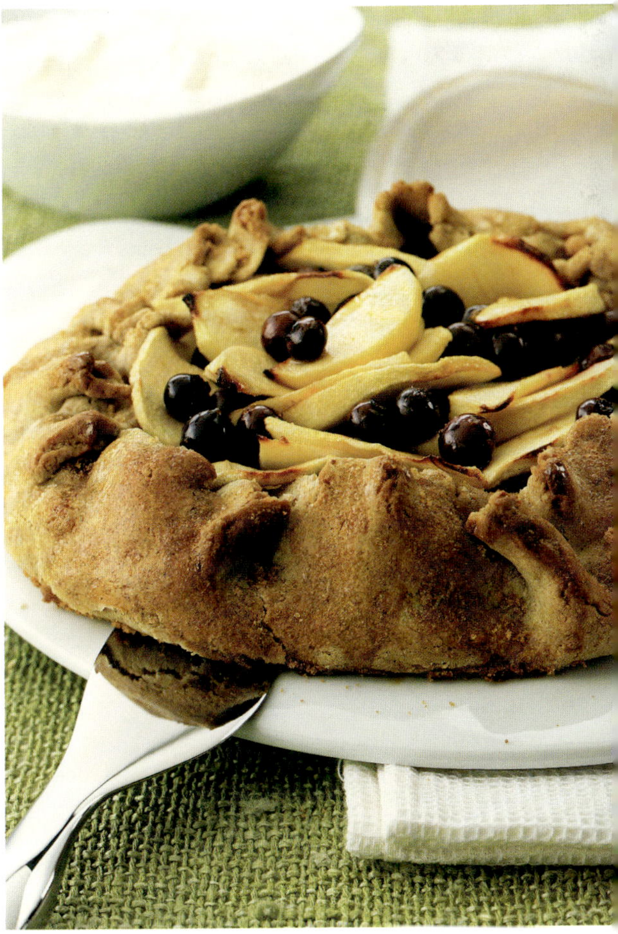

Chock-Full Chocolate Chip Cookies

MAKES 5 DOZEN

- 1 1/2 cups **whole-wheat pastry flour**
- 1 cup whole **oats**, ground
- 1/3 cup **cocoa powder**
- 1 teaspoon baking soda
- 1/2 teaspoon salt
- 1 cup nonhydrogenated butter-replacement stick margarine
- 1/2 cup granulated sugar
- 1 cup firmly packed light brown sugar
- 2 eggs
- 1 tablespoon vanilla extract
- 1 cup bittersweet **chocolate** chips (60% or higher cocoa content)
- 1 cup **raisins**
- 1 cup **walnuts**, coarsely chopped

1. Preheat the oven to 350°F. In a medium bowl, whisk together the flour, oats, cocoa powder, baking soda, and salt.

2. In a large bowl, with an electric mixer at medium speed, beat the margarine with the granulated and brown sugar until light and fluffy, 2 minutes. Add the eggs and vanilla and beat until smooth.

3. On low speed, beat in the flour mixture until combined. Stir in the chocolate chips, raisins, and walnuts.

4. Drop by teaspoons onto a baking sheet. Bake until browned, 10 minutes. Let cool on the baking sheet for 2 minutes, then transfer to a rack and let cool completely.

Per cookie: 97 calories, 1 g protein, 12 g carbohydrates, 1 g fiber, 5 g total fat, 2 g saturated fat, 7 mg cholesterol, 77 mg sodium.

Orange-Glazed Roasted Plums

SERVES 4

- 1 teaspoon freshly grated orange zest or grated fresh ginger
- 1/4 cup fresh orange juice
- 3 tablespoons firmly packed brown sugar
- 2 teaspoons unsalted butter
- 4 medium **plums** or **pluots** (1–1 1/4 pounds), halved and pitted
- 2 tablespoons slivered **almonds**
- 1/2 cup vanilla fat-free yogurt

1. Preheat the oven to 400°F. Coat an 8-inch square baking dish with nonstick spray.

2. Combine the orange zest or ginger, orange juice, and brown sugar in a small saucepan. Bring to a simmer, stirring to dissolve the sugar. Remove from the heat, add the butter, and stir until melted.

3. Place the plums or pluots, cut side up, in the prepared baking dish. Pour the orange juice mixture over the plums. Cover with aluminum foil and bake until the plums are almost tender, 20 to 25 minutes.

4. Baste the plums with the orange syrup and sprinkle with the almonds. Bake, uncovered, until the plums are tender and glazed, 10 to 15 minutes, basting once or twice.

5. Serve the plums warm or chilled, drizzled with the syrup and accompanied by a dollop of yogurt.

Per serving: 151 calories, 3 g protein, 28 g carbohydrates, 1 g fiber, 4 g total fat, 1 g saturated fat, 6 mg cholesterol, 25 mg sodium.

BRAIN FOOD

Fruit provides a sweet ending to your meal—and countless **phytochemicals** that protect precious brain cells.

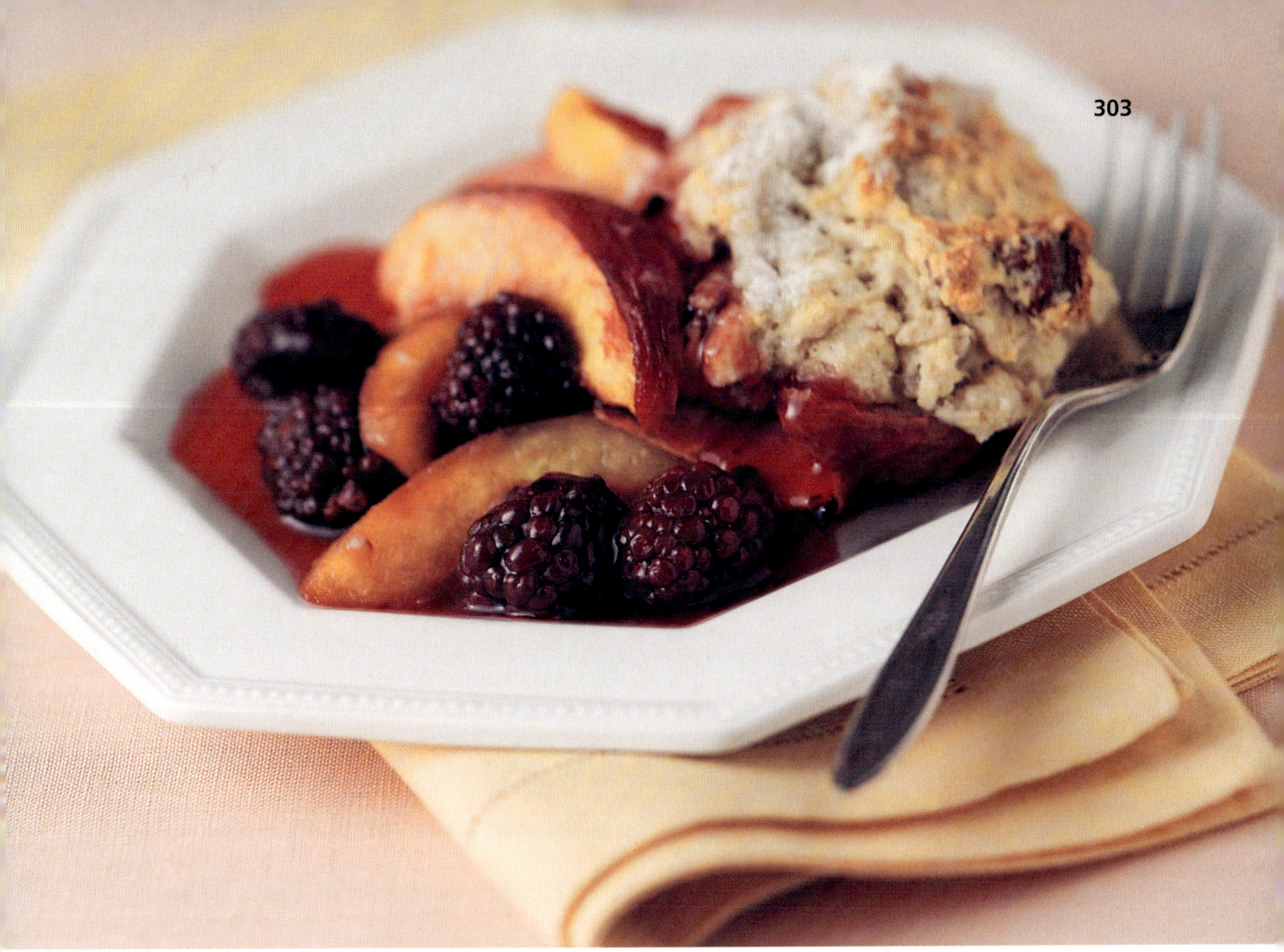

Peach-Berry Cobbler

SERVES 12

- 3 pounds peaches (about 8), peeled, pitted, and sliced
- 2 pints blackberries
- 3/4 cup firmly packed light brown sugar
- 1 tablespoon cornstarch
- 2 tablespoons fresh lemon juice
- 2 cups self-rising flour
- 1/3 cup pecans, toasted and chopped
- 1/4 teaspoon ground nutmeg
- 6 tablespoons cold margarine, cut into pieces
- 3/4 cup plus 2 tablespoons reduced-fat (2%) milk
- 2 tablespoons granulated sugar

1. Preheat the oven to 375°F. Coat a 13 x 9-inch baking dish with nonstick cooking spray.

2. Toss the peaches, blackberries, 1/2 cup of the brown sugar, the cornstarch, and the lemon juice in large bowl. Turn into the prepared baking dish and bake for 30 minutes.

3. Combine the flour, pecans, the remaining brown sugar, and the nutmeg in a large bowl. Cut in the margarine with a pastry blender or two knives until the mixture resembles very coarse crumbs. Add 3/4 cup of the milk and stir with a fork until a thick batter forms, adding water, if necessary.

4. Drop the batter on top of the fruit, spacing evenly, to make 12 dumplings. Lightly brush the dumplings with the remaining milk and sprinkle with the granulated sugar.

5. Bake until a toothpick inserted in center of a dumpling comes out with moist crumbs clinging, 25 to 30 minutes. Serve warm or at room temperature.

Per serving: 292 calories, 4 g protein, 52 g carbohydrates, 6 g fiber, 9 g total fat, 1 g saturated fat, 4 mg cholesterol, 346 mg sodium.

cooking tip

If you don't have self-rising flour, substitute 2 cups sifted all-purpose flour mixed with 1/4 tablespoon baking powder and 1/4 teaspoon salt. When fresh berries are scarce, use a 20-ounce package of frozen blackberries.

index

A

B

D

E

N

Q

R

T

V

W

CREDITS

Page 25, 26—illustrations ©Studio MacBeth Inc.; page 39, 262—illustrations ©Adam Raiti; page 263—illustration ©Dave Phillips. Additional photos courtesy Jupiter Images, Masterfile, RD Images, Veer.

Your Best Resource for Everyday Advice Is Reader's Digest

Every month, more than 100 million people around the globe turn to Reader's Digest books and magazines for clever, proven advice on managing their health, home, kitchen, and yard. The following Reader's Digest books are available by calling 1-800-846-2100 or visiting readersdigeststore.com.

Home Advice

Extraordinary Uses for Ordinary Things

2,001 Amazing Cleaning Secrets

Long Life for Your Stuff

Forbidden Advice

Early Bird Specials

Reader's Digest Complete Do-It-Yourself Manual

Super Salads

Extraordinary Meals from Ordinary Ingredients

Save $20,000 with a Nail

Baking Soda, Banana Peels, Baby Oil and Beyond

1,519 All-Natural All-Amazing Gardening Secrets

Health Advice

Magic Foods for Better Blood Sugar

Foods That Harm Foods That Heal

30 Minutes a Day to a Healthy Heart

Cut Your Cholesterol

What Works What Doesn't

Reverse Diabetes

Disease Free

Long Life Prescription

759 Secrets for Beating Diabetes

1,801 Home Remedies

Best Remedies

Stealth Health

Reader's Digest Guide to Drugs and Supplements

Food Cures

Cooking Smart for a Healthy Heart